W9-BXU-132

Ethnocultural Factors in Substance Abuse Treatment

Ethnocultural Factors in Substance Abuse Treatment

Edited by
Shulamith Lala Ashenberg Straussner

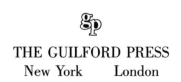

THE GUILFORD PRESS
New York   London

© 2001 The Guilford Press
A Division of Guilford Publications, Inc.
72 Spring Street, New York, NY 10012
www.guilford.com

Paperback edition 2003

Printed in the United States of America

This book is printed on acid-free paper.

Last digit is print number: 9   8   7   6   5   4   3   2

Library of Congress Cataloging-in-Publication Data

Ethnocultural factors in substance abuse treatment / edited by
  Shulamith Lala Ashenberg Straussner.
     p. cm.
  Includes bibliographical references and index.
  ISBN 1-57230-630-0 (hc.)   ISBN 1-57230-885-0 (pbk.)
    1. Substance abuse—Treatment—Cross-cultural studies.   2. Drug
  abuse—Treatment—Cross-cultural studies.   3. Cross-cultural
  counseling.   I. Straussner, Shulamith Lala Ashenberg.

RC564 .E785 2001
616.86′06—dc21   00-067723

About the Editor

Shulamith Lala Ashenberg Straussner, DSW, CSW, CEAP, BCD, CAS, is a tenured full professor at the Shirley M. Ehrenkranz School of Social Work at New York University and coordinator of its Post-Master's Program in the Treatment of Alcohol- and Drug-Abusing Clients. She was a visiting professor at the Tel Aviv School of Social Work during 1994 and at the Omsk State Pedagogical University in Siberia, Russia, during Spring 2000.

Dr. Straussner has written numerous publications dealing with substance abuse and with occupational social work and Employee Assistance Programs. Among her eight books are *Gender and Addictions: Men and Women in Treatment* (coedited with Elizabeth Zelvin; 1997, Jason Aronson) and *Clinical Work with Substance-Abusing Clients* (1993, The Guilford Press), both of which were chosen as main selections of the Psychotherapy Book Club.

Dr. Straussner is a founding board member of the New York State Addictions Institute, has served on the National Center on Substance Abuse Treatment panel on workforce issues, and is the past chair of the National Association of Social Workers Section on Alcohol, Tobacco, and Other Drugs. She serves as a consultant to various hospitals, agencies, and other organizations in New York and lectures on a variety of topics throughout the United States and abroad. She also has a private therapeutic and supervisory practice in New York City, with particular focus on couple treatment and the treatment of recovering men and women.

Contributors

Ann A. Abbott, PhD, LSW, LCSW, Associate Dean, School of Social Work, Rutgers University, Camden, New Jersey

Nuha Abudabbeh, PhD, Clinical and Forensic Psychologist, NAIM Foundation for Health-Social Care, Washington, DC

Louis R. Alvarez, MD, MPH, Instructor, Department of Psychiatry, Harvard Medical School, Boston, Massachusetts

Mary Ann Bromley, PhD, LICSW, Professor, Rhode Island College, School of Social Work, and consultant and clinician, Socio-Economic Development Center for Southeast Asians, Providence, Rhode Island

Jim Gilbert, PhD, CSW-R, CASAC, Social Work Supervisor, Division of Substance Abuse, Albert Einstein College of Medicine, Bronx, New York

Andrew Hamid, PhD, Assistant Professor, School of Social Work, Columbia University, New York, New York

Eda F. Harris-Hastick, EdD, Associate Professor, Department of Social and Behavioral Sciences, Medgar Evers College, City University of New York, Brooklyn, New York

Helen Kagan PhD, CSW, Director of Substance Abuse Services for Russian-Speaking Immigrants, Educational Alliance, Incorporated, New York, New York

Young Hee Kwon-Ahn, DSW, CSW, Adjunct Professor, Hunter College School of Social Work, City University of New York, and private practice, New York, New York

Ting-Fun May Lai, MSW, CASAC, Director, Chinatown Alcoholism Services, Hamilton–Madison House, New York, New York

Jan Langrod, PhD, CSW-R, CASAC, Director of Admissions, Division of Substance Abuse, Albert Einstein College of Medicine, Bronx, New York

Ruby Malik, PhD, private practice, New York, New York

Pia Marinangeli, CSW, CASAC, Adjunct Instructor, New York University, Shirley M. Ehrenkranz School of Social Work, and private practice, New York, New York

Jun Matsuyoshi, CSW, Program Director, Assessment and Referral Team, Medical and Health Research Association of New York City, Incorporated, New York, New York

Catherine Medina, MSW, Clinical Assistant Professor, New York University, Shirley M. Ehrenkranz School of Social Work, New York, New York

Philip O'Dwyer, EdD, Adjunct Lecturer, Department of Counseling, Oakland University, Rochester, Michigan, and Clinical Director, Brookfield Clinics, Garden City, Michigan

Eugenio M. Rothe, MD, Director, Child and Adolescent Psychiatry Outpatient Clinic and School Consultation Programs, Jackson Memorial Hospital, and Associate Professor of Psychiatry, University of Miami School of Medicine, Miami, Florida

Pedro Ruiz, MD, Professor and Vice Chair for Clinical Affairs, Department of Psychiatry and Behavioral Sciences, and Medical Director, Mental Sciences Institute, University of Texas at Houston, Houston, Texas

Daya Singh Sandhu, EdD, NCC, Professor and Chair, Department of Educational and Counseling Psychology, University of Louisville, Louisville, Kentucky

Kathryn C. Shafer PhD, LCSW, CAP, Director of Clinical Services, Limitless Potentials, Incorporated, West Palm Beach, Florida

S. K. Chhem Sip, MA, Deputy Director, United Cambodian Community Development Foundation, San Francisco, California

Shulamith Lala Ashenberg Straussner, DSW, CSW, CEAP, BCD, CAS, Professor and Coordinator, Post-Master's Program in the Treatment of Alcohol- and Drug-Abusing Clients, New York University, Shirley M. Ehrenkranz School of Social Work, New York, New York

Katherine Stuart van Wormer, PhD, Professor of Social Work, University of Northern Iowa, Cedar Falls, Iowa

Hilary N. Weaver, DSW, Associate Professor, School of Social Work, State University of New York at Buffalo, Buffalo, New York

Ednita M. Wright, PhD, CSW, MSW, CAC, Counselor/Therapist and Diversity Coordinator, Cornell Gannett Health Center, Ithaca, New York

Preface

What does it mean to an Irish American to drink to excess? How do Korean Americans make sense of drug abuse in their families and communities? What effect does shame or fear of deportation have on an immigrant's motivation to seek professional help for an addiction? What does it take to engage an addict who is African American in an ongoing treatment regimen? How can substance abuse treatment providers earn the trust of people they seek to serve when these professionals' ethnocultural backgrounds differ radically from those of their clients?

The contributors to this book explore practical questions and issues in their discussions of treating substance abuse across racial, cultural, and ethnic lines. I chose each contributor because of his or her familiarity with and/or track record of working effectively with a particular ethnocultural group. The various chapters in this book discuss the roots of culturally idiosyncratic attitudes toward, and use of, alcohol and other drugs. The authors describe the hurdles in working with each population, but more important, they offer specific guidelines for treatment that will increase the likelihood of success.

Having grown up on three different continents and having been at different times both a member of a severely discriminated-against ethnoreligious minority and a member of a powerful majority, I have been acutely conscious of ethnic, cultural, and religious issues throughout my life. Yet I was unaware of the importance of these issues to the treatment of substance abuse until I started working on my 1993 book, *Clinical Work with Substance-Abusing Clients* (New York: Guilford Press). It was only then that I became aware that traditional treatment of substance-abusing clients has ignored gender, life cycle, and, particularly, ethnocultural issues.

Having addressed the gender issues in my 1997 book, *Gender and Addictions: Men and Women in Treatment* (coedited with Elizabeth Zelvin, Northvale, NJ: Jason Aronson), I decided that my next book had to focus on ethnicity, without fully appreciating how difficult and time consuming this task would be. Finding authors who were knowledgeable about both substance abuse treatment and the various ethnic cultures was just the first hurdle. Another was the struggle between my desire to include chapters on many other ethnocultural groups and to offer a comprehensive and balanced exploration of the issues in each chapter and the need to operate within real constraints on the length of the manuscript.

Therefore, though the scope of this book embraces only some of the numerous ethnic and cultural groups in the United States, I nonetheless hope it will serve as a beginning guide to exploring the various aspects of culture and ethnicity that are important in understanding our clients and in offering culturally competent substance abuse treatment. Because it is difficult to avoid some generalization in a project such as this, it is important that the reader does not interpret any statements regarding dynamics or general trends as fully characterizing specific populations.

The focus of this book is on applying the current state of knowledge to treatment. It attempts to move beyond ethnic sensitivity to address the delivery of ethnoculturally competent treatment of individuals with alcohol and other drug (AOD) problems. In order to achieve this, each chapter identifies the unique beliefs, customs, and values of an ethnocultural group as they relate to AOD issues and how they can be applied to treatment. Wherever possible, each chapter explores issues related to women and adolescents and provides available data regarding HIV/AIDS. Most important, the book identifies the numerous gaps in our current state of knowledge about the impact of ethnicity and culture on substance use, abuse, and treatment—gaps that I hope will be filled by future research studies.

This book is the outcome of a collaboration of many people: my students, supervisees, and patients who sensitized me to their diverse cultures and ethnicities; all the wonderful authors, most of whom had to rewrite their chapters a number of times to meet my own need for perfection and who had to wait a long time to see their work in print; the staff of The Guilford Press, particularly Kristal Hawkins and Jim Nageotte; and my friends and colleagues at the Shirley M. Ehrenkranz School of Social Work at New York University. I particularly want to thank Dean Thomas Meenaghan, who provided the institutional support that made this book possible, and my friends at NYU and elsewhere, RoseMarie Perez Foster,

Norma Phillips, Jeff Seinfeld, and Eileen Wolkstein, who gave me feedback on my chapters and who listened during my struggles to complete this book. Most of all I want to thank my family—my sister, Lusia; my children, Adam and Sarina; and particularly, my husband, Joel, who has had to deal with our own ethnocultural differences on top of my preoccupation with this book. Thank you all for your love and support.

SHULAMITH LALA ASHENBERG STRAUSSNER

Contents

I

Introduction

1

Ethnocultural Issues in Substance Abuse Treatment

An Overview

Shulamith Lala Ashenberg Straussner

America is the melting pot where nothing melted.
—TONY KUSHNER, *Angels in America*

The traditional view of the United States as an "ethnic melting pot" (Glazer & Moynihan, 1970; Park, 1950) in which all ethnic and cultural groups lose their cultural identifications and form a new American ethnocultural "puree" has changed. This change is a reflection of what had been termed the "unmeltable ethnics" (Novak, 1973) and the desire of different ethnic groups "to affirm their right to a separate identity within the framework of a pluralistic nation" (Steinberg, 1981, p. ix). The current view may be best conceptualized as having the various ethnocultural groups in the United States form a "mosaic," or better yet, an "ethnocultural salad"—a mixture in which all the ethnic and cultural ingredients of various groups are tossed together while still retaining their unique "flavor and taste." It is those unique ethnocultural "flavors" that make working with substance-abusing clients today so fascinating, yet so challenging.

The increase in ethnic pride among Blacks and Hispanics during the 1960s and 1970s (Steinberg, 1981; Sue & Sue, 1990), combined with the diversity among immigrants during the past two decades, has led to a renewed interest in the uniqueness of different ethnocultural groups in the United States. As pointed out by Hayton (1994), "One of the ironies of our time is that the unique customs, values and traditions of cultural groups have become more important as the world has become smaller and the inhabitants of the planet realize that they live in a global village" (p. 99). Yet, despite the growing recognition of the need for ethnoculturally sensitive provision of services and a tremendous increase in the literature on this topic among all mental health professions, the application of such knowledge to the field of addictions remains limited, with much of it focused on prevention of substance abuse among people of color—a reaction to the earlier focus on substance abuse among Whites (Amodeo & Jones 1997, 1998; Amodeo, Robb, Peou, & Tran, 1996; Bennett & Ames, 1985; de la Rosa & Recio Adrados, 1993; Gordon, 1994; Griffith et al., 1996; Maddahian, Newcomb, & Bentler, 1988; Mayers, Kail, & Watts, 1993; National Institute on Drug Abuse [NIDA], 1995; Orlandi, Weston, & Epstein, 1992; Philleo, Brisbane, & Epstein, 1995; Szapocznik, 1995; Trimble, Bolek, & Niemcryk, 1992; Tucker, 1985; Turner & Cooper, 1997).

This chapter provides an introduction to ethnocultural issues as they apply to alcohol and other drug (AOD)-related problems and treatment approaches. It explores such concepts as race, culture, and ethnicity. And, in order to avoid stereotyping, it focuses on variables such as social class, encounters with prejudice, migration, acculturation, language, socioeconomic status, family roles, and gender—factors that create diversity even among specific ethnic and cultural groups. The relationship of these variables to substance abuse problems and the implications for treatment with alcohol- and drug-abusing individuals and their families are considered.

THE MEANING AND IMPORTANCE OF RACE, ETHNICITY, AND CULTURE

As pointed out by Hays (1996), "despite distinct differences in their meanings, the terms *race, ethnicity*, and *culture* continue to be used interchangeably and in ways that reinforce Eurocentric assumptions" (p. 333). Thus it is important to have a clear understanding of these concepts and the impact they have on the treatment of those affected by substance abuse problems.

Definition of Race

Although awareness of racial differences has existed for ages, the modern notion of "race" originated in the 17th century as an attempt to classify people on the basis of genetically transmitted physical characteristics, such as skin color and hair texture (Hays, 1996; Orlandi et al., 1992). Although most scientists today agree that the concept of race has no scientific meaning, it remains a powerful sociopolitical construct that plays an important role in understanding social attitudes, prejudice, stereotypes, and discrimination, as well as in the interactions between patients and clinicians (Davis & Proctor, 1989; Lu, Lim, & Mezzich, 1995; McGoldrick, Giordano, & Pearce, 1996).

Moreover, what may be viewed as racial characteristics are frequently manifestations of socioeconomic and cultural differences, thereby confounding the use of race an explanatory factor in behavior—particularly in relationship to the use and abuse of alcohol and other drugs. Thus the typical classification of substance use and abuse within such population categories as "White, Black, and Hispanic" and the more recently added "Asian/Pacific Islanders" is not helpful because it obscures the ethnic and cultural background of those so classified. Such classification is particularly problematic in relation to those of Hispanic/Latino background, because a substance-abusing "Hispanic" client can be of Black, White, or of Native American or other indigenous racial background, representing a variety of different cultures. Furthermore, such classification negates the identification of the growing number of people of mixed racial backgrounds.

Definition of Culture

As stated by Devore and Schlesinger (1996), "culture is a commonly used concept that is difficult to define. It revolves around the fact that human groups differ in the way they structure their behavior, in their world view, in their perspectives on the rhythms and patterns of life, and in their concept of the essential nature of the human condition" (p. 43). In essence, culture is the sum total of life patterns passed on from generation to generation within a given community. It includes institutions, language, religious ideals, artistic expressions, and patterns of social and interpersonal relationships. Culture also includes values, attitudes, customs, and beliefs that are shared by group members (Lu et al., 1995; Lum, 1996; Sue & Sue, 1990). Cultural beliefs, moreover, determine who will be oppressed and who will benefit from socioeconomic and political privileges in any given society.

It is within a cultural context that attitudes and reactions to the use and abuse of alcohol and other drugs are formed. And it is only within such a context that we can understand the differential meaning of the snorting of methamphetamine by a group of White upper-class teens at a private club, the drinking of beer at a local bar by a group of Polish American working-class men, or the passing of a bottle of wine by a group of underemployed African American men on an inner-city street corner. As found by Maddahian and colleagues (1988) in their exploration of risk factors for adolescent substance abuse: "One of the most interesting findings of our research was that the same behavior [drug use] may have different causes among different demographic groups or populations because of their unique traditions, cultures, and expectations from life" (p. 12).

Definition of Ethnicity

Whereas the concept of *culture* is a global one, the concept of *ethnicity* is more narrow: "Ethnicity refers to the sense of peoplehood experienced by members of the same ethnic group" (Devore & Schlesinger, 1996, p. 45). The term "ethnicity" comes from the Greek work *ethnos,* meaning "people" or "nation," and refers to the notion that members of an ethnic group share common identity, ideals, and aspirations and a sense of continuity (Gordon, 1964). These commonalities provide an individual with an "ethnic identity"—a major form of group identification. According to Alba (1985), it is the "self-definition in terms of the past [that] makes an ethnic group different from most other kinds of social groups and constitutes the sine qua non of its existence" (p. 17).

Ethnic values and identification are retained for many generations: "Second-, third-, and even fourth-generation Americans, as well as new immigrants differ from the dominant culture in values, life-style and behavior. . . . Ethnicity patterns our thinking, feeling and behavior in both obvious and subtle ways. It plays a major role in determining what we eat, how we work, how we relax, how we celebrate holidays and rituals, and how we feel about life, death and illness" (McGoldrick, 1982, p. 3). Thus, although the surrounding culture may affect an individual's access to a given substance such as alcohol, crack cocaine, or Ecstasy, one's ethnic identity plays an important role in when and how a substance is used and in one's reactions to these substances.

Ethnocultural Awareness

Although an exclusive focus on the ethnic and cultural backgrounds of people can readily lead to stereotyping of individuals and communities, ignoring them can lead to inadequate understanding of a client and inappropriate provision of services. As pointed out by Cunningham (1994):

The cultural beliefs of a group of people are directly related to how alcohol and other drug problems are defined. The very definition of health differs by ethnicities and cultures. Therefore, it is of critical importance to understand how the members of an ethnic group define alcohol and other drug problems; what is considered to be a positive outcome; and what they feel are appropriate ways to prevent these problems from occurring. (p. viii)

Moreover, because ethnicity and culture interact and influence each other, clinicians and agencies need to focus on both the specific ethnicity and the broader cultural context, that is, to become *ethnoculturally competent,* in their delivery of substance abuse services.

ETHNOCULTURAL COMPETENCY

Ethnocultural competency can be defined as the ability of a clinician to function effectively in the context of ethnocultural differences. Ethnocultural competency has been shown to influence client–clinician communication and trust (Tirado, 1998) and is a crucial component in the effective provision of substance abuse services and the retention of clients. It includes awareness and acceptance of differences—differences that need to be explored respectfully, nonjudgmentally, and with curiosity (Dyche & Zayas, 1995).

Ethnocultural competency is a developmental process that moves beyond "cultural sensitivity" and includes cognitive, affective, and skills dimensions (Orlandi, 1992). It includes an understanding of one's own ethnocultural background and values; a basic knowledge about the ethnoculture of clients with whom one is working; a commitment to working with diverse clients; and an ability to adapt practice skills to fit the client's ethnocultural background, including flexibility in reaching out to appropriate cultural resources in a given ethnic community (Amodeo & Jones, 1998; Center for Mental Health Services, 1997; Gordon, 1994; Hays, 1996; Lum, 1996; Orlandi et al., 1992).

Ethnocultural competence includes not only the individual clinician but also the setting in which the individual works (Tirado, 1998). A substance abuse clinician cannot provide ethnoculturally competent services in a setting that does not support and validate such values. The agency should strive to include some recognition and celebration of ethnocultural holidays, customs, and rituals—including food, music, and art—of the diverse ethnic groups seen in the agency; to hire professional and paraprofessional staff that reflect the ethnic and linguistic diversity of clients; and to provide ongoing training and supervision to help the counseling staff understand their clientele and their own countertransferential reactions to them.

Establishing close linkages with community groups that represent the ethnocultural background of clients and cross-training of staff can be extremely beneficial to all. For example, a substance abuse clinic with a number of Russian or Dominican immigrant clients may offer to provide a lecture on the signs and symptoms of AOD addictions to an ethnic Russian or Dominican community organization while inviting staff from such an organization to offer in-service training regarding issues that affect the particular ethnic group.

In addition, ethnoculturally competent organizations use computerized management information systems that have the capacity to record data regarding clients' ethnicity, migration and immigration information, religious and spiritual beliefs, and languages spoken. They also track information regarding accessibility to and frequency of the need for interpreters (Tirado, 1998). Moreover, an ethnoculturally competent organization makes use of treatment outcome research in order to identify its abilities and deficits in providing ethnoculturally competent treatment services to its clientele.

SUBSTANCE ABUSE AMONG DIFFERENT ETHNOCULTURAL AND RACIAL GROUPS

Recognition of variation in substance abuse patterns among different ethnocultural groups is not new; neither are its political implications. As pointed out by Room (1985),

> The social sciences have considered ethnic differences in the United States at least as far back as the Progressive era, when the descendants of earlier immigrants became concerned about the living conditions and cultural patterns of the new waves of immigrants crowding into American cities. Not least among the concern, both of "know-nothing" nativists and of well-wishing social reformers were the drinking patterns and problems of the new immigrants. . . . (pp. xi–xii)

Consequently, the early years of the 20th century saw numerous studies focusing on drinking patterns among different ethnic groups and on the interplay of ethnicity and alcoholism. Most sociological studies of ethnic variations dropped out of favor following World War II because "such a focus went against the prevailing melting-pot ideology of American society . . .

[and] any emphasis on ethnic differentiation was uncomfortably reminiscent of the Nazis' racist ideology and its genocidal consequences" (Room, 1985, p. xii). Nevertheless, studies of ethnic difference in drinking patterns continued. These studies were viewed, in today's terminology, as "politically correct," because their findings "cut against the grain of racist and nativist assumptions of cultural superiority. In terms of their drinking practices, ethnicities that had borne the brunt of racist and nativist attacks—such as Italians, Jews, and the Chinese—could be presented as paragons others might aspire to copy" (Room, 1985, p. xii). Thus it is evident that the use of substances is not just an individual or even a familial dynamic but an issue that has important sociocultural meanings for different ethnic groups and for society as a whole. Consequently, research and discussion of substance abuse among different ethnic groups has been and continues to be a highly charged social and political issue.

Current State of Knowledge

Despite the long-standing awareness that the use and abuse of alcohol and other drugs is governed by specific ethnocultural norms and values, current national databases that survey alcohol and other drug abuse in the United States tend to aggregate individuals into global racial or ethnocultural categories, such as Black, White, Hispanic, Asian, or Native American. Such classifications tend to ignore the distinctions in the drinking and drug use patterns among the various subgroups within each ethnocultural category. Consequently, there is limited data regarding alcohol and other drug problems among various Asian/Pacific Islander populations or the numerous European American groups or within the various subgroups classified as Native American or Black. Moreover, due to the absence of an appropriate category, there is total lack of information about substance abuse among people of Middle Eastern background. Fortunately, the most recent federal analysis of data obtained from the national household surveys during 1991–1993 has recognized some subcategories within the Hispanic grouping, providing much needed information (Substance Abuse and Mental Health Services Administration [SAMHSA], 1998).

As reflected in Table 1.1, the prevalence of alcohol and drug problems does vary among different ethnic and racial groups. Alcohol dependence is more of a problem among Native Americans and those of Mexican background, whereas other drug problems (see the column "Need for drug abuse treatment") are higher among Native Americans, Blacks, and those of Mexican and Puerto Rican background when compared with the "total

TABLE 1.1. Prevalence of Substance Use and Abuse

Race/ethnicity	Alcohol use past year	Any illicit drug use past year	Marijuana use past year	Cocaine use past year	Need drug abuse treatment	Alcohol dependence	Cigarette use past year
			Substance used				
Total surveyed population	66.4%	11.9%	9.0%	2.5%	2.7%	3.5%	30.9%
White (non-Hispanic)	68.9%	11.8%	8.9%	2.4%	2.5%	3.4%	31.5%
Native American	63.7%	19.8%	15.0%	5.2%	7.8%	5.6%	52.7%
Black (non-Hispanic)	55.4%	13.1%	10.6%	3.1%	3.9%	3.4%	29.9%
Asian/Pacific Islander	53.2%	6.5%	4.7%	1.4%	1.7%	1.8%	21.7%
Hispanic–Caribbean	60.8%	7.6%	5.6%	1.5%	1.6%	1.9%	21.2%
Hispanic–Central American	51.1%	5.7%	2.7%	1.1%	1.5%	2.8%	17.9%
Hispanic–Cuban	65.7%	8.2%	5.9%	1.7%	2.6%	0.9%	27.3%
Hispanic–Mexican	63.7%	12.7%	9.1%	3.9%	3.6%	5.6%	29.1%
Hispanic–Puerto Rican	59.5%	13.3%	10.8%	3.7%	3.7%	3.0%	32.7%
Hispanic–South American	74.1%	10.7%	8.4%	2.0%	1.7%	2.1%	31.3%

Source: Office of Applied Studies, Substance Abuse and Mental Health Services Administration, National Household Survey on Drug Abuse, 1991–1993.

surveyed population." Asians/Pacific Islanders tend to have an almost equal problem with drugs as compared with alcohol, with all substances being abused to a much lower degree than among the other populations studied.

It is important to note that, whereas our culturally approved substance, alcohol, is a bigger problem nationwide and particularly among the White population in the United States than is other drug use, illegal drugs are more of a problem among Native Americans, Blacks, Cubans, and Puerto Ricans. The implications of these differences are profound both in terms of social policy and clinical practice. The negative consequences of using a substance that is culturally defined as "illegal" are reflected in legal, familial, social, and economic sequelae and affect the availability of quality treatment and on the recovery process:

> Since the time and effort necessary to obtain drugs and to pay for the addiction are considerable, the lifestyle associated with opiate [and crack] addiction is highly unstructured and generally characterized by poverty and illegal activities, which tend to have a severe negative impact on family life. Numerous live-in partners, prostitution and incarcerations are common. . . . The use of crack in the United States has had a particularly destructive and tragic impact on black families and communities, due in part to the high rate of use among black women, thereby diminishing their availability to maintain familial and community life. (Straussner, 1994, pp. 394–395)

Moreover, African American and Hispanic communities have been severely affected by AIDS resulting from intravenous drug use or sexual relations with HIV-infected individuals (Friedman, 1997; Strom, 1993). According to Day (1999), during 1997, AIDS was the leading cause of death among African Americans between the ages of 25 and 44, with over 60% of these deaths being injection related: "Among those who inject drugs, African Americans are five times as likely as whites to get AIDS" (p. 1). For Latinos in the same age group, AIDS was the second leading cause of death, with over half of the deaths related to drug injection compared with less than one quarter for Whites. Both African American and Latino women suffer disproportionately from this epidemic: African American women, who represent only 12% of the population, account for over half of all injection-related AIDS cases among women, whereas Latino women, who represent 10% of the female population in the United States, account for 20% of all injection-related AIDS cases (Day, 1999).

Given the differential patterns and impact of alcohol and other drug use among different ethnic and cultural groups, it is evident that ethnocultural dynamics have to be taken into account during substance abuse treatment process.

ETHNOCULTURALLY COMPETENT TREATMENT

Ethnoculturally competent substance abuse treatment, like any effective substance abuse treatment, must begin with a comprehensive assessment of the client's alcohol and other drug use and its impact on the client and his or her family (Straussner, 1993) and with the utilization of good counseling skills. However, to make it ethnoculturally competent, treatment must take into account the client's ethnocultural beliefs, customs, and values, particularly as they relate to AOD issues, as well as the social conditions that have an impact on the client's ethnocultural group.

The disease concept of addiction is often unknown to many immigrants, who are more likely to see the abuse of alcohol and other drugs as immoral behavior reflecting a weakness of character; as mental illness requiring institutionalization; as a sinful or criminal behavior; as a reflection of cosmic or supernatural forces; as an understandable reaction to life stressors or social oppression; as a harmless use of a substance that is widely used in one's culture; or even as a helpful way of coping with psychic pain (Amodeo & Jones, 1997). Most, however, see it as a shameful, stigmatizing issue that has to be kept secret from the outside world. An open admission of such problems may be considered a disgrace not just for the individual but for the whole family and community. For many individuals from traditional cultures, particularly those in which marriages are arranged, admitting that a family member has a substance abuse problem may make not only this individual but others in the family unmarriageable. In addition, fear of deportation may also keep many immigrants and refugees from admitting to having a problem, whereas a general distrust of authority may make many African Americans reluctant to admit the truth about their substance use (Debro & Conley, 1993). Thus an important aspect in ethnoculturally competent substance abuse treatment is an assessment of how AOD problems are viewed not only by the individual client and his or her family but also by the client's ethnic culture. For example, a Jamaican-born male referred for treatment by his Employee Assistance Program (EAP) due to a positive marijuana screen may come from a very different ethnocultural context of substance use and beliefs about such use and thus have different treatment needs than his Greek American coworker who also tested positive for the same substance. Moreover, cultural rituals and celebrations provide a context for the use and abuse of alcohol and other drugs. Drinking may be an expected ritual during a wake in an Irish American family but totally unacceptable during a funeral, or even a birthday party, in a traditional Anglo-Saxon Southern Baptist family.

Ethnoculturally Competent Assessment of Substance Abusers

It is evident, without minimizing genetic, health, familial, and personality dynamics (Straussner, 1993), that ethnocultural factors play an important role in the development and in the consequences of AOD problems in the United States. The following are among the most important ethnoculturally affected dynamics that must be taken into account during assessment.

Ethnic, Racial, and Religious Identification

Ethnic and racial identification are not always clearly evident when a counselor first sees a client, and most intake forms do not allow for mixed racial or ethnic identifications. Thus it is important to ask clients how they identify themselves, rather than assume a certain classification based on the client's physical looks or place of birth. For example, Lynda, a cocaine- and heroin-snorting 24-year-old daughter of an African American father and a White Jewish mother, identified herself as a "Black Jew" even though she looked White and put down "agnostic" as a religious identification on the intake form. Angelo, a 38-year-old alcohol- and marijuana-abusing client, identified himself as Italian American Roman Catholic, the ethnic and religious background of his foster mother who raised him from age 4, even though he and his birth parents were born in Puerto Rico and his family there is still involved with a Pentecostal church.

Because much of current substance abuse treatment in the United States remains spiritually focused, clinicians will find it helpful to assess the role that religion and spirituality play in the current life of the client and his or her family. For example, a middle-aged client who identifies himself as Catholic but who has not been in a church since being expelled from parochial school for smoking pot in the sixth grade may feel more negatively about religion and spirituality than a client who has never been involved in any formal religion but who recently had been reading about Zen Buddhism and meditation. A Muslim male client from Pakistan may resist participating in an Alcoholics Anonymous (AA) meeting that ends with the Lord's Prayer, whereas an African American woman may find the spiritual aspect of her Narcotics Anonymous (NA) meeting of crucial importance in her recovery.

Religious rituals provide important affirmations of one's ethnocultural identity and may offer an important source of support during recovery for some clients; however, they also may provide a dangerous context for the use of substances. For example, a Jewish client trying to maintain her recovery from alcohol dependence may find it difficult to deal with the offer of wine, an important aspect of Jewish religious services and holiday rituals. Thus it is crucial that clinicians assess both the benefits and potential dangers when encouraging clients to reconnect with their religious upbringing.

Encounters with Prejudice and Discrimination

Encounters with discrimination based on one's ethnic or racial identity are part of both past and current reality of many clients. It may be racism based on skin color, such as that experienced by African Americans, Black Caribbeans, or the more recent African immigrants; it may be based on differences in physical characteristics and historical stereotypes as experienced by Asians or Native Americans; it may be anti-Semitic Jewish or anti-Muslim prejudice due to religious differences; or it may be prejudice and discrimination based on country of origin, such as that historically experienced by Irish, Polish, and Italian immigrants in the United States. In all these cases cultural memories and the impact of such experiences remain long after the experience ends. When prejudicial experiences are institutionalized and continue to affect the daily lives of our clients today, as reflected in the experience of many Black, Native American, and some Latino, Asian, and Middle Eastern clients, it is even more critical that clinicians assess the impact of such experiences on a given client, their connection to AOD problems, and their effect on the client–clinician relationship.

Circumstances of Migration and Immigration Status

The abuse of AOD has been long associated with loss, grief, and mourning (van Wormer, 1995). For many immigrants, the process of migration to a new country is connected to numerous losses: the loss of one's homeland, of friends and loved ones, of familiar food, sounds, and smells. Moreover, many immigrants, particularly refugees who escaped or who were expelled from their country of origin, have suffered trauma prior to or during their process of migration to the United States (Castex, 1997; Lu et al., 1995; Marsella, Friedman, & Spain, 1994). These dynamics need to be clearly understood if treatment is to be effective, because using alcohol and other drugs may be one way of self-medicating for posttraumatic stress disorder or of numbing the pain of homesickness and loneliness (Westermeyer, 1993b).

In addition, clinicians need to be sensitive to the current antirefugee and anti-immigrant sentiment in the United States that may lead clients to increased feelings of alienation from the mainstream culture, thereby contributing to substance abuse, while at the same time making it more difficult to seek and obtain treatment. In many immigrant communities, fear of possible deportation leads to greater tolerance for pathological behavior both within the family and the community, so that the individual is often sheltered from the consequences of his or her drug use until it is out of control ("Abused Illegal," 1999).

Acculturation and Assimilation

As indicated previously, ethnocultural mores and norms regulate the behaviors of individuals, including the use and abuse of alcohol and other drugs. In general, the further removed in generation from the country of origin, the more assimilated one becomes to the mainstream or dominant culture. This dynamic and highly complex process is called "acculturation."

For many immigrants, the acculturation process is a very painful one. Adapting to a new cultural environment, different lifestyles, and a new language can lead to increased personal stress and interpersonal conflicts (Akhtar, 1995; Gaw, 1993; Lu et al., 1995; Sandhu, Portes, & McPhee, 1996). Difficulties with the process of acculturation and assimilation have been linked to the development of emotional and behavioral problems, including mental illness, delinquency, and substance abuse (Oetting & Beauvais, 1991; Rogler, Cortes, & Malgady, 1991). Moreover, because different generations and genders assimilate at different rates (Rotheram-Borus & Wyche, 1994), risk of AOD problems vary among different people in a family and in immigrant communities. According to researchers (Kim, McLeod, & Shantzis, 1992; Oetting & Beauvais, 1990), those at highest risk of AOD problems are individuals who lack connections to both their original culture and to the mainstream one and who have access to a substance. For example, Karin, a 38-year-old German-born woman who was isolated from both her family of origin and her German culture and at the same time disconnected from any supportive network in the United States, quickly slid from social drinking to alcohol dependence and pill abuse following her divorce from her American husband. A similar dynamic played a role in the abuse of drugs and gang membership for Da Wai (David), a 15-year-old U.S.-born adolescent whose parents fled from China shortly before his birth. Disconnected from his parents' culture yet not assimilated to the adolescent culture in the United States, Da Wai feels closest to his gang peers, who form their own subculture with their own rituals, values, and norms.

Language

An important aspect of ethnocultural assessment is an exploration of the language or languages spoken by the client in childhood and the client's current level of verbal, comprehension, and writing proficiency in both English and the native language. In addition, many individuals, although fluent in English, may feel stigmatized by their foreign accent. Moreover, from an ethnocultural perspective, language refers not only to different spoken words but also to nonverbal communication such as physical gestures, distance between speakers, and eye contact (Lu et al., 1995). It also includes different usages and meanings of the same language by people of different ethnocultural and social class backgrounds. For example, the idioms and nonverbal modes of expression used among a group of substance-abusing Spanish-speaking Chicano former gang members may be as foreign to their upper-class, well-educated, Spanish-speaking Argentinean-born group therapist as to a non-Spanish-speaking clinician.

Moreover, it is through the use of language that experiences, memories, and perceptions are coded and organized (Buxbaum, 1949; Greenson, 1950; Perez Foster, 1996). Thus a French-born alcohol-dependent woman who was sexually abused during childhood by her father may be devoid of affect when talking in English about her early life experiences. For such a bilingual client, the second language can be used to intellectualize the emotional content—the emotional content can be recaptured only by shifting to the original language in which it was stored (Perez Foster, 1996). Although it is not possible to provide a bilingual clinician for every bilingual client, it is important that substance abuse clinicians have an understanding of the client's language dominance and the language used during the traumatic experience in order to understand their client's current reactions.

Although studies of native language speakers indicate "an almost complete breakdown in the transmission of non-English language between the second and third generations" of immigrants (Steinberg, 1981, p. 45), certain emotionally laden words continue to be transmitted from one generation to another and may play an important role in emotional communication about the use of substances. They can also be triggers for resumption of substance abuse. For example, Peter, the grandson of Swedish immigrants, vividly remembered certain Swedish words and sayings his bilingual alcoholic father used to put him down during his childhood. Although Peter never learned to speak Swedish, hearing these words while on a business trip was enough of a trigger for him to resume drinking after months of sobriety.

Educational Attainment

The level of educational attainment, both abroad and in the United States, provides important cues in assessment and in terms of appropriate interventions. An immigrant with a third-grade education in his native Ecuador will have a hard time following the literature given out in his treatment program, even though it may be in Spanish. On the other hand, the Croatian woman who works as an office cleaner may have been trained as a physician prior to her migration. A realistic assessment of her retraining potential and educational and professional opportunities may play a crucial role in her recovery from her alcohol abuse and coexisting depression.

Past and Current Socioeconomic Status

Although often related to level of education, clients' current socioeconomic status in comparison with their previous one is an important factor to assess. Such assessment not only offers important clues in the possible downhill progression due to substance abuse but is also a crucial factor in understanding immigrant clients who may have held high educational and economic status in their homelands but are reduced to poverty level or low-status positions in the United States. These are factors that may play a role in their substance abuse.

Unfortunately, "many cultural attributes commonly associated with ethnicity are not rooted in ethnicity as such, but are artifacts of social class" (Steinberg, 1981, p. 67). Consequently, the therapist must separate attitudes resulting from physical and environmental adversity from cultural or individual traits of the client (Sue & Sue, 1990). As pointed out by Orlandi (1992), "It is very important to distinguish between the culture of the underclass in our society . . . and the culture of the ethnic/racial subgroups. The experience of being poor in our society is different, for example, from that of being Hispanic, and these conditions must be further distinguished from the experience of being both poor *and* Hispanic" (p. 295).

Unemployment has been correlated with substance abuse, both among native and immigrant populations (NIDA, 1995), and lack of economic resources may interfere with accessing treatment resources or obtaining high-level treatment. In addition, some individuals, particularly inner-city African American and Latino adolescents and young adults, may turn to selling and then using illicit substances as a form of compensation for the scarcity of opportunity to attain economic independence through traditional means (Johnson, Williams, Dei, & Sanabria, 1990).

Socioeconomic dynamics also affect many immigrants who may work long hours in menial jobs, supporting not only their immediate families but also their extended family members in their native countries (Kim, McLeod, & Shantzis, 1992). Their lack of time to monitor their children may play a role in the abuse of substances by their adolescent children.

Family Structure and Roles

An important aspect of ethnocultural assessment is understanding the client's family structure and role expectations and the relationship of substance abuse to these characteristics. As pointed out by Kim and colleagues (1992), "In families in which the parents do not speak English, children who do may be forced to accept certain adult responsibilities—e.g. spokesperson for the family. This is a clear role reversal for the father in his traditional role as the source of authority in the family" (p. 223). This is a particularly painful situation for those families, such as Asians and Latinos, whose culture emphasizes a clear hierarchy of family roles and respect for the older generations. Such role reversal can lead to a loss of respect of children for their parents, which in turn contributes to alienation of the children from their ethnic culture and to intergenerational conflict within the family (Kim et al., 1992; Lu et al., 1995)—all risk factors for substance abuse. It is also important to keep in mind the findings of Maddahian and colleagues (1988) that, compared with White, Hispanic, and Asian adolescent substance abusers, "the single salient high-risk factor for blacks . . . was poor relationship with family members" (p. 20).

Another factor is the cultural variation in child-rearing practices, including the use of physical force. For many families who migrated to provide a better life for their children, having children who are exhibiting academic, emotional, or substance abuse problems may be viewed as a personal failure on the part of the parents, leading to feelings of depression, helplessness, and rage against the child (McQuiston, 1996). Most clinicians are mandated to report cases of child abuse; however, it is also important to help parents understand cultural differences in child-rearing practices, as well as their own expectations of their children and the best ways of dealing with them.

Gender-Related Issues and Roles

Available data indicates that in most ethnic cultures men are more likely to use alcohol and other drugs than women but that substance abuse among women is more stigmatizing than for men (Rebach, 1992). However, such findings may be changing with the latest national data indicating that Hispanic Caribbean women are as likely as Caribbean men to use cocaine (SAMHSA, 1998, Table 4.6), whereas Native American women are even more likely than men to use alcohol, as well as illegal drugs (SAMHSA, 1998, Tables 4.3 and 4.4). The implications of these dynamics for a particular ethnic group and for society in general call for further research.

According to Coll (1992), "gender differences have been noted in the processes of migration, acculturation, and adaptation" (p. 7). Women have been found to see their ethnic identity as more important than do men; at the same time, however, they tend to acculturate more rapidly than men (Coll, 1992). Because the role of women in U.S. society often differs from that in more traditional and more patriarchal cultures, couple and familial conflicts may increase as immigrant women become acculturated to the U.S. norm and more independent of the men in their lives. Such change in familial dynamics can lead not only to the abuse of substances but also to an increase in domestic violence—an issue that must be explored during the assessment process.

Beliefs about homosexuality and about individuals with gender identity disorders are important dynamics among many ethnic groups. Although gays and lesbians are stigmatized in most ethnic cultures, in some cultures they are more likely to be ostracized than in others. Because recovery often requires acceptance of one's sexuality, the impact of open admission of such identity within one's ethnocultural group must be fully explored.

Coexisting Disorders

Not much is known regarding coexisting disorders and ethnocultural differences, particularly as they relate to both mental illness and substance abuse. As discussed previously, it is likely that many immigrants suffer from mood and anxiety disorders, as well as adjustment and posttraumatic stress disorders (Marsella et al., 1994; Westermeyer, 1993b). It also appears that, regardless of culture, the prevalence of psychopathology is higher among female substance abusers than among males, although research data are limited

(Robins & Regier, 1991). A culturally sensitive mental health assessment should be part of every substance abuse assessment.

Ethnoculturally Competent Intervention Approaches

The literature on specific ethnoculturally competent substance abuse treatment skills and techniques is limited. Most substance abusers who do enter treatment, regardless of their ethnic group, receive the same treatment approach. Given the possible difference in treatment expectations among various ethnocultural groups, the clinician should carefully describe the rationale for recommending a particular treatment approach and its goals. Providing clients with or helping them share positive information about their ethnic history, cultural values, traditions, and contributions enhances their self-worth and potential for recovery (see Gilbert & Langrod, Chapter 12, this volume; Gordon, 1994). Moreover, helping clients connect to recovering peers from the same ethnocultural group can provide essential role models and support.

As indicated previously, some ethnic groups, particularly those among the newer immigrant groups, may be unfamiliar with the disease model of addiction that is commonly used in many treatment settings. There are two different approaches in dealing with this issue. One is to help clients and their family members become more familiar with the disease model, thereby helping them better utilize the treatment process and at the same time removing some of the stigma of having an AOD problem (Straussner, 1993). Such an approach is best done by using a psychoeducational didactic model of group lecture or on a more private basis during individual or family sessions. Depending on the literacy level of the client and his or her family members and on the availability of literature in the native language, providing take-home literature is usually helpful.

A different approach is based more on the harm-reduction model, which emphasizes limiting the negative consequences of substance use while at the same time utilizing more ethnoculturally congruent treatment approaches. Such treatment methods may include using culturally appropriate case management to help the client and family meet their basic needs before addressing the substance abuse (see Bromley & Sip, Chapter 16, this volume); focusing on medical problems associated with AOD abuse and working together with medical personnel to address the impact of AOD on the body (see Matsuyoshi, Chapter 19, this volume); and/or recruiting native healers or religious, cultural, and community leaders to provide support and address specific life issues affecting the individual and his or her family (see Weaver, Chapter 4, and Medina, Chapter 7, this volume).

Whether one or a combination of the two approaches may be best for a given individual is highly variable. It depends on the client's entry point into the treatment system, on the client's openness to address AOD problems directly, on the availability of specific ethnic and general community resources, and on specific agency philosophy.

It is important to note that the use of family and group confrontation—a common treatment approach in many settings—may not be effective for those ethnic groups, such as Asians or Native Americans, for whom confrontation is not a culturally common method of communication (Amodeo et al., 1996). Moreover, individual counseling or the use of more ethnically homogeneous treatment groups may be a better treatment approach for some populations, such as Hispanics (Booth, Castro, & Anglin, 1990; Prendergast, Hser, & Gil-Rivas, 1998), than for others.

Studies of family rituals point out their preventative and therapeutic functions in substance abuse problems (Bennett, Wolin, & Reiss, 1988). Therefore, identifying and restoring ethnoculturally appropriate rituals may play an important role in treatment (Harvey & Rauch, 1997; Weaver, Chapter 4, this volume). Connecting or reconnecting to religious and ethnic holiday celebrations while also adapting new rituals, such as anniversary celebrations in 12-step programs, may provide important linkages between past and present cultures. However, for many individuals whose cultural values emphasize the family more than the individual, traditional 12-step programs may be less beneficial than other treatments, such as cognitive behavioral approaches or support groups that include the family or other significant individuals (Draguns, 1995).

Use of interpreters is often a necessary but a complicating factor. Family members, especially children, are usually not appropriate or reliable interpreters. Moreover, even when using a trained interpreter, it is not uncommon to find biases, distortions, and limitations in such communications (Amodeo et al., 1996; Westermeyer, 1990).

Intervention with Women

Given the previously discussed greater stigma regarding substance-abusing women, clinicians need to pay attention to the special issues that bear on women of diverse ethnocultural groups. Depending on ethnic culture and immigration status, women may find themselves with fewer support systems than men, more endangered in terms of losing their children, and more trapped in destructive lifestyles and relationships (for a fuller discussion of women's issues, see Straussner & Zelvin, 1997). Concrete needs such as housing, child care, or vocational training have to be addressed. The possibility for special outreach to, or protection from, the men in their lives must be an important consideration during the treatment process of women; at the same time clinicians must be cognizant of any ethnocultural conflicts that this consideration may cause the client.

ETHNOCULTURAL ISSUES
IN CLIENT–WORKER INTERACTIONS

A crucial issue in offering ethnoculturally competent services is the question of matching the ethnocultural characteristics of the staff with those of the clients (Sue, 1998). Clinicians bring their own cultural assumptions, both conscious and unconscious, into the treatment arena (Perez Foster, 1998). The difficulties in working with clients of different cultural groups from the clinician was recognized as early as 1918 by Freud in his classic case of the Russian "Wolf Man," when he noted that not only the "personal peculiarities" in the patient but also "a national character different from ours made the task of feeling one's way into his mind a laborious one" (1918/1955, p. 7). More recently, in an exploratory study of seven prevention and treatment programs for childbearing and pregnant substance-abusing women, Kirk and Amaranth (1998) found that staff that reflected the client's culture, race, socioeconomic level, and community:

> provided a much needed role model for a population that was poor, undereducated, unemployed and the target of racism and sexism . . . staff who were immediately recognizable as a member of the client's own race or culture had a much easier time and were more successful in engaging and retaining the clients. . . . The agencies contended that staff who did not share the cultural heritage of the participants could be effective, but that the engagement process with the program participants would be longer. (p. 263)

Based on such findings, confirmed by my own supervisory work with a wide variety of clinicians, it becomes crucial that those working with clients who are unlike themselves become aware that they may need to work harder and longer to engage these clients in treatment.

Moreover, staff members may act out what has been termed as "cultural countertransference" (Perez Foster, 1998; Westermeyer, 1993a), communicating their ethnic prejudice to their clients, thereby undermining treatment. Furthermore, "politically correct" clinicians may be afraid to explore the interrelationships between their own ethnocultural values and those of the clients, thereby driving "away those clients who we do not want to treat, covertly betraying and deftly blaming the patient for their lack of 'suitability' to the treatment process" (Perez Foster, 1999, p. 18). For example, a White clinician may be afraid of confronting a Black client for fear of being called a racist, at the same time blaming the client for denying the impact of his or her substance abuse problems on his or her life.

Although clinicians who are themselves from the same ethnocultural background as their clients may find it easier to initially connect with their clients, it does not mean that they may not have their own negative countertransferential reactions and prejudices toward their clients that result from internalized shame of or discomfort with their own ethnocultural background. At the same time, it is important to realize that clients may have their own prejudices and transferential reactions toward the ethnocultural background of the staff, as well as toward other clients. Thus it is crucial that the power and impact of ethnicity and culture be recognized in every treatment encounter.

CONCLUSION

The provision of ethnoculturally competent substance abuse services is no longer an option but a necessity. As pointed out in this chapter and as elaborated on in the chapters that follow, different ethnocultural groups have different experiences and values and different worldviews. Much research needs to be done on substance abuse among specific ethnocultural populations, not just global ethnic and racial categories: We need to know more about what specific treatment and prevention efforts are most effective for different ethnocultural groups, how to engage diverse clients in treatment, and what is the best way to educate staff to be ethnoculturally competent.

In the meantime, clinicians must learn to walk the fine line between ethnocultural awareness and stereotyping of individual clients and groups. They must be careful to assess each individual client, determining the client's views regarding his or her ethnocultural background and current identification and the connection of the substance abuse problem to the client's ethnicity and culture, and must utilize appropriate ethnoculturally competent intervention skills. Most of all, they must remain aware of their own feelings and reactions to their own and their clients' ethnic and cultural backgrounds and make sure that their agencies and communities recognize and value the wonderful diversity of the "ethnocultural salad" that comprises the population of the United States—and our clients—today.

REFERENCES

Abused illegal residents fear spouses and law. (1999, April 18). *The New York Times*, pp. 37, 41.

Akhtar, S. (1995). A third individuation: Immigration, identity and the psychoanalytic process. *Journal of the American Psychoanalytic Association, 43*(4), 1051–1083.

Alba, R. D. (1985). *Italian-Americans: Into the twilight of ethnicity*. Englewood Cliffs, NJ: Prentice Hall.

Amodeo, M., & Jones, L. K. (1997, May/June). Viewing alcohol and other drug use cross-culturally: A cultural framework for clinical practice. *Families in Society, 78*(3), 240–254.

Amodeo, M., & Jones, L. K. (1998). Using AOD cultural framework to view alcohol and other drug issues through various cultural lenses. *Social Work Education, 34*(3), 387–399.

Amodeo, M., Robb, N., Peou, S., & Tran, H. (1996). Adapting mainstream substance-abuse interventions for Southeast Asian clients. *Families in Society, 77*(7), 403–412.

Bennett, L. A., & Ames, G. M. (1985) *The American experience with alcohol: Contrasting cultural perspectives*. New York: Plenum Press.

Bennett, L. A., Wolin, S. J., & Reiss, D. (1988). Deliberate family process: A strategy for protecting children of alcoholics. *British Journal of Addiction, 83*, 821–829.

Booth, M. W., Castro, F. G., & Anglin, M. D. (1990). What do we know about Hispanic substance abuse? A review of the literature. In R. Glick & J. Moore (Eds.), *Drugs in Hispanic communities* (pp. 21–43). New Brunswick, NJ: Rutgers University Press.

Buxbaum, E. (1949). The role of the second language in the formation of the ego and superego. *Psychoanalytic Quarterly, 18*, 279–289.

Castex, G. M. (1997). Immigrant children in the United States. In N. K. Phillips & S. L. A. Straussner (Eds.), *Children in the urban environment: Linking social policy and clinical practice* (pp. 43–60). Springfield, IL: Thomas.

Center for Mental Health Services. (1997). *Cultural competence standards in managed mental health care for four underserved/underrepresented racial/ethnic groups*. Boulder, CO: Western Interstate Commission for Higher Education.

Coll, C. G. (1992). *Cultural diversity: Implications for theory and practice* (Work in Progress No. 59). Wellesley, MA: Wellesley College, Stone Center.

Cunningham, M. S. (1994). Foreword. In J. U. Gordon (Ed.), *Managing multiculturalism in substance abuse services* (pp. vii–ix). Thousand Oaks, CA: Sage.

Davis, L. E., & Proctor, E. K. (1989). *Race, gender, and class: Guidelines for practice with individuals, families, and groups*. Englewood Cliffs, NJ: Prentice Hall.

Day, D. (1999). *Health emergency 1999: The spread of drug-related AIDS and other deadly diseases among African Americans and Latinos*. Princeton, NJ: Dogwood Center.

Debro, J., & Conley, D. J. (1993). School and community politics: Issues, concerns and implications when conducting research in African-American communities.

In M. R. de la Rosa & J.-L. Recio Adrados (Eds.), *Drug abuse among minority youth: Advances in research and methodology* (NIDA Research Monograph No. 130, pp. 298–307). Rockville, MD: U.S. Department of Health and Human Services, Public Health Service, National Institutes of Health, National Institute on Drug Abuse.

de la Rosa, M. R., & Recio Adrados, J.-L. (Eds.). (1993). *Drug abuse among minority youth: Advances in research and methodology* (NIDA Research Monograph No. 130). Rockville, MD: U.S. Department of Health and Human Services, Public Health Service, National Institutes of Health, National Institute on Drug Abuse.

Devore, W., & Schlesinger, E. G. (1996). *Ethnic-sensitive social work practice* (4th ed.). Boston: Allyn & Bacon.

Draguns, J. (1995). Cultural influences upon psychopathology: Clinical and practical implications. *Journal of Social Distress and the Homeless, 4*(2), 79–103.

Dyche, L., & Zayas, L. H. (1995). The value of curiosity and naivete for the cross-cultural psychotherapist. *Family Process, 34,* 389–399.

Freud, S. (1955). From the history of an infantile neurosis. In J. Strachey (Ed. & Trans.), *Standard edition of the complete psychological works of Sigmund Freud* (Vol. 17, pp. 3–122). London: Hogarth Press. (Original work published 1918)

Friedman, E. G. (1997). The impact of AIDS on the lives of women. In S. L. A. Straussner & E. Zelvin (Eds.), *Gender and addictions: Men and women in treatment* (pp. 197–222). Northvale, NJ: Jason Aronson.

Gaw, A. (Ed.). (1993). *Culture, ethnicity and mental illness.* Washington, DC: American Psychiatric Press.

Glazer, N., & Moynihan, D. P. (1970). *Beyond the melting pot: The Negroes, Puerto Ricans, Jews, Italians, and Irish of New York City* (2nd ed.). Cambridge, MA: MIT Press.

Gordon, J. U. (Ed) (1994). *Managing multiculturalism in substance abuse services.* Thousand Oaks, CA: Sage.

Gordon, M. (1964). *Assimilation in American life.* New York: Oxford University Press.

Greenson, R. R. (1950). The mother tongue and the mother. *International Journal of Psycho-Analysis, 31,* 18–23.

Griffith, E. E., Chung, H., Foulks, E., Lu, F., Ruiz, P., Wintrob, R., & Yamamoto, J. (Eds.). (1996). *Alcoholism in the United States: Racial and ethnic considerations.* Washington, DC: American Psychiatric Press.

Harvey, A. R., & Rauch, J. B. (1997). A comprehensive Afrocentric rites of passage program for black male adolescents. *Health and Social Work, 22,* 30–37.

Hays, P. A. (1996). Addressing the complexity of culture and gender in counseling. *Journal of Counseling and Development, 74*(4), 332–338.

Hayton, R. (1994). European American perspective: Some considerations. In J. U. Gordon (Ed.), *Managing multiculturalism in substance abuse services* (pp. 99–116). Thousand Oaks, CA: Sage.

Johnson, B., Williams, T., Dei, K., & Sanabria, H. (1990). Drug abuse and the inner city: Impact on drug users and the community. In M. Tonry & J. Q. Wilson (Eds.), *Drugs and crime* (pp. 9–67). Chicago: University of Chicago Press.

Kim, S., McLeod, J. H., & Shantzis, C. (1992). Cultural competence for evaluators working with Asian-American communities: Some practical considerations. In M. A. Orlandi, R. Weston, & L. G. Epstein (Eds.), *Cultural competence for evaluators: A guide for alcohol and other drug abuse prevention practitioners working with ethnic/racial communities* (pp. 203–260). Rockville, MD: U.S. Department of Health and Human Services, Public Health Service, Alcohol, Drug Abuse, and Mental Health Administration, Office for Substance Abuse Prevention, Division of Community Prevention and Training.

Kirk, C., & Amaranth, K. (1998). Staffing issues in work with women at risk for and in recovery from substance abuse. *Women's Health Issues, 8*(4), 261–266.

Lu, F. G., Lim, R. F., & Mezzich, J. E. (1995). Issues in the assessment and diagnosis of culturally diverse individuals. In J. Oldham & M. Riba (Eds.), *Review of psychiatry* (Vol. 14, pp. 477–510). Washington, DC: American Psychiatric Press.

Lum, D. (1996). *Social work practice and people of color: A process-stage approach* (3rd ed). Pacific Grove, CA: Brooks/Cole.

Maddahian, E., Newcomb, M. D., & Bentler, P. M. (1988) Risk factors for substance abuse: Ethnic differences among adolescents. *Journal of Substance Abuse, 1*(1), 11–23.

Marsella, A. J., Friedman, M. J., & Spain, E. H. (1994). Ethnocultural aspects of posttraumatic stress disorder. In J. Oldham, M. B. Riba, & A. Tasman (Eds.), *Review of psychiatry* (Vol. 12, pp. 157–181). Washington, DC: American Psychiatric Press.

Mayers, R. S., Kail, B., & Watts, T. D. (Eds.). (1993). *Hispanic substance abuse.* Springfield, IL: Thomas.

McGoldrick, M. (1982). Ethnicity and family therapy: An overview. In M. McGoldrick, J. K. Pearce, & J. Giordano (Eds.), *Ethnicity and family therapy* (pp. 3–30). New York: Guilford Press.

McGoldrick, M., Giordano, J., & Pearce, J. K. (Eds.). (1996). *Ethnicity and family therapy* (2nd ed.). New York: Guilford Press.

McQuiston, J. T. (1996, April 18). Six-month term for immigrant who shot son. *The New York Times*, p. B2.

National Institute on Drug Abuse. (1995). *Drug use among racial/ethnic minorities* (NIH Publication No. 95–38888). Rockville, MD: Author.

Novak, M. (1973). *The rise of the unmeltable ethnics: Politics and culture in the seventies.* New York: Macmillan.

Oetting, E. R., & Beauvais, F. (1991). Orthogonal cultural identification theory: The cultural identification of minority adolescents. *International Journal of the Addictions, 25*(5/6), 655–685.

Orlandi, M. A. (1992). Defining cultural competence: An organizing framework. In M. A. Orlandi, R. Weston, & L. G. Epstein (Eds.), *Cultural competence for evaluators: A guide for alcohol and other drug abuse prevention practitioners working with ethnic/racial communities* (pp. 293–299). Rockville, MD: U.S. Department of Health and Human Services, Public Health Service, Alcohol, Drug Abuse, and Mental Health Administration, Office for Substance Abuse Prevention, Division of Community Prevention and Training.

Orlandi, M. A., Weston, R., & Epstein, L. G. (Eds.). (1992). *Cultural competence for evaluators: A guide for alcohol and other drug abuse prevention practitioners working with ethnic/racial communities.* Rockville, MD: U.S. Department of Health and Human Services, Public Health Service, Alcohol, Drug Abuse, and Mental Health Administration, Office for Substance Abuse Prevention, Division of Community Prevention and Training.

Park, R. (1950). *Race and culture.* Glencoe, IL: Free Press.

Perez Foster, R. M. P. (1999). An intersubjective approach to cross-cultural clinical work. *Smith College Studies in Social Work, 69,* 269–291.

Perez Foster, R. M. P. (1998). The clinician's cultural countertransference: The psychodynamics of culturally competent practice. *Clinical Social Work Journal, 26*(3), 253–270.

Perez Foster, R. M. P. (1996). Assessing the psychodynamic function of language in the bilingual patient. In R. M. P. Foster, M. Moskowitz, & R. Javier (Eds.), *Reaching across boundaries of culture and class: Widening the scope of psychotherapy* (pp. 243–263). Northvale, NJ: Jason Aronson.

Philleo, J., Brisbane, F. L., & Epstein, L. G. (Eds.). (1995). *Cultural competence for social workers: A guide for alcohol and other drug abuse prevention professionals working with ethnic/racial communities* (National Association of Social Workers/Center for Substance Abuse Prevention Monograph No. SMA 95-3075). Rockville, MD: U.S. Department of Health and Human Services, Public Health Service, Substance Abuse and Mental Health Services Administration, Center for Substance Abuse Prevention.

Prendergast, M. L., Hser, Y.-I., & Gil-Rivas, V. (1998). Ethnic differences in longitudinal patterns and consequences of narcotic addiction. *Journal of Drug Issues, 28*(2), 495–516.

Rebach, H. (1992). Alcohol and drug use among American minorities In J. E. Trimble, C. S. Bolek, & S. J. Niemcryk (Eds.), *Ethnic and multicultural drug abuse: Perspective on current research* (pp. 23–57). New York: Haworth.

Robins, L. N., & Regier, D. A. (1991). *Psychiatric disorders in America.* New York: Free Press.

Rogler, L., Cortes, D., & Malgady, R. (1991). Acculturation and mental health status among Hispanics. *American Psychologist, 46*(6), 585–597.

Room, R. (1985). Foreword. In L. A. Bennett & G. M. Ames (Eds.), *The American experience with alcohol: Contrasting cultural perspectives* (pp. xi–xvii). New York: Plenum Press.

Rotheram-Borus, M. J., & Wyche, K. F. (1994). Ethnic differences in identity development in the United States. In S. Archer (Ed.), *Interventions for adolescent identity development* (pp. 62–83). Thousand Oaks, CA: Sage.

Sandhu, D. S., Portes, P. R., & McPhee, S. A. (1996). Assessing cultural adaptation: Psychometric properties of the Cultural Adaptation Pain Scale. *Journal of Multicultural Counseling and Development, 24,* 15–25.

Steinberg, S. (1981). *The ethnic myth: Race, ethnicity and class in America.* New York: Atheneum.

Straussner, S. L. A. (1993). Assessment and treatment of clients with alcohol and other drug abuse problems: An overview. In S. L. A. Straussner (Ed.), *Clinical work with substance-abusing clients* (pp. 3–30). New York: Guilford Press.

Straussner, S. L. A. (1994). The impact of alcohol and other drug abuse on the American family. *Drug and Alcohol Review, 13,* 393–399.

Straussner, S. L. A., & Zelvin, E. (1997). *Gender and addiction: Men and women in treatment.* Northvale, NJ: Jason Aronson.

Strom, D. P. (1993). AIDS and intravenous drug users: Issues and treatment implications. In S. L. A. Straussner (Ed.), *Clinical work with substance-abusing clients* (pp. 330–350). New York: Guilford Press.

Substance Abuse and Mental Health Services Administration. (1998). *Prevalence of substance use among racial and ethnic subgroups in the United States: 1991–1993* [Online]. Available: http://www.samhsa.gov/oas/nhsda/ethn/ETHN-Allb.htm

Sue, D. W., & Sue, D. (1990). *Counseling the culturally different: Theory and practice* (2nd ed.). New York: Wiley.

Sue, S. (1998). In search of cultural competence in psychotherapy and counseling. *American Psychologist, 53*(4), 440–448.

Szapocznik, J. (Ed.). (1995). *A Hispanic/Latino family approach to substance abuse prevention* (Cultural Competence Series No. SMA 95-3034). Rockville, MD: Center for Substance Abuse Prevention.

Tirado, M. D. (1998, December). *Monitoring the managed care of culturally and linguistically diverse populations.* Vienna, VA: National Clearinghouse for Primary Care Information.

Trimble, J. E., Bolek, C. S., & Niemcryk, S. J. (Eds.). (1992). *Ethnic and multicultural drug abuse: Perspectives on current research.* New York: Haworth Press.

Tucker, M. B. (1985). U.S. ethnic minorities and drug use: An assessment of the science and practice. *International Journal of Addictions, 20,* 1021–1047.

Turner, S., & Cooper, M. (1997). Working with culturally diverse substance abusers and their families. In E. P. Congress (Ed.), *Multicultural perspectives in working with families* (pp. 236–251). New York: Springer.

van Wormer, K. (1995). *Alcoholism treatment: A social work perspective.* Chicago: Nelson-Hall.

Westermeyer, J. J. (1993a). Cross-cultural psychiatric assessment. In A. C. Gaw (Ed.), *Culture, ethnicity, and mental illness* (pp. 125–144). Washington, DC: American Psychiatric Press.

Westermeyer, J. J. (1993b). Substance use disorders among young minority refugees: Common themes in a clinical sample. In M. R. de la Rosa & J.-L. Recio Adrados (Eds.), *Drug abuse among minority youth: Advances in research and methodology* (NIDA Research Monograph No. 130, pp. 308–320). Rockville, MD: U.S. Department of Health and Human Services, Public Health Service, National Institutes of Health, National Institute on Drug Abuse.

Westermeyer, J. J. (1990). Working with an interpreter in psychiatric assessment and treatment. *Journal of Nervous Mental Disease, 178,* 745–749.

II

Working with Clients
of African Background

The two chapters in this section address the substance abuse issues that affect descendants of the African diaspora. The authors reflect the cultural diversity of people whom we often group together under the single category of "Black." Yet, despite the common legacy of slavery, it is evident that the historical background and its impact on the use of substances varies greatly for African Americans whose families have lived in the United States for generations and for those who emigrated from the Caribbean. Moreover, it is important to note that even among African Americans there is a tremendous difference in patterns of alcohol and drug use and in the resources, both internal and external, that are available to address substance abuse problems. The following two chapters provide some guidelines as to how these differences can be addressed during the treatment of alcohol and other drug problems.

2

Substance Abuse in African American Communities

Ednita M. Wright

African Americans are diverse in socioeconomic status and have origins in many different countries (various areas of Africa, South and Central America, the Caribbean, and so forth), each country having its own unique history of substance use and abuse. Even within the United States, the experiences of African Americans vary according to region of the country and geographic location (e.g., urban, rural, suburban) in which they reside. Despite their diversity, experiences such as a history of slavery and ongoing racism are pervasive influences for virtually all African Americans, and substance abuse is a problem for many individuals, families, and African American communities (McNeece & DiNitto 1994).

Clinicians working with substance-abusing clients need to understand the cultural context of African American life and how it has shaped their relationship with substances. They need to understand that for many African Americans alcohol and other drugs are used as an elixir for the emotional pain and stress of living in an oppressive environment. Such understanding will better inform strategies that are aimed at motivating substance-abusing clients toward healthy choices and, at the same time, will foster the creation of environments that promote cultural dignity.

This chapter addresses the issues of substance abuse in the African American community and provides a brief overview of the historical background, cultural norms and values, and the quintessential connection between substance abuse and racism, White privilege, oppression, poverty, and sexism. Patterns of substance use and abuse and implications for treatment, prevention, and research are discussed.

HISTORIC BACKGROUND
OF AFRICANS IN AMERICA

According to African American scholars, most African Americans can trace their ancestry to West Africa (Baker, 1988; Pinderhughes, 1982). In the African homeland it was customary to use fermented grains and palm sap for the making of beer and wine. Drinking was tribally regulated and accepted only as part of ceremonial practices. Drinking to excess was strongly discouraged (Umunna, 1967). Drinking problems among tribal Africans were therefore rare.

Slavery, the African holocaust (Asante, 1991), resulted in the kidnapping and sale of millions of Africans as a means of cheap labor for the economic development of America and other developing countries. There are varied accounts of alcohol use during the period of slavery. Some accounts describe alcohol as being used as a daily reward given by the "master" for good hard work (Wright, Kail, & Creecy, 1990). Alcohol is also believed to have been used as a means of controlling slaves, especially on weekends and special holidays, by rendering them incapable of escape (Joyner, 1991). Alcohol is also said to be used as a deterrent to organized rebellion (Herd, 1993). At the same time, slaves may have discovered that the effects of alcohol helped them to cope with the daily trauma of their intolerable existence. Nevertheless, there appears to be agreement among historians that there were no significant alcohol-related problems during the period of slavery. The absence of alcohol-related problems was so pervasive that it was even hypothesized that African Americans were physiologically immune to alcoholism (Brown & Tooley, 1989; Herd, 1993; Philleo, Brisbane, & Epstein, 1995).

Following World War I, migration brought freed Blacks from Southern rural areas, in which family and religion were the major influences on codes of conduct, to urban inner-city communities, in which norms regarding behavior were not yet established. The urban environment offered greater economic opportunities, but it was relatively impersonal. Weekend drinking, developed during slavery and carried to the North, emerged as a means of coping with the environment—an environment devoid of any traditional support (Davis, 1974).

African Americans have also been affected by the 19th-century temperance movement (Brown & Tooley, 1989). Although at this time African Americans "had the lowest mortality rate due to alcoholism of any ethnic group" (Brown & Tooley, 1989, p. 117), African Americans intensely supported this movement because of its antislavery platform. But as the temperance movement's political base changed from Northern abolitionists to poor rural Southerners, so did their ideology. The liquor issue became the backdrop for the promotion of White supremacy. Violence against African Americans intensified. Blacks became the "scapegoats" for political agitation and economic strain (Philleo et al., 1995) and the symbolic illustration of much larger issues inherent in the structure of the United States. The legacy of this role continues to challenge our society as it moves into the 21st century.

CULTURAL NORMS AND VALUES

Knowledge of cultural norms and values of African Americans, whose tradition is a mixture of values brought from the continent of Africa and the adaptations required in order to survive slavery and oppression in the United States, is crucial if clinicians are to provide an environment in which African Americans can feel welcomed. Such understanding can be useful in removing some of the barriers that may inhibit active engagement in the therapeutic process.

Worldview

Consideration of cultural similarities that identify African Americans as a group with bonds of African kinship (Butler, 1992) are relevant to enhancing practitioners' knowledge of this resilient group of people. Value themes carried from Africa still influence the contemporary African American at an unconscious level. These values—oneness with nature and spirituality, mutual aid aimed at survival of the group, importance of the extended family, and a present orientation and spiral concept of time—came primarily from West Africa, and their vestiges can be readily found within the African American community today (Bell & Evans, 1981; Brisbane, 1992; Butler, 1992; Jackson, 1995).

The Value of Oneness with Nature and Spirituality

This African value asserts that all things in the universe are interconnected and mutually dependent on one another for existence. It is through religion, in most instances, that this value is expressed. The value of oneness with nature and spirituality is also founded on the notion that there is no separation between what one believes and how one acts. For African Americans, spirituality and its expression have deep historical roots and are well established in the activities of daily living (Asante, 1988). The emphatic belief that there is always hope is the cornerstone of African Americans' spirituality and has enabled them to survive horrendous adversity.

The Concept of Mutual Aid

The identity and survival of African American individuals are defined through relationships with family and groups and through mutual aid. A modern example of this theme is the *Nguzo Saba* (seven principles) developed by Maulana Karenga (1977). These principles are: (1) *umoja* (unity)—to strive for and maintain unity in the family, community, nation, and race; (2) *kujichagulia* (self-determination)—to define ourselves, name ourselves, create for ourselves, and speak for ourselves; (3) *ujima* (collective work and responsibility)—to build and maintain our community together and to solve our problems together; (4) *ujamaa* (cooperative economics)— to build and maintain our own stores, shops, and other businesses and to profit from them together; (5) *nia* (purpose)—to make our collective vocation the building and developing of our community in order to restore our people to their traditional greatness; (6) *kuumba* (creativity)—to do always as much as we can, in the way we can, in order to leave our community more beautiful and beneficial than it was when we inherited it; and (7) *imani* (faith)—to believe with all our hearts in our people, our parents, our teachers, our leaders, and the righteousness and victory of our struggle (Karenga, 1977).

These seven principles promote mutual aid through working collectively and support the value of dependence on mutual support in order to be self-sufficient. In Africa it was expected that each community member share resources so that all members' basic needs were met. In America the poverty experienced by many African American individuals renders them incapable of fulfilling traditional community obligations, thereby resulting in a sense of inadequacy. This sense of powerlessness and frustration may contribute to the abuse of substances.

The Extended View of Family and Focus on Children

The African concept of family includes extended members who may or may not be related by blood. Elders are to be respected for their spirituality, age, and wisdom. It is expected that they are addressed by their titles—*Dr.*, *Ms.*,

Miss, Mr., Mrs., Aunt, Uncle, or *Rev.* Although this practice is not as evident now as it has been in the past, it is still considered a sign of disrespect to address elders by their given names without their permission.

Children in African culture are viewed as the link between the past and the future and are seen as either reflecting or possessing the wisdom of their ancestors. *Umoja,* the first principle referenced earlier, states that striving and maintaining unity in the family and community is an obligation for every African American community member. Children should be infused with a sense of ethnic pride and positive self-esteem. Children are seen as a gift from God and need to be provided with an environment that will enhance their belief in themselves. Many African Americans, however, feel impotent in their ability to create such an environment for their children. Some, such as African American Muslims in inner-city areas, are actively challenging felt hopelessness by developing community services that create life-sustaining environments.

Present Orientation and the Spiral Concept of Time

For Africans and African Americans time is perceived as supple—much like the Native American belief system. Time is marked by events, with its focus on relationships between people. Events begin when all participants arrive rather than at a designated time.

The apparent orientation toward living in the present could represent the vestiges of historical events that conditioned African Americans not to ponder the future or consider the past. Furthermore, in today's inner-city environment, in which the death tolls among young African Americans are extremely high, living moment by moment is a viable coping skill.

CURRENT ISSUES AFFECTING
THE USE OF SUBSTANCES

African Americans are not a monolithic group, but they do share a common cultural heritage rooted in the historical backdrop of slavery, the Northern migration, urban living, the civil rights movement, and the continuing undercurrent of racism. The substance abuse pattern that exists today among African Americans is thus clearly influenced both by history and by current societal conditions.

Among the various explanations for contemporary substance abuse patterns in the African American communities are the following:

• Historical patterns of alcohol use and abstinence by African Americans have played a significant part in influencing their current drinking practices and their current attitudes toward drinking. According to this explanation, the use and abuse of substances by some African Americans on the weekends is reminiscent of the days when slaves were rewarded with alcohol or drank excessively after payday once they moved North. Others, primarily women, do not drink at all, due to early prohibitions against drinking by African Americans and to religious beliefs, role expectations and family responsibilities.

• There is an overabundance of available alcohol and other drugs in African American communities in which liquor stores and drug dealers are readily accessible. Whereas in White communities liquor stores are, generally, located in commercial areas, liquor stores are ever present in African American residential neighborhoods (Brown & Tooley, 1989).

• Economic frustration over not being able to get a job to fulfill their financial responsibilities is a factor in the use and abuse of substance for many African Americans, especially men. Although a discussion of the complex issues girdling the position of African American men is beyond the scope of this chapter, the clinician needs to take into account the social and economic dynamics that have an impact on the ability of these men to fulfill the role of breadwinner.

• Racism and discrimination provide the backdrop for substance use and abuse as a means for African Americans to escape unpleasant feelings or to fulfill psychological needs. The pain associated with the African American experience may be mitigated, at least temporarily, by using substances. In most instances, substances are an available, affordable, and predictable (at least initially) stress reducer for social and recreational purposes and, for some, the major strategy for coping with the untenable circumstance of being Black in America.

Racism and Internalized Oppression

The insidious nature of racism and its effect on African Americans cannot be emphasized enough. Using and/or abusing substances provides a brief yet costly escape from the feelings of anger, guilt, alienation, isolation, and self-hatred engendered by the practice of racism.

Oppression continues to permeate American society. Internalized oppression results when the person who is oppressed internalizes, or embraces, the negative images promoted by the oppressor. Thus self-hatred and lack of trust for other group members emerges. For African Americans, internalized oppression destroys self-confidence and obstructs the development of a healthy self-image, which severely impairs achievement and performance potential.

"Double Consciousness"

Basic to substance abuse treatment is the establishment or redevelopment of a healthy self-concept. For African Americans, developing a healthy self-concept is an arduous task, considering their history and the reality of a racist environment (Boyd-Franklin, 1989; Gary & Gary, 1985; Pena & Koss-Chiono, 1992). Bell and Evans (1981) suggest that strategies aimed at assisting African Americans in self-empowerment must include an understanding of "double consciousness"—the awareness of being Black in a White society. For African Americans the stress of living in such a dual reality is overwhelming because it is coupled with their ongoing experience of racism. This factor complicates the establishment of trust in the social service system, in mental health services, and in substance abuse treatment regimens.

Poverty and Violence

Although historically there has been a decrease in the overall level of poverty among African Americans, according to the 1990 census, the poverty rate for African Americans was 33.1% compared with 10.1% for European Americans (Queralt, 1996). Poverty increases the likelihood of violence and limits life chances and the opportunities for positive living conditions (Queralt, 1996). Use and abuse of alcohol and other drugs have, in many instances, become a response to these conditions.

Violence, initiated by alcohol and drug use and abuse and correlated with drug sales, has gripped the African American community in the last two decades. In some African American communities, the sale and distribution of illegal drugs is a major source of income. Whitehead, Patterson, and Kaljee (1994) observed that drug trafficking is viewed as a means of economic support of one's family, as well as a vehicle to enhance one's masculine image (reputation, status, and respect). At the same time, the correlation between substance abuse, criminal behavior and the African American population (Harper & Dawkins, 1976; Staples, 1988) has created another stereotype that serves to undermine prevention and intervention strategies and treatment approaches.

African Americans are more likely to be arrested than to be treated for substance-related disorders. The average African American person is between three to six times more likely to be arrested than the average White person. According to the Sentencing Project (D'Souza, 1995), about 25% of young African American men are in prison, on probation, or on parole on any given day, compared with about 6% of Whites. Most are young men between the ages of 18 and 35 (D'Souza, 1995).

Lack of Positive Role Models

African American substance abusers have limited role models. As William Julius Wilson (1987) observed in *The Truly Disadvantaged*: "The exodus of black middle-class professionals from the inner city has been increasingly accompanied by a movement of stable working-class blacks to higher-income neighborhoods in other parts of the city and to the suburbs" (p. 143). In the past, the presence of working- and middle-class African Americans in urban communities promoted strong norms and sanctions against aberrant behaviors, as well as on enhanced sense of community, social organization, and positive neighborhood identification. The loss of these role models in inner-city African American communities has had a lasting negative impact on individuals and communities.

Although Alcoholics Anonymous (AA) and other 12-step programs offer a fellowship based on role models who are in recovery, African Americans are often underrepresented in these self-help programs. Many African Americans who join such programs become discouraged because there is no one who can relate to their personal experience. This discouragement often results in limited attendance or leads to dropout, further perpetuating such lack of support. Pairing clients with positive role models in their own community, whether in recovery or not, is a vital step to ensure positive outcomes.

Advertising

Many African American communities, particularly in the inner city, are inundated with billboard messages that clearly link drinking and smoking with social power and influence. In many inner-city communities a 40-ounce bottle of beer is cheaper to buy than a loaf of bread and is more readily available. Because recovery depends on the ability of the substance abuser to sustain abstinence, these environmental factors affect treatment outcomes by acting as relapse "triggers." Most African Americans do not have the option to change "people, places and things," as suggested by 12-step recovery programs (Alcoholics Anonymous, 1976); therefore, they are often at a disadvantage due to environmental influences beyond their control.

Ideology of Conspiracy

The failure of our society in fulfilling the promises of opportunity and equality anticipated by the civil rights movement perpetuates the anger and frustration felt in African American communities. The resulting despair contributes to the emergence of "conspiracy theories" that promote a link between unfulfilled promises and the annihilation of the Black race by the U. S. government (Thomas & Quinn, 1991).

During the 1960s it was postulated that the government was aware of undercover activity by the FBI to infuse the African American community with heroin and other substances in order to undermine civil rights activities. This belief reemerged in the mid-1980s with the advent of crack and AIDS.

The 1956 Narcotics Drug Control Act sanctioned the death penalty for the sale of heroin, which was believed to be a "Black problem" (Philleo et al., 1995). More recent federal policies have carried more severe penalties for possession of crack, which is more common in Black communities, than of the cocaine from which it is derived, which is more commonly used by Whites. Policies such as these contribute to the perpetuation of conspiracy ideologies. On an individual level, such beliefs exacerbate feelings of hopelessness and may ultimately sabotage self-improvement efforts. These beliefs still permeate African American communities and must be addressed during treatment.

PATTERNS OF SUBSTANCE USE AND ABUSE

Alcohol use among African Americans is an established and accepted practice. For most African Americans, drinking in groups is still preferred to solitary drinking, and the brand names and amount of alcohol drunk are often status symbols (Bell & Evans, 1981; Brown & Tooley, 1989; Philleo et al., 1995). In some African American communities offering a drink or other substance is often considered a symbol of wealth, sophistication, and status, but, in general, the inability of an individual to control himself or herself while using substances is perceived as a sign of weakness rather than as a health issue.

Three subgroups of African Americans require further examination of their patterns of use and abuse: women, adolescents, and gay and lesbian persons. A case example, which is a compilation of various individual cases, is presented for each subgroup to focus the examination.

Women

Alcohol use patterns for African American women tend to be polarized, with women either abstaining or drinking heavily (Gary & Gary, 1985; Jackson, 1995; Straussner, 1985). African American women are still either idealized as superwomen or stereotyped as women who emasculate men (Boyd-Franklin, 1989; Devore & Schlesinger, 1991). These myths influence and limit African American women's options in addressing and coping with stress. Consequently, substance use is seen as an expedient and efficient coping strategy with limited repercussions. In reality, African American women suffer disproportionately from health consequences associated with alcohol and other substances. These consequences include cancer, obstructive pulmonary disease, severe malnutrition, hypertension, and birth defects as well as HIV/AIDS (Friedman, 1997).

At the same time, requesting assistance—putting personal business out on the street—is seen as compromising one's status with family and community. Many African American women fail to pursue treatment because of financial resources, child-care responsibilities, lack of support from their significant others, fear of abuse from their partners, and/or fear of losing their children. The following case exemplifies only a few of the hurdles faced by African American women who become trapped in addiction due to poverty and lack of social supports.

> Dawn, a 23-year-old African American mother of three, entered an outpatient treatment agency in upstate New York. She was an admitted crack user and alcoholic. Her current live-in lover was the father of her youngest child and a substance abuser himself. Dawn wanted treatment for her addictions but could not enter an inpatient rehabilitation facility because she had no family or friends to care for her young children. Although she continued to come to outpatient treatment, she complained that her boyfriend was becoming abusive because he thought she would leave him if she got straight. She could not afford to move to her own apartment and felt trapped in her current life circumstance. The clinician urged her to become involved with AA, where she would find support during her recovery process. Dawn attended meetings for several months, then stopped going, claiming that there were very few Black women to whom she could relate and that she couldn't find a reliable baby-sitter. After a few more weeks of abstinence, she relapsed. The clinician tried to make referrals for child care so that Dawn could enter inpatient treatment but was unsuccessful in her efforts. Dawn stopped showing up for sessions shortly afterward.

Three specific issues are highlighted in Dawn's story:

1. The history of oppression has left many African American women residing in poverty and in abusive relationships. It is difficult to consider leaving a destructive relationship or entering a treatment program for substance abuse when basic needs such as housing or safe child care have not been realized.
2. The social support necessary for a successful treatment outcome is severely limited for many African American women. Therefore, treatment programs that emphasize separation from significant relationships as a primary vehicle for complete recovery may lead to treatment dropout.
3. Lack of positive role models and continuing stereotypes limit the utilization of clients' strengths.

Adolescents

Adolescence is a time of multiple transformations. This developmental stage demands an increased ability to form healthy relationships with family, community, and society at large. Ingredients necessary for a successful passage through adolescence include a healthy self-esteem, a sense of competence, and a supportive, nurturing environment in which various roles and capacities can be practiced. Although the tasks involved in this stage of development are the same for all adolescents, African American adolescents healthy passage to adulthood is severely compromised by the reality of racism. According to the National Institute on Drug Abuse, 20.4% of African American adolescents (12–17 years old) reported that they had used illicit drugs within the past year and 7% had used them in the past month.

The following case example illustrates some of the difficulties encountered by a low-income African American adolescent in the process of developing a healthy self-image.

George was a 13-year-old African American boy who lived within an inner-city low-income housing project in Chicago. He attended a public junior high school with other students from his neighborhood. Until this year, George was described by his teachers as a bright and quiet student who excelled at academics, although his teachers were quick to add that his African American classmates teased him about being "too White." Recently, George was referred to the school counselor because he had missed many classes and hadn't seemed to be able to concentrate on his studies. Because there were rumors that George was involved with drugs, the counselor asked him about it. George denied using any substances and stated that the reason he couldn't do his schoolwork was because he had been busy working. The counselor stated that he didn't believe his story and told him to come back when he was willing to tell the truth about his drug use.

Two weeks later, George was picked up by the police for selling marijuana outside the school. Upon arrest, George began to cry, stating that he was trying to get money to get his mother out of jail. Further investigation uncovered that George's mother had been incarcerated for stabbing her boyfriend, who was beating her. George, as the oldest, was attempting to support and care for his 9-year-old twin sisters. George was taken to a juvenile detention center, and his sisters were remanded to temporary custody of the social services department.

Lesbians and Gay Men

Homophobia is one of the most complex issues that African Americans must face and resolve. Even though lesbians and gay men have greatly contributed to the African American community, they still remain ostracized from African American communities at large. According to Keith Boykin (1996), "being gay and Black involves shuttling back and forth between two identities and searching to make peace between them" (p. 92).

> Bill is a 48-year-old African American gay man in recovery who lives in a small town in California. He was married for 20 years and has been divorced for 3 years. The major reason for his divorce was that his wife felt he was having extramarital affairs. Bill denied these allegations. At the recommendation of their pastor, Bill and his wife went to see a marriage counselor. After several months, Bill's wife decided that the problem was not with her and stopped going. She accused Bill of being more interested in being with his best male friend than with her. During one of their arguments she even accused Bill of being a "faggot." Bill continued for a couple more sessions until he revealed that, although he had not had any affairs, he was not feeling sexually interested in his wife and was very concerned about this. He went further, saying that he did enjoy the company of his best friend more than that of his wife and felt confused about why he had such strong feelings for his friend. The clinician responded with a prescription for a quiet, seductive evening with his wife. Bill left the session and ended up in a neighborhood bar. It was only a year later, after his divorce and admission of his being gay, that he was able to address his drinking problem.

Substance Use and HIV/AIDS

The use of alcohol and drugs is viewed as a cofactor in the transmission of the HIV virus because of their frequent pairing with sexual activity. Substance use has the potential to lower inhibitions and impair judgment, which in turn reduces the likelihood of individuals practicing safe sex (Hoffman, 1996).

For African Americans, HIV/AIDS and substance abuse are intimately connected. The Centers for Disease Control and Prevention reported that in 1997 African Americans made up 52.1% of all new HIV cases and that the fastest growing group was African American intravenous drug users.

TREATMENT ISSUES AND APPROACHES

Paramount to effective treatment is the consideration of all possible barriers to the proper utilization of treatment services and to recovery. The following section underscores barriers to treatment utilization, to quality assessment, to intervention approaches, and to the client–clinician relationship.

Barriers to Treatment

Given that most substance abuse prevention and treatment programs are based on European American values (Philleo et al., 1995), it is reasonable to suggest that the majority of treatment models are not only culturally insensitive to African Americans but may also, in fact, be culturally inappropriate for most of them. Fortunately, many education and training curriculums are now including material to expand the knowledge base of clinicians in this area.

Culturally Biased Diagnostic Tools

The majority of the standardized assessment tools currently used in the substance abuse field are derived from studies of European American clients. Clinicians thus need to administer and interpret diagnostic scales and tests with a critical eye. The use of qualitative approaches in conjunction with traditional diagnostic tools can offset the bias inherent in culturally insensitive measurements and allow for modifications in treatment approaches more appropriate to the African American cultural context.

Biased Clinicians

One of the primary barriers to treatment is the clinician's attitude, or countertransference, toward the African American client. For both the African

American and the non-African American clinician it is imperative that supervision be utilized regularly as a means of self-examination and honest discussion of challenges met in the treatment of clients. Cultural competence is an evolutionary process. As clinicians become increasingly self-aware of their biases, racism, internalized oppression, power dynamics, and classism, their cultural competency will also be enhanced.

Clinicians' Fear of Client Rage

The outward expression of anger and rage by a substance abuse client is challenging for even the most experienced clinician. Persons involved in substance abuse treatment often get in touch with repressed rage. This is especially true of African Americans, who have suffered from extended exposure to the effects of racism and oppression. Clinicians need to invite the expression of these intense emotions (within practical parameters) so that the client can begin to understand the origins and full scope of these emotions and their connection to substance abuse and recovery.

Reactions of Non-African Clinicians

Bell and Evans (1981) defined five possible reactions of White clinicians to African American clients. These responses may be generalized to other non-African American clinicians. First, the clinician may use her or his power and privilege to exercise *overt racism* and hostility, thereby dehumanizing the client. Second, the clinician may be aware of personal prejudices but may realize that that disclosure will alienate the client. This reaction is considered *covert prejudice*. The third type of reaction is the *culturally ignorant* one, in which the clinician feels insecure regarding his or her ability to relate to the client. In the fourth type, the *color-blind* reaction, the clinician attempts to create common boundaries with her or his African American clients while negating the ethnicity and cultural uniqueness of the clients, which subsequently reinforces oppression. Fifth, the *culturally liberated* reaction represents an informed practitioner who does not fear differences, is able to express positive regard, confronts honestly, and does not allow the realities of racism and oppression to excuse a client's inappropriate behavior.

The establishment of a therapeutic relationship through trust is based on the honesty of both parties. Therefore, it is incumbent on clinicians to examine and acknowledge their own prejudices, stereotypes, racist attitudes, and power issues and how these are manifested in practice. It may, at times, be desirable for the practitioner to concede the difference in racial background and to be willing to discuss the client's feelings on this matter early in the relationship. Clinicians who have dealt with their own feelings about race and feel comfortable working with culturally different clients will be better able to distinguish whether race is their own issue or the client's.

Reactions of African American Clinicians

African American clinicians are not exempt from their own struggles with racism and cultural identity. It is essential for African American clinicians to be vigilant in examining their own internalized racism and their own use of power and to acknowledge how these issues manifest themselves in their work. It is important to be aware of the differences between themselves and their clients and to be willing to discuss how these differences might influence the client–clinician relationship. This becomes crucial in situations in which African American clients feel betrayed by "one of their own." Some African American clinicians may feel trapped between their identification with their clients and the requirements of the treatment facility.

Assessment of African American Clients

In addition to the utilization of culturally appropriate assessment tools, the following questions can be used to guide the assessment of substance-abusing African American clients:

1. What does the substance mean to the person?
2. Is the client showing resistance or denial or a difference in language and behavioral style?
3. Is the treatment regimen empowering the individual or maintaining him or her in an inferior and dependent position?

Furthermore, assessing spiritual beliefs and practices provides an important lens through which substance abuse among African Americans can be understood and utilized to expand the resources for support. Questions may include:

4. Do you have any religious practice?
5. Did you grow up with any religious practices?
6. Do you believe in a higher power?
7. Do your spiritual beliefs help you cope in life?

A basic task for the clinician is to engage the client in a healthy therapeutic alliance. Such an alliance is influenced by the client's reaction to the treatment milieu. Bell and Evans (1981) defined four interpersonal styles that African Americans may exhibit and that should be assessed by clinicians during substance abuse treatment:

1. *Acculturated* African Americans have consciously or unconsciously made a decision to reject Africentric culture in order to escape the oppression, racism, and rejection that is inherent in being African American in the United States. Therefore, their social, emotional, economic, and at times spiritual needs are met outside the African American community, and their relationships with other African Americans may be uncomfortable or unpleasant. Such clients may resist being placed in a group with other African American clients or may prefer to have a non-African American clinician. Such wishes need to be understood and addressed respectfully.

2. *Bicultural* African Americans have pride in their culture and at the same time can function and fulfill their needs in both African and European American communities. Their emotional, educational, economic, and spiritual needs are usually fulfilled in a diverse integrated living environment. For some, however, this interpersonal style can result in "cultural or racial schizophrenia" (Bell & Evans, 1981, p. 21)—the feeling of not belonging to either community. A client exhibiting this style could appear at ease within the clinical setting while feeling emotionally isolated from both Black and White clients and staff.

3. *Culturally immersed* African Americans have rejected European values and culture and made the promotion of Africentric living central to their lives. Their emotional and spiritual needs are exclusively met in the African American community. Peter Bell (1990) divided the culturally immersed interpersonal style grouping into the "culturally immersed conformists" (p. 60) and the "culturally immersed Afrocentric" (p. 61). The former group has a strong sense of their heritage. They live within and predominately meet their needs in African American communities. The latter group was described as the "new black intelligentsia" (p. 61). This group is not only committed to the promotion of Africentric values in this country but also has a strong association with traditional African peoples. Although such a sense of self may serve as a protective factor against substance abuse, for those who do develop a substance abuse problem, the success of treatment would depend on the ability of the clinician to be emotionally available as the client worked through his or her rage at being an African American in America.

4. *Traditional* African Americans are defined as having "a strong Christian spiritual base" and are represented among the elders and carriers

of African American tradition. They are neither overtly accepting nor rejecting of their African American identity. Traditional persons have met most of their emotional, spiritual, and, to some degree, educational, needs within the African American community. Although their economic needs are primarily met in a European American context, they are usually fraught with extreme power imbalances, leaving them distrustful of non-African Americans and African Americans outside their immediate community. For such individuals, coming into a mainstream substance abuse treatment program is usually a foreign and frightening experience that calls for extreme sensitivity by treatment staff.

The heterogeneity of African Americans emphasizes the need for careful assessment of clients' interpersonal styles. This care in assessment allows for a more culturally appropriate intervention and focuses on the importance of matching client and worker according to interpersonal styles, not just race (Philleo et al., 1995).

Intervention Approaches with African American Clients

An essential aspect of working with African American clients is the issue of respect. Respect can be shown in a variety of ways: by addressing the client by his or her full name and title (*Mr., Mrs., Ms., Dr.*) until given permission to do otherwise; by requesting personal information in private; and by understanding the issue of White privilege. In order to further increase cultural competence and strengthen positive relationships with African American clients, clinicians need to:

- Recognize that an Africentric perspective values the interpersonal relationship between people (client and clinician) above other motivations for change.
- Express genuine interest in and become familiar with cultural norms.
- Dispense with assumptions of racial and cultural identity based on appearance.
- Ask the client how he or she identifies culturally.
- Be careful not to assume privilege by using the client's first name prematurely, particularly when addressing elderly clients or members of the client's family.
- Express a willingness to understand the language of the client.
- Gradually request pertinent personal information, creating an environment conducive to relationship building. Even in this era of brief

treatment, time is needed to establish trust. Clinicians need to look for openings to obtain desired information rather than to force an agenda of data gathering.

- Solicit the client's definition of family. Inquire about who is considered as part of the family, who lives in the home, and who can be depended upon when help is needed.
- Be sensitive to use of words that imply that family members are defective in some way.
- Recognize the role of elders by extending opportunities for collaboration in assessment, intervention, and treatment.

CONCLUSION

The issues that contribute to and perpetuate substance abuse in the African American community are as complex and diverse as the community itself. To decrease substance abuse problems among African Americans will require strategies that are sensitive to the multiple realities that challenge the survival of African Americans in general. We must educate clinicians to the issues of racism and the socioeconomic factors that contribute to substance abuse among African American individuals. We must promote the inclusion of child-care services to augment treatment programs for women. Finally, advertisers must be pressured to cease the glamorization of substance use.

Current research methods do not capture the extensive environmental or possible biological, economic, political, and cultural factors linked to alcohol and drug use and abuse among African Americans (Straussner, 1993). There is a desperate need for research that is conducted utilizing cultural theories, ethnographic approaches, and involvement of African American researchers (Beatty, 1994). Finally, research studies need to explore the relationship between substance abuse and the trauma associated with racism, the impact of the acculturation and socialization process, the effects of poverty, and other issues that perpetuate substance abuse in African American communities.

Treatment and prevention programs must ensure that services are accessible to the African American community via flexible hours, outreach services, and an approach that considers the total individual and their life circumstances. This means that clinicians and treatment programs need to address areas outside the traditional substance abuse arena, such as housing, employment, child care, and other health concerns. Substance abuse services must be made available for that segment of the African American community currently disengaged from services because of limited or nonexistent health insurance and those incarcerated or recently released.

Forming a respectful, informed relationship with the substance-abusing client is paramount to successful outcomes. Utilizing culturally appropriate approaches that are based on Africentric values will strengthen the treatment efforts and illicit positive outcomes. In addition, clinicians must advocate for an increase in prevention, intervention, and treatment research efforts.

ACKNOWLEDGMENT

I wish to thank Rhonda Stanford-Zahn, MSW, CSW, for her assistance in the preparation of this chapter.

REFERENCES

Alcoholics Anonymous: The story of how many thousands of men and women have recovered from alcoholism (3rd ed.). (1976). New York: Alcoholics Anonymous World Services.

Asante, M. K. (1988). *Africentricity*. Trenton, NJ: Africa World.

Asante, M. K. (1991). The Afrocentric idea. *Journal of Negro Education, 60*(2), 170–180.

Baker, F. M. (1988). Afro-Americans. In L. Comas-Díaz & E. E. H. Griffith (Eds.), *Clinical guidelines in cross-cultural mental health* (pp. 151–181). New York: Wiley.

Beatty, L. A. (1994). Issues in drug abuse prevention, intervention, and research with African Americans. In P. Bell, *Chemical dependency and the African-American: Counseling strategies and community issues.* Center City, MN: Hazelden.

Bell, P. (1990). *Chemical dependency and the African-American: Counseling strategies and community issues.* Center City, MN: Hazelden.

Bell, P., & Evans, J. (1981). *Counseling the Black client: Alcohol use and abuse in Black America.* Minneapolis, MN: Hazelden.

Boyd-Franklin, N. (1989). *Black families in therapy: A multisystems approach.* New York: Guilford Press.

Boykin, K. (1996). *One more river to cross: Black and gay in America.* New York: Anchor Books/Doubleday.

Brisbane, F. (1992). *Working with African Americans: The professional handbook.* Chicago: HRDI International.

Brown, F., & Tooley, J. (1989). Alcoholism in the black community. In G. W. Lawson & A. W. Lawson (Eds.), *Alcoholism and substance abuse in special populations* (pp. 115–130). Rockville, MD: Aspen.

Butler, J. (1992). Of kindred minds: The ties that bind. In M. A. Orlandi, R. Weston,

& L. G. Epstein (Eds.), *Cultural competence for evaluators: A guide for alcohol and other drug abuse prevention practitioners working with ethnic/racial communities* (pp. 23–54). Rockville, MD: U.S. Department of Health and Human Services, Public Health Service, Alcohol, Drug Abuse, and Mental Health Administration, Office for Substance Abuse Prevention, Division of Community Prevention and Training.

Davis, F. (1974). Alcoholism among American Blacks. *Addiction, 3*, 8–16.

Devore, W., & Schlesinger, E. G. (1991). *Ethnic-sensitive social work practice* (3rd ed.). New York: Macmillan.

D'Souza, D. (1995). *The end of racism: Principles for a multiracial society.* New York: The Free Press.

Friedman, E. G. (1997). The impact of AIDS on the lives of women. In S. L. A. Straussner & E. Zelvin (Eds.), *Gender and addictions: Men and women in treatment* (pp. 197–222). Northvale, NJ: Jason Aronson.

Gary, E., & Gary, R. B. (1985). Treatment need of Black alcoholic women. In R. L. Brisbane & M. Womble (Eds.), *Treatment of black alcoholics* (pp. 97–114). New York: Haworth Press.

Harper, F. D., & Dawkins, M. (1976). Alcohol and blacks: Survey of periodical literature. *Journal for Specialists in Groupwork, 9*(1), 38–43.

Herd, D. (1993). Ambiguity in Black drinking norms: An ethnohistorical interpretation. In L. Bennett & G. Ames (Eds.), *The American experience with alcohol: Contrasting cultural perspectives* (pp. 149–170). New York: Plenum Press.

Hoffman, M. A. (1996). *Counseling clients with HIV disease: Assessment, intervention, and prevention.* New York: Guilford Press.

Jackson, M. S. (1995). Afrocentric treatment of African American women and their children in a residential chemical dependency program. *Journal of Black Studies, 26*(1), 17–29.

Joyner, C. (1991). The world of the plantation slaves. In E. D. C. Campbell, Jr. & K. S. Rice (Eds.), *Before freedom came: African-American life in the antebellum south* (pp. 51–99). Charlottesville: University Press of Virginia.

Karenga, M. (1977). *Kwanzaa: Origin, concepts, practice.* Inglewood, CA: Kawaida.

McNeece, C. A., & DiNitto, D. M. (1994). *Chemical dependency: A systems approach.* Englewood Cliffs, NJ: Prentice-Hall.

Pena, J., & Koss-Chiono, J. (1992). *Ethnic and multicultural drug abuse.* Binghamton, NY: Haworth Press.

Philleo, J., Brisbane, F. L., & Epstein, L. G. (1995). *Cultural competence for social workers: A guide for alcohol and other drug abuse prevention professionals working with ethnic/racial communities.* Rockville, MD: U.S. Department of Health and Human Services, Public Health Service, Substance Abuse and Mental Health Services Administration, Center for Substance Abuse Prevention.

Pinderhughes, E. (1982). Afro-American families and the victim system. In M. McGoldrick, J. K. Pearce, & J. Giordano (Eds.), *Ethnicity and family therapy* (pp. 29–39). New York: Guilford Press.

Queralt, M. (1996). *The social environment and human behavior: A diversity perspective.* Boston, MA: Allyn & Bacon.

Staples, R. (1988). The Black American family. In C. Mindel (Ed.), *Ethnic families in America* (pp. 303–324). New York: Elsevier.

Straussner, S. L. A. (1985). Alcoholism in women: Current knowledge and implications for treatment. In D. Cook, S. L. A. Straussner, & C. H. Fewell (Eds.), *Psychosocial issues in the treatment of alcoholism* (pp. 61–77). New York: Haworth Press.

Straussner, S. L. A. (Ed.). (1993). *Clinical work with substance-abusing clients.* New York: Guilford Press.

Thomas, S. B., & Quinn, S. C. (1991). Public health then and now. The Tuskegee syphilis study, 1932 to 1972: Implications for HIV education and AIDS risk education programs in the Black community. *American Journal of Public Health, 81*(11), 1498–1505.

Umunna, I. (1967). The drinking culture of a Nigerian community. *Quarterly Journal of Studies on Alcohol, 28,* 529–596.

Whitehead, R. L., Patterson, J., & Kaljee, L. (1994). The "hustle": Socioeconomic deprivation, urban drug trafficking, and low-income, African-American male gender identity. *Pediatrics, 93*(6), 1050–1054.

Wilson, W. J. (1987). *The truly disadvantaged: The inner city, the underclass, and public policy.* Chicago: University of Chicago Press.

Wright, R., Kail, B., & Creecy, R. (1990). Culturally sensitive social work practice with Black alcoholics and their families. In S. Logan, E. Freeman, & R. McCray (Eds.), *Social work practice with black families* (pp. 203–222). White Plains, NY: Longman.

3

Substance Abuse Issues among English-Speaking Caribbean People of African Ancestry

Eda F. Harris-Hastick

> Black Americans are not homogeneous. There is a rainbow of skin tones, and a range of class differences, educational and cultural differences, regional and economic variables, in addition to the infinite host of individual personalities.
> —LONESOME (1985/86, p. 68)

Categorization makes people easily identifiable, for example, "Irish Americans," "Italian Americans," "African Americans," and so forth. However, categorization is not without risks. In the United States, for example, there is a tendency to put all Black people into a single category—African Americans—as if all Blacks belonged to one single monolithic ethnocultural group. Labels such as "African American," "Afro-American," or "Black" have a positive, unifying effect and represent an acknowledgement of the history of Blacks in the United States: brutalized and commonly separated from their nuclear families during the centuries of enslavement; disenfranchised, oppressed, and marginalized despite their emancipation. At the same time, unfortunately, labels deny the diversity that exists among Blacks, who vary greatly in cultural identity, family structure, socioeconomic status, educational levels, and even reactions to racism. Relevant to the context of this book, labeling inhibits the potential for understanding the cultural context within which alcohol and other drugs are used and/or abused by ethnically different groups of Blacks and, consequently, the potential for designing treatment that is culturally responsive and more likely to be effective. This chapter focuses on alcohol and other drug problems in the community of Black English-speaking[1] immigrants to the United States with distinct cultural and historical roots in the Caribbean region—a group frequently undifferentiated in the literature from Blacks born and raised in the United States (i.e., African Americans). This demographic "oversight" seems particularly disturbing because Black West Indian immigrants are in many ways culturally distinct from Blacks born in the United States, and their subculture in this country is both sizable and visible. Given the complexity of this group and the general lack of information about it, the goals of this chapter are threefold: to provide a frame of reference for understanding Black Caribbean immigrants to the United States, to identify the cultural factors that are likely to affect recruitment and retention of such individuals in alcoholism and other drug treatment programs, and to offer culturally sensitive strategies for providing assessment, counseling, and clinical intervention to substance-abusing members of this immigrant group.

UNDERSTANDING THE WEST INDIAN IMMIGRANT

This section is designed to offer insight into the background factors necessary to understanding the Black, English-speaking immigrant from the West Indies, particularly as such factors may have contributed to his or her abuse of alcohol and/or other drugs. It provides an overview of the Caribbean region and an examination of the historical and cultural factors that distinguish immigrants from this region from Blacks from the United States. It also examines the attitudes of Caribbean immigrants toward the use and abuse of alcohol and other drugs, as well as behaviors consequent to their use and abuse.

---

[1]The decision to limit the discussion of this chapter to English-speaking immigrants only is a practical one: The goals of this chapter far exceed the space allotted it without having to examine the problems encountered by immigrants whose need to master the English language significantly impedes their acculturation process consequent to immigration. Although their acculturation process after they arrive in this country is similar to that of individuals from the British West Indies, individuals who move to the mainland from the United States West Indies are also excluded from discussion based on their being free from having either to struggle for legal immigration status or to worry about deportation as "illegals."

The Caribbean

In order to understand an immigrant group, it is necessary to understand something about the place that they have left. Although it is beyond the space limitations of this chapter to provide an extensive history of the Caribbean, I offer a brief geographical, historical, and social overview of the area.

The "Caribbean" refers to that section on the map called the Caribbean Basin: an intricate chain of hundreds of islands approximately 1,500 miles long and between 400 and 7,600 miles in width, stretching from the coast of Venezuela in South America to southern Florida in North America. Although these islands share a common heritage of slavery and colonization, they are distinguished from each other by differences in language and by the influences on the cultures of their individual colonizers: French, Dutch, Spanish, East and South Asian, and English. Although people of African ancestry predominate throughout the Caribbean, its population also includes people from a broad spectrum of other races and ethnic groups, including Garifunda (Afro-Amerindian), Asian Indians, Chinese, Europeans, and those of Arab descent.

The term "West Indian" describes the people from the English-speaking Caribbean region that was settled mainly by the English in the 17th century. Commonly known as the British West Indies, this region is made up of 19 scattered islands with a shared history of enslavement and colonization (Gopaul-McNicol, 1993). Among the largest and/or most familiar of the English-speaking islands are Jamaica (with a population estimated in 1995 at 2,574,291), Trinidad and Tobago (1,280,000), the Bahamas (273,055), Guyana (735,000), Barbados (264,000), Belize (205,000), St. Vincent and the Grenadines (109,900), Grenada (97,400), Antigua and Barbuda (65,000), and the Cayman Islands (33,200; Bureau for International Narcotics and Law Enforcement Affairs, 1996a, 1996b, 1997a, 1997b, 1997c, 1997d, 1997e, 1997f, 1997g, 1997h, 1997i). These islands have close links with one another because of their linguistic, ethnic, and cultural commonalities. However, each of the islands has its own distinct personality, conditioned by history as well as local geography and topography.

Historical and Cultural Perspectives of the English-Speaking Caribbean

A historical and cultural perspective contributes to our understanding of the differences between American-born Blacks and Caribbean Blacks who migrate to the United States, bringing with them a different frame of reference. To understand this phenomenon, we must first examine the historical perspective of enslavement. Although both groups share a common history of struggle and enslavement, there were distinct differences between slavery in the United States and slavery in the Caribbean.

Different Social Structures of Slavery in the Caribbean and the United States

The basic social divisions in the structure of enslavement in the Caribbean were extremely simple and similar to those in the United States: White owners and overseers occupied the top of a pyramid, at the base of which were the Negro slaves (Higman, 1984; Williams, 1976). However, the social structure of slavery in the Caribbean was organized differently from that in the United States. Slaveholders in the United States tended to assimilate everyone (including the newly arrived slaves) into their "American" culture, leading to a loss of ethnic identity by the African slave (Williams, 1976). Slaves were prevented from associating with other slaves of their tribe, and according to Williams, American slave owners assured the separation of families and shipmates as soon as they arrived in the United States by insisting that members of these units were purchased by different slaveholders. The practice in the West Indies was very different. British slaveholders, for example, often identified their slaves by tribe and encouraged the maintenance of a collective identification (Williams, 1976).

According to Mullin (1992), searching for ways to reduce expenses, the Caribbean slave owner permitted slaves to grow their own food at the cost of giving them land and time off to do so. This method of "slave maintenance" became the slave institution in the Caribbean, especially in the mountainous and volcanic islands of Jamaica: Only a portion of land was suitable for sugarcane, so the remainder—the slopes and the ridges of the interior spine—was given over to the slaves as their "mountain," where they grew their own food. Mullin believes that this enterprise provided the base for the modern internal marketing system commonly found in the West Indian islands. Slaves, who grew their own food and marketed the surpluses, traveled constantly and readily beyond their plantation boundaries. By contrast, the mass of slaves in the southern United States did not grow or market their food and were therefore more susceptible to the stifling socioeconomic structure that made plantations the only homes they knew. Slaves in the South were fed "allowances," that is, food doled out to slaves by their masters in arbitrarily determined amounts. For the Caribbean slaves, the process of growing their own food and feeding themselves "diluted white power and slaves acted as if planters (slave masters) owned only their labor, not their lives or personalities" (Mullin, 1992, p. 127).

Another critical difference between slavery in the Caribbean and in the United States was the way in which new slaves in the Caribbean were introduced to plantation slavery: not by Whites but by Africans who were often countrymen of the new arrivals. According to Mullin (1992), seasoned Africans boarded slave ships or went into the merchant yards where newly arrived slaves were held in order to quiet their fears and tell the new slaves, in their own language, what to expect. This West Indian practice of acclimating newcomers stands in direct opposition to the dehumanizing methods practiced in the United States, which had been devised especially to keep slaves divided and subservient by stripping them of their cultural identities.

The practice of keeping slaves together, coupled with their increasing numbers, served to foster resistance and rebellion among slaves in the West Indies. Whereas slaves in the United States were greatly outnumbered by Whites, slaves in the West Indies greatly outnumbered their slave masters. Ironically, the West Indian plantation owners were themselves responsible for maintaining their status as a minority and thus vulnerable to rebellion.

The social structure of slavery in the West Indies differed from that in the United States in another way. In the United States, plantation life existed within the context of a New World made up of family-based communities. At the same time, for young men of the merchant class or younger sons of aristocrats in Europe, trapped by a highly stratified, largely impenetrable class system and the strictures of primogeniture (according to which, by law, all inherited property passed to the eldest son), travel to the West Indies provided one of the few opportunities to make their fortunes. In the absence of an established European community to impose its morality and an overabundance of single, White males, a pattern of forced "socialization" evolved between White masters and their Black slave women, resulting in an elite population of racially mixed Blacks known as "mulattos" (Williams, 1976).

Mulattos in the Caribbean were viewed and treated differently by their slave masters than were their counterparts in the United States. In the absence of a self-righteous, White social elite to voice its condemnation of the practice, mulatto children in the Caribbean were afforded special privileges not afforded to mulatto children in the United States (and certainly not to children of Black slaves either in the United States or the Caribbean). Many West Indian mulattos were allowed to learn to read and write. Some attended European universities, becoming doctors, lawyers, and other professionals, and then returned to their native lands to practice their professions.

This concept of mulattos as a "privileged" class formed the basis of the colored middle class in the Caribbean (Williams, 1976).

One of the roles assigned to Caribbean mulattos was to prevent potential uprisings by collaborating with their White owners and informing against conspiracies among the field slaves. This historical approach of "divide and conquer" is viewed as resulting in the development of the contempt among middle-class mulattos for their blacker brothers and sisters (Williams, 1976). Division of class and economic power correspond to relative degrees of lightness or darkness, with Whites at the top of the hierarchy and dark-skinned Blacks at the bottom. Some researchers maintain that this "divide and conquer" attitude persists even today in many of the Caribbean islands, creating division and serving as a barrier to keep groups apart by race and color.

Another important difference between enslavement in America and in the Caribbean was the lack of overt, legalized discrimination, Jim Crow laws, and lynching in the latter (Williams, 1976). Unburdened by the oppressive legal structure devised to keep slaves in the United States apart, the slave culture in the Caribbean engendered a collective consciousness that was characterized by hope for empowerment in the future.

BLACK IMMIGRATION FROM THE
CARIBBEAN TO THE UNITED STATES

The migration from the West Indies to the United States began in the early 1900s, when the introduction of European beet sugar triggered a severe depression in the Caribbean sugar industry (Gopaul-McNicol, 1993), and continued during World War II and throughout the postwar decades. Traditionally, the primary reasons for Caribbean immigration to the United States have been geographic proximity, poverty, and unemployment in the home countries. Two almost simultaneous political events in the 1960s provided further impetus for emigration: the closing by Britain of its doors to immigration from the Black Commonwealth countries in 1960s (Bureau for International Narcotics and Law Enforcement Affairs, 1996a; Gopaul-McNicol, 1993) and the passage of the U.S. Immigration Act of 1965, which allowed persons of all nations, including those previously discriminated against such as those of the West Indies, to compete equally for entry into this country.

According to the U.S. Bureau of the Census (1993), Caribbeans made up almost 30% (893,000) of the 3,130,000 immigrants who arrived in the United States between 1980 and 1990. More than 20,000 Jamaicans alone

immigrate to the United States annually, principally to large cities such as
New York, Miami, Chicago, and Hartford, Connecticut (Bureau for International Narcotics and Law Enforcement Affairs, 1996a). According to a
release from the New York City Department of Planning's Office of Immigrant Affairs (Dugger, 1997), individuals from the English-speaking countries in the West Indies accounted for more than 15% of the 563,000 immigrants who settled in New York City between 1990 and 1994.

Black West Indian immigrants to the United States are notable because
of their sizable presence on all points in the socioeconomic spectrum. At
one end are the West Indians in professional occupations, who, according
to Sowell (1982), represent a disproportionately large segment of the number of Black professionals in this country. At the other end are the West Indian women who work at low-skilled, low-paying jobs, such as domestic
work and child care, that are available to them but not to men. In between
these two groups are large numbers of Caribbean immigrants of both sexes
who have achieved middle-class status as civil servants. Appointments to
these jobs are based on merit exams, on which Caribbean immigrants tend
to score well, presumably due to the focus on good education that is relatively universal throughout the West Indies.

The terms "Afro-American" or "African American" imply a distinct
cultural and ethnic identity influenced by three sources: (1) cultural rites
and practices passed down from Africa, (2) identification with mainstream
United States, and (3) adaptations and responses to the "victim" system
that is a product of racism, poverty, and oppression (Pinderhughes, 1982).
However, Black immigrants from the West Indies view themselves differently from Blacks whose history of slavery is based here. West Indians associate their history of enslavement and discrimination with their home country, not the United States, to which they have come in search of a "final
frontier" offering educational, occupational, and economic opportunities
(Brice-Baker, 1996). Sowell (1982), the conservative African American historian, believes that Blacks who move here from the Caribbean differ from
those born in this country because they come to the United States with the
drive to succeed that is a tradition among individuals from all cultures who
immigrate here. Moreover, West Indians commonly retain an ethnic identity associated with their island or region, and they continue to view themselves as immigrants long after establishing themselves in this country both
socially and professionally (Brice-Baker, 1996). In recent years, the lower
costs of transportation have made it possible for West Indians to return
home relatively often, and many retain a stronger tie to "home" politics
than to those in the United States (Basch, 1992).

Black West Indian immigrants have different life experiences from

Blacks in the United States as a result of having lived in predominantly Black societies in which they had been accustomed to seeing Blacks in positions of respect as lawyers, doctors, politicians, and civil servants (Green & Wilson, 1990). This educated professional class is available to serve as positive role models even for those Blacks in the Caribbean who grow up in poverty. By contrast, athletes and other celebrities are often the only examples of Black success available in some poor Black communities in the United States.

Arriving in the United States, Black immigrants from the Caribbean are often mistakenly accused of elitist styles of behavior and socialization. In the West Indies, it is common practice to socialize only with one's extended family and peers from one's social class. Those who continue to do so after settling in the United States, however, are often accused of being unwilling or uninterested in "making new friends." Similarly false interpretations are drawn when West Indian immigrants, working at several jobs in order to have money to send back to family members, are not free to participate in after-work activities (Brice-Baker, 1994). Often, these behaviors are interpreted by Blacks in this country as unfriendly or even arrogant, lacking in appreciation for the civil rights struggles that opened up the door of opportunity for mass migration to the United States. Brice-Baker (1994) refers to the issue of "double discrimination" (p.146), that is, Black West Indian immigrants, although commonly surprised by the intensity of the personal and institutional racism they encounter from the White community in the United States, are almost always unprepared for a negative response from the African American community.

Many Black English-speaking immigrants from the Caribbean often experience language problems due to the West Indian or Creole dialects they speak. "[While] West Indians do not experience the same sort of language barrier as do non-English-speaking clients, they do encounter difficulty when they speak only West Indian dialect or English Creole" (Gopaul-McNicol, 1993, p.7). However, not all islands have the same dialect, and some speech patterns are easier to understand than others. Nonetheless, clinicians may find it difficult to understand a client from the West Indies, either because of speech patterns or because of particular sayings that are unique to the Caribbean. For example, there is a favorite saying among Jamaicans that "everything is irie," which means "everything is fine"—whether things are going well or not. Substance abuse counselors accustomed to clients who avoid looking at their feelings are likely to perceive a client's claim that "everything is fine" as an indication that he or she is "in denial" or at best minimizing the severity of his or her problems. A client who says, "everything is irie" may not be "in denial" of his or her feelings but may be using a culturally familiar phrase with which to engage in conversation.

THE USE OF ALCOHOL AND
OTHER DRUGS IN THE CARIBBEAN

As in the United States, the sale and consumption of alcohol is legal in the Caribbean, whereas the sale and use of other mood-altering drugs is illegal. The effect of this distinction is also similar to that in this country: Alcohol abuse—and denial of its negative effects—is pervasive, and the abuse of other drugs is accompanied by criminal, often violent, elements. At the same time, attitudes among some members of the Caribbean population appear to be more positive toward marijuana, which often is used as an herbal remedy. However, possession and distribution of this drug is as illegal in the Caribbean just as it is in the United States.

The Use of Alcohol

The manufacture, sale, and use of rum played an integral role in the history of slavery in the Caribbean. Beginning with the first plantations, the economy in the West Indies revolved around the rum business, and slavery was a critical component in its operation. Rum is also part of the region's social fabric. The name "rum" evolved from its West Indian name, *rumbullion* (Taussig, 1928). According to Taussig, both male and female slaves were known to indulge in excessive amounts of rum, sometimes to the point at which drinking contributed to their deaths. Heavy drinking was seen as a way of life, to pass the time, to avoid boredom, and, most likely, to escape the cruel, inhuman horror of slavery.

Alcohol is still very much an integral part of the Caribbean economic structure. Liquor production is a major industry throughout the Caribbean, and West Indian rums and other liquors are exported all over the world. Alcohol is a vital component of the all-important tourism industry in the islands. Drinking is a 24-hour-a-day activity at the resorts, casinos, and nightspots at which large numbers of West Indians work. Favorable duty-free prices on alcoholic beverages have been a traditional lure for U.S. tourists to the West Indies. Mosher and Ralston (1982) criticize such policies because they encourage a continued reliance on the alcohol industry.

Alcohol is also used by many West Indians in cultural ceremonies, at celebrations of births and weddings, for special holidays, and at special events. According to O'Brien, Cohen, Evans, and Fine (1992), over-consumption of alcohol in Jamaica is a serious problem among individuals of all classes but appears to be more prevalent among the lower socioeconomic group. A social worker who emigrated from Barbados describes her childhood impressions of the attitudes prevalent there toward heavy drinking—or at least heavy drinking by men:

"When I think back, I realize that what I now know as 'alcoholic' drinking was not uncommon at home—we just didn't have a name for it. I had one uncle who must have had a drinking problem because I can't remember seeing him when he wasn't drinking. He shifted from job to job. He was always promising his wife that he would never drink again, only to see him drunk again a few days later. He even tried what Alcoholics Anonymous calls 'geographic'— moving to Trinidad to see if the change of scene would help him change. I think we all accepted heavy drinking as a part of the culture of poverty—you know, the only escape open to a poor man. Looking back, it's almost hard to believe the denial we practiced but we did not see it as denial. We thought it was normal behavior, sort of. I can't remember anyone ever blaming alcohol for an accident that happened, or a fight that broke out."

Whereas it is acceptable for Caribbean men to drink, drinking by women, especially in public places, is frowned upon even today. It always has been and still is perfectly acceptable for men to drink in the "rum shops" (small establishments along the side of the road, particularly in rural areas); however, it is considered "unladylike" for women to be seen in such establishments. A man can stop at the rum shop on the way home to have a "drink with the boys," but the employed woman is expected to go home after work to care for the children and prepare the meals. (Women professionals, who are able to afford maids, are not free of these expectations: They are required to go home as soon as the work day is finished in order to oversee the preparation of the evening meal).

The Use of Marijuana

Marijuana was first introduced to the West Indies by way of Jamaica sometime in the 19th century, a by-product of the migration of large numbers of Indians from Asia who were lured to the Caribbean in order to work in sugar plantations after the emancipation of African slaves in 1838. Locally, marijuana is called by its Indian name, *ganja,* and the manner in which it is prepared is likewise Indian in origin (Chevannes, 1988). Chevannes (1988) reports that *ganja* smoking is socially acceptable and widely used by Caribbean people. In Jamaica, for example, as in India, it is used in a variety of ways and for a variety of purposes. *Ganja* is one of the many natural ingredients used by local herbalists, who are often the primary healers in communities in which medical practitioners are scarce. *Ganja* is highly rated as a cure for the common cold, stomachaches, fever, colic, and other ailments. It is given to babies to ward off evil spirits; in some instances, it is prepared as a vegetable or boiled in soup. *Ganja* is also added to overproof rum; after burying the mixture in the ground for several days, it is taken, a spoonful at a time, as a powerful tonic. *Ganja* appeals strongly to working-class youth and persons who espouse the Rastafari ideology, which considers *ganja* a holy weed and promotes its use. According to Chevannes, this ideology appeals especially to the unemployed and school dropouts. It has been glamorized in the music of reggae artists such as the late composer/singer Peter Tosh, whose popular song, "Legalize It," claims that all sections of Jamaican society use marijuana. Because of its notoriety, the song was eventually banned.

Over the past 100 years, the use of *ganja* has proliferated in Caribbean society and has become well integrated into the life styles of the working class—both men and women—with its ritual, medicinal, and recreational value. It is said that it is so entrenched in the culture of Jamaica and so accepted by some individuals from all socioeconomic classes that, despite government efforts, eradication of *ganja* use appears almost impossible (Broad & Feinberg, 1995; Rubin & Comitas, 1975).

The Use of Narcotics

Over the past 10 years, drug-related problems in the West Indies have increased significantly. This shift is due, at least in part, to the deportation from the United States of Caribbean citizens who are convicted of drug-related felonies (Bureau for International Narcotics and Law Enforcement Affairs, 1997; Rohter, 1997). These deportees commonly continue their patterns of drug abuse and/or the criminal activities necessary to their habits once they are returned to the Caribbean region. Even a drug-addicted deportee who wants to change his or her lifestyle has a hard time doing so, given the paucity of drug treatment facilities (as we know them) in the West Indies.

During the past 10 to 15 years, the islands of the West Indies have become major centers for the transshipment of cocaine and some heroin from South American suppliers to distributors in the United States and Europe. It is believed that this new routing, which is a consequence of the policies of the "War on Drugs" being waged by the U.S. Drug Enforcement Agency and its cooperating countries, has fueled a wave of addiction, crime, and violence in these small, largely poor Caribbean islands (Hamid, 1994). Widespread social and economic dysfunction and the absence of culturally generated parameters that channel and control drug consumption have resulted in a growing number of persons getting caught up in the illegal distribution of and addiction to crack cocaine. Drehner and Hudgins (1992) report on drug trends in Jamaica at the time when crack cocaine had only recently become the illegal drug most disturbing to government officials. Moreover, there is an increasing trend of crack cocaine use, once primarily a male activity, by women of childbearing age (Drehner & Hudgins, 1992).

TREATMENT ISSUES OF SUBSTANCE-ABUSING INDIVIDUALS FROM THE CARIBBEAN IN THE UNITED STATES

Because epidemiology studies on substance abuse lump Blacks of all cultural backgrounds into a single category, it is virtually impossible to state with certainty the true number of Caribbean immigrants in the United States suffering from alcohol and other drug problems. Despite the large Caribbean population in the United States, particularly in the New York region and parts of the southern United States, Caribbean immigrants are noticeably underrepresented in substance abuse treatment facilities. It is tempting to interpret these statistics positively, that is, as proof of a low rate of alcohol and other drug-use problems. Unfortunately, oral interviews and ethnographic research indicate that the rate of chemical dependency problems among West Indians is at least equal to that of other groups in the United States (Broad & Feinberg, 1995; Hamid, 1994).

A particularly disturbing explanation for the underrepresentation of Caribbean immigrants in substance abuse treatment facilities is that such individuals are reluctant to enter and stay in treatment programs that are insensitive to their culture. Black West Indian immigrants enrolling in treatment for problems with alcohol or other drugs too often encounter personnel who are unfamiliar with issues related to the immigrant experience and/ or cultural differences between Caribbean clients and Blacks whose roots are in the United States. Speaking anonymously, a clinician working for a New York City substance abuse treatment agency comments about what she feels are some of the fundamental problems that clients from the West Indies often encounter at her agency:

"Where I work—and I don't think the situation is very different from agencies almost anywhere in the country—we use a treatment model that is based on key principles that often run counter to fundamental cultural behaviors and attitudes of our clients from the Caribbean. At the heart of our treatment is a belief in the curative power of the group process. Many West Indian clients have been raised not to discuss their problems outside their immediate family (or not at all), and here we are, using what amounts to peer pressure to 'get them' to talk. Also, many clients enter treatment because they have been mandated, due to a urine test at their job that is positive for marijuana (which they don't see as a drug) or a DWI [driving while intoxicated]. They enter the program feeling humiliated, like they've fallen from some special place into what they feel is the American mainstream. According to them, now they're labeled for life as 'alcoholics' or 'drug addicts.' They're too ashamed to speak to their families, but we press them to bring their wives and/or the parents they revere into treatment. They also can't understand the bureaucracy here, and the power it has on their lives. Like all clients, we send them to Alcoholics Anonymous 'to find spirituality' when many of these clients have been spiritual all their lives."

Incorporating the information discussed previously about Black immigrants from the Caribbean, this section offers a blueprint for substance abuse treatment that is sensitive to the special needs and experiences of such clients. It identifies the elements of culturally sensitive assessment and treatment, effective use of group modalities (including referrals to 12-step programs), clinical issues specific to working with women from the Caribbean, and common transference and countertransference reactions that can arise due to cultural factors.

Issues in Assessment and Early Treatment

Clinicians' awareness of clients' cultural backgrounds is a critical factor in the formation of accurate diagnoses and appropriate treatment planning, and it can make the difference between clients' commitment to treatment or premature termination. Culturally sensitive clinicians must always remember the dangerous potential for stereotyping under the guise of awareness.

Assessments of clients from the West Indies should explore their attitudes about drinking and the use of other drugs (particularly marijuana), because many of these individuals hold attitudes that are culturally informed and different from what is acceptable in the United States. It is not uncommon to hear stories of drinking alcohol as a child with parental consent as part of the "special" Sunday meal or to hear men talk about daily drinking sessions with the guys in which "a man is expected to hold his liquor." Some Caribbean clients may need help adjusting to the more openly negative laws about and attitudes toward marijuana.

A number of other culturally related issues are likely to affect the treatment outcome of Black immigrant clients from the Caribbean: use of language; attitudes about gender and about child rearing; the level of the client's awareness of and/or identification with the history of enslavement in his or her country (and especially how those factors may be different from those of Blacks in the United States); the client's socioeconomic, educational, and career background, reasons for migration, and expectations of his or her future in this country; location of immediate family members; and lack of family or other sources of emotional support in the United States. One way of finding and maintaining friendships and emotional support that is commonly used by immigrants from the Caribbean is through the African custom called *susu* that is still practiced today. *Susu* is a West African custom of pooling money from members of a trusted group of persons, usually friends (Warner-Lewis, 1991). Customarily, the money is held by one member of the group, who ensures that over a period of time the entire fund will be at the disposal of each contributor in turn. It is a unique method of assessing funds and postponing gratification in order to make large purchases or to provide an education for their children. According to Kasinitz (1992), the *susu* concept is practiced throughout the Caribbean, where it performs a vital economic service, that is, the creation of rotating credit associations. Of importance to clinicians is the reality that this practice offers a mutual support system for clients who may be separated from family and loved ones. The social benefits of membership in a *susu*—friendship, companionship, and the sharing of information—are as valuable as the economic benefits (Kasinitz, 1992).

The following vignette demonstrates the extraordinarily powerful meaning that the *susu* holds for its members.

Mrs. H is a Barbadian-born lawyer in her mid-30s, divorced and the mother of a teenage daughter, who came to an outpatient substance abuse clinic treatment at the suggestion of a friend who thought that she had a drinking problem. During the intake, Mrs. H revealed that, a few days before, she had stopped for a drink at a bar on her way home. While she was drinking, the $1,400 that she had received in her *susu* turn, money with which she had intended to pay two months' back rent, disappeared. She remembered being on the way to the ladies' room when she realized that she did not have her pocketbook, which she had placed on the floor beside her seat. When she returned to her seat, the pocketbook was open and her wallet, containing all the money, was gone. Hearing what happened, her friend, a partner in the *susu* who works as a nurse's aide in a local hospital, loaned her the money with which to pay her back rent. It was this friend who had strongly encouraged Mrs. H to contact the clinic. Mrs. H told the intake worker that she was not worried about repaying her friend because she earns a substantial income as an attorney. She also insisted that she does not have a drinking problem, that it was just "that one time when [she] was socializing with friends that [she] had had a little too much to drink." Her immediate concern was to save face and she was fearful that she might lose the trust of her *susu* partners and become an outcast.

Clinicians must also be sensitive to a variety of other special issues, such as the problems faced by a man in treatment for drug abuse who moved to a large American city after a farming life in Guyana, where he had never learned to read or write. His literacy problem and his sense of inferiority because of it came to light during an assessment. It is likely that his treatment would have failed had not his problem been picked up and addressed at the very beginning.

Awareness of Gender Role

In most of the islands of the Caribbean, both men and women ascribe to a more rigid and traditional concept of gender roles than found in the United States today. Men are masters in the home and the primary breadwinners. Women, even those who are highly educated and work as professionals, are considered mistresses of the household, fully responsible for its upkeep (cooking, cleaning, child care, etc.) During the assessment interview, the clinician should be alert to how these gender-role expectations may affect a client's sense of well-being and treatment expectation. For example, a male client who had arrived from Antigua felt demeaned and ashamed when he could not find a job equal to his qualifications, even after he was informed about the tightness of the job market in his field. A female client from Belize, where she was raised to value privacy, reacted with confusion, anger, and embarrassment whenever the women in her treatment group talked openly about their sex lives.

Later Treatment Issues

Once the treatment process has begun, counselors should be flexible in the approach they use with West Indian clients. In the case of culturally based differences in attitudes toward marijuana, for example, a confrontational approach on the part of the counselor can result in a therapeutic impasse.

The client in the following case, who was mandated by his job to treatment for marijuana use, entered treatment staunchly defending the medicinal powers of marijuana, a major component, he said, in the herbal remedies he had been given as a child. The culturally sensitive approach employed by the counselor was able to break through the client's resistance in a way that a hard-line antidrug argument was unlikely to have accomplished:

> Mr. R, a Bahamian-born bus driver, initially denied using marijuana, claiming that there had been a mix-up in the drug reports. Later he admitted that he smokes marijuana on occasion with his friends, but never when he is driving the bus. He did not see a problem with "an occasional joint. Marijuana is better than alcohol," he argued, "but the White, American liquor lobby is too powerful for anyone to take on—that's why it's okay to drink but not to smoke." Instead of confronting him directly, Mr. R's counselor eventually broke through his resistance to treatment by focusing on the impact on Mr. R's family should he lose his job. After several weeks of venting anger at the "system," Mr. R noted with surprise that he had not missed smoking marijuana—and had, in fact, rather enjoyed not having to worry about testing positive on random drug tests given at work. He also noticed a new clarity of thought, improved relations with his wife and children, and having more pocket money between paydays.

Some clients from the West Indies require basic education about the effects of alcohol and other drug use. Individuals from areas in which heavy drinking by men is an accepted behavior enter treatment unaware of the risk of severe organ damage from alcohol abuse. Clients may not know "obvious" things. For example, to check the labels of over-the-counter medications for alcoholic content or that nontraditional remedies such as stout (which contains yeast and is used as a tonic or aphrodisiac) contain alcohol or that remedies purchased from a local herbalist may contain detectable amounts of cannabis or other natural but controlled substances. Two clients in Mr. R's treatment group almost lost their jobs because of ignorance. One client tested positive for alcohol after taking Nyquil cold treatment syrup (12.5%, or 25 proof, alcohol), and the other was shocked when he tested positive for marijuana after drinking a "cleansing tea" given to him by a West Indian herbalist.

Use of Group Treatment and 12-Step Programs

Group therapy is almost universally the modality of choice in the treatment of chemical dependency. However, talking about their problems in a group may be extremely difficult for many clients who emigrate from the Caribbean. Privacy is highly valued, and for many individuals problems are not discussed at all—not even with close family members. Techniques that can be used to diminish the level of discomfort West Indian clients may experience include providing an orientation that includes didactic groups that explain the treatment process and/or provide basic education about alcohol and other drugs, scheduling individual sessions for a limited time until they are comfortable talking about themselves, and/or assigning them to groups with other Caribbean members.

Another area requiring special sensitivity is how and when to refer West Indian clients to 12-step programs. Many clients may be resistant to attending such meetings, although in cities with large Caribbean populations clinicians may be able to enlist other West Indian members to take Caribbean newcomers to their first 12-step meetings. For example, one counselor got nowhere as long as she insisted that a female client from Trinidad go to an Alcoholics Anonymous (AA) meeting. On her own, however, the client sought out the support of the pastor of her church, and through him got involved with an AA group that met regularly at his church.

Use of Language

Clinicians must pay attention to the use of language. Counseling sessions must include opportunities for discussion of unfamiliar sayings and statements (like the saying "everything is irie" previously discussed); otherwise, the client may well feel frustrated and misunderstood. In such situations, just as one would with any client, the therapist needs to seek clarification of any statements he or she does not understand and to let clients know when he or she cannot understand the client's accent. It is important to recognize that sayings and proverbs are philosophical and "rich in precept, instruction, advice, admonition, and judgment" (Blackman, 1982, p. vi). These proverbs contain varying degrees of "relevant information on the mentality, manners, world view and moral framework of the social group which uses them" (p. vi). One in particular, "Drunk or sober, mind yah business," should have special meaning to the chemical dependency clinician: Clients from the West Indies who are reluctant to share information about themselves may be acting from a sense of privacy that is culturally imbued and not, as it would be easy to assume, out of resistance to treatment.

The following case study highlights the need for clinicians to explore culturally rooted factors—such as the client's perception of the nature of the problem, his or her reaction to a particular treatment modality, and discrepancies in communication styles between the counselor, the client, and/ or his or her peers—and, when and where possible, to encourage discussion of practices rooted in African culture that have some relevance to greater understanding of Caribbean clients' lifestyles.

Dr. W is a 34-year-old married father of four children whose family was waiting in St. Lucia until he could afford to pay for them to join him in Miami. Dr. W was referred to an alcohol outpatient program following his arrest for driving while intoxicated. On intake, Dr. W revealed that he had a PhD in sociology from the University of the West Indies but had been unable to find work in his field since entering the United States 2 years previously. Apparently he was expecting his PhD to secure him a job immediately upon arrival in the United States, and he seemed baffled by the responses of potential employers, several of whom questioned the validity of the credentials he had earned at a university with which they were unfamiliar. Some seemed to have trouble understanding his accent, a problem that upset him a great deal because he was very proud of his ability to use language well. Dr. W eventually took a job driving a cab. At intake, he denied having a drinking problem and expressed anger about being mandated to get treatment "for a problem I do not have." He was also concerned about the temporary loss of his driver's license, without which he would have no means of support.

Although Dr. W kept his appointments, he continued to deny having a drinking problem, always appeared well dressed in a suit and tie, and was always polite, though reserved and standoffish. He spoke English with a slight British accent and was reluctant to engage in dialogue with other clients or with clinic staff, most of whom perceived him as "haughty." His denial of his drinking problem frustrated the agency staff and other clients and resulted in his being scapegoated in therapy groups. Treatment was half over before a breakthrough occurred. Hearing another member of his group describe her parents' disappointment with her failure at school, Dr. W admitted that he also felt like a failure. The success he had anticipated when he emigrated had not materialized, and he had not fulfilled the great promise his family had always attributed to him. He revealed too that he had been lying to his friend from St. Lucia who sometimes dropped him off at the treatment center, saying that he was teaching in a school at the treatment facility because he was ashamed to admit that he had a problem with alcohol. In the weeks that remained in his treatment, the counselor and the other members of his group helped him work through his frustrations in his job search, described as "degrading." When the time came to send for his wife and children, the group gave him their support and helped him to face the shame he experienced at not having accomplished "enough" since arriving in this country.

Caribbean Women in Treatment

Generally, very few Caribbean women are seen in treatment, and most of the women who do enter treatment have been mandated to do so by a child welfare or other public agency. Several factors contribute to the paucity of female clients. As previously discussed, drinking is viewed as more acceptable for men than women. Shame and fear of what might happen were they to admit to having a problem keep many Caribbean women from getting help. Others are "protected" by the Caribbean social structure itself from acknowledging the need to seek treatment. With extended families to assist them with the care of their children and to serve as substitute parents when their problems with alcohol and/or other drugs interrupt their ability to parent, some women may not feel the need to stop or to seek treatment. Moreover, because women in the traditional Caribbean culture are not supposed to complain about their marriages, women who are victims of domestic violence may find in drinking the comfort they cannot get from their family and friends. These women may be even more reluctant to enter substance abuse treatment because doing so would lead to facing up to their domestic situations.

> Mrs. T, a Trinidadian-born, married mother of a 9-year-old in her late 30s, came to the United States 3 years previously by way of Canada, where she had lived for several years while her husband sought work in the United States. She was referred to an outpatient treatment clinic by a local child welfare agency after the placement of her son in foster care due to child abuse. In her intake interview, Mrs. T said that she had been drinking heavily since arriving in the United States. Despite her drinking problem, Mrs. T had maintained her job at a local nursing home. A year before, she had stopped drinking for approximately 3 months but had started to drink again after a fight with her husband that resulted in his injuring her so badly that she had been forced to miss work. Mrs. T was assigned to a women's early recovery group that met three times weekly. Although she was the only Caribbean immigrant in the group, she was not alone in being a victim of domestic violence. Initially, Mrs. T defended her husband, a nonunion construction worker from St. Kitts who sometimes went months between work assignments. It was a blow to his Caribbean male ego, she explained, that they often had to live on her salary and depended on the health benefits from her job. With the support of her group, Mrs. T stopped drinking and

learned that nothing justified her husband's occasional violence. She was referred to a Victims Services agency where she learned about options for temporary shelter and legal interventions.

Transference and Countertransference

The client–counselor relationship often raises transference–countertransference issues related to cultural differences. In any situation, the issues of power and authority are major influences on the feelings of the client toward the therapist (transference) and the feelings of the counselor toward his or her client (countertransference). Traditionally, transference and countertransference have been viewed as related exclusively to reactions to early childhood experiences with parental authority figures. Currently, race and gender, key factors in determining power, are considered equal influences on these reactions.

Arriving in the United States, Black immigrants from the Caribbean are forced to deal with the dominance of White culture, and this imbalance of power plays a role in their transferential reactions. These reactions depend on the gender of the client, the race and gender of the counselor, and qualities and experiences that are unique to each partner in the dyad. For example, male West Indian clients accustomed to authority based on gender may be more likely to accept a female counselor who is White (e.g., culturally empowered) than one who is African American. On the other hand, Black Caribbean women clients may react with either passivity or anger at both White and African American male counselors in response to the perception of them as authority figures. Caribbean men who are accustomed to being authority figures may also feel somewhat intimated by an African American male counselor. Similarly, an African American male counselor may need to address his own transferential issues in supervision. For example: Dr. W's male African American substance abuse counselor admitted in supervision that he found Dr. W, with his formal attire and speech, to be "uppity." The counselor's supervisor helped him to look at some of his own feelings of inadequacy and to consider returning to school for an advanced degree. He admitted to his supervisor that he had always been too frightened to return to school, feeling that he could not measure up to the task.

The Latina counselor for Mrs. T, the battered nursing-home aide, had a negative countertransference to her client, whom she viewed as weak and passive for not standing up to her husband. In supervision she examined her strong reaction, which she connected to her own marriage to an abusive man.

CONCLUSION

The literature on substance abuse reflects increased recognition of the critical role of culturally sensitive counseling. To be effective, counseling must take into account the client's particular world and perceptions of himself or herself (Brice-Baker, 1996), as well as historical and cultural differences that are unique to that individual. To deny or negate such differences fosters "ethnocentric bias" (Sue & Sue, 1990) and impedes the helping process.

As with any immigrant group, immigrants from the West Indies often experience problems with communication, a loss of community, family, and/or support system, the need to adjust to a new climate and different foods, new models of family living, immigration difficulties, and so forth. Black English-speaking immigrants from the Caribbean also are confronted with the realities of elitism and racial stereotyping. The difference in gender-role expectations in the United States is often another source of confusion and alienation. Any or all of these factors may play a role in the development of substance abuse problems and in treatment.

Rum and tourism are intrinsic to the history, culture, and economy of the Caribbean. The use of other drugs, particularly marijuana, appears to play a different role than it does in the United States. These powerful realities can have significant impact on the substance abuse counseling process with Black, English-speaking immigrants who migrate to the United States from the West Indies. Further research is needed to understand more fully the attitudes of Caribbean immigrants on the use, abuse, and treatment of alcohol and other drugs. The results of this research must then be applied to developing specific strategies to identify, assess, and treat this clientele.

REFERENCES

Basch, L. G. (1992). The politics of Caribbeanization: Vincentians and Grenadians in New York. In C. R. Sutton & E. M. Chancy (Eds.), *Caribbean life in New York City: Sociocultural divisions* (pp. 147–166). New York: New York Center for Migration Studies.

Blackman, M. (Ed.). (1982). *Bajan proverbs*. Barbados, West Indies: Caribbean Graphics and Letchworth.

Brice, J. (1982). West Indian families. In M. McGoldrick, J. Giordano, & J. K. Pearce (Eds.), *Ethnicity and family therapy* (2nd ed., pp. 123–133). New York: Guilford Press.

Brice-Baker, J. R. (1994). West Indian women: The Jamaican woman. In L. Comas-

Díaz & B. Greene (Eds.), *Women of color: Integrating ethnic and gender identities in psychotherapy* (pp. 139–160). New York: Guilford Press.

Broad, K., & Feinberg, B. (1995). Perceptions of ganga and cocaine in urban Jamaica. *Journal of Psychoactive Substances, 27,* 261–276.

Bureau for International Narcotics and Law Enforcement Affairs. (1996a, May). *Background notes: The Cayman Islands.* Washington, DC: U.S. Department of State.

Bureau for International Narcotics and Law Enforcement Affairs. (1996b). *Background notes: Jamaica.* Washington, DC: U.S. Department of State.

Bureau for International Narcotics and Law Enforcement Affairs. (1997a, April). *Background notes: Antigua and Barbuda.* Washington, DC: U.S. Department of State.

Bureau for International Narcotics and Law Enforcement Affairs. (1997b, April). *Background notes: The Bahamas.* Washington, DC: U.S. Department of State.

Bureau for International Narcotics and Law Enforcement Affairs. (1997c, April). *Background notes: Barbados.* Washington, DC: U.S. Department of State.

Bureau for International Narcotics and Law Enforcement Affairs. (1997d, March). *Background notes: Belize.* Washington, DC: U.S. Department of State.

Bureau for International Narcotics and Law Enforcement Affairs. (1997e, April). *Background notes: Grenada.* Washington, DC: U.S. Department of State.

Bureau for International Narcotics and Law Enforcement Affairs. (1997f, April). *Background notes: Guyana.* Washington, DC: U.S. Department of State.

Bureau for International Narcotics and Law Enforcement Affairs. (1997g, April). *Background notes: St. Vincent and the Grenadines.* Washington, DC: U.S. Department of State.

Bureau for International Narcotics and Law Enforcement Affairs. (1997h, April). *Background notes: Trinidad and Tobago.* Washington, DC: U.S. Department of State.

Bureau for International Narcotics and Law Enforcement Affairs. (1997i). *International Narcotics Control Strategy Report, 1996.* Washington, DC: U.S. Department of State, Drug Enforcement Administration.

Chevannes, B. (1988). *Background to drug use in Jamaica* (Working Paper No. 34). Institute of Social and Economic Research, University of West Indies, Mona Campus, Jamaica, West Indies.

Drehner, V., & Hudgins, A. (1992). *Women and crack.* Unpublished manuscript.

Dugger, C. W. (1997, January 12). For half a million, this is still the new world. *The New York Times,* p. 27.

Gopaul-McNicol, S.-A. (1993). *Working with West Indian families.* New York: Guilford Press.

Green, C., & Wilson, B. (1990). Socio-political relations between African-Americans and African-Caribbeans in New York City. In J. A. G. Irish & E. W. Riviere (Eds.), *Political behavior and social interaction among Caribbean and African American residents in New York* (pp. 125–138). New York: Caribbean Research Center.

Hamid, A. (1994). Marijuana and cocaine in the Caribbean since the 1960s: The complementary nature of rapid assessment and epidemiologic monitoring of drug abuse. In *Community Epidemiology Work Group, Vol. 2, Epidemiological trends in drug abuse* (NIH Publication No. 95-3989, pp. 306–313). Washington, DC: U.S. Government Printing Office.

Higman, B. W. (1984). *Slave population of the British Caribbean, 1807–1834*. Baltimore: Johns Hopkins University Press.

Kasinitz, P. (1992). *Caribbean New York: Black immigrants and the politics of race*. Ithaca, NY: Cornell University Press.

Lonesome, R. B. (1985/86). Inpatient rehabilitation for the black alcoholic. In F. L. Brisbane & M. Womble (Eds.), *Treatment of Black alcoholics* (pp. 67–81). New York: Haworth Press.

Mosher, J. F., & Ralston, L. D. (1982). *Tourism, alcohol problems and the international trade in alcoholic beverages*. Geneva, Switzerland: World Health Organization.

Mullin, M. (1992). *Africa in America: Slave acculturation and resistance in the American South and the British Caribbean, 1736–1831*. Urbana: University of Illinois Press.

O'Brien, R., Cohen, S., Evans, G., & Fine, J. (1992). *The encyclopedia of drug abuse* (2nd ed.). New York: Facts on File.

Pinderhughes, E. (1982). Afro-American families and the victim system. In M. McGoldrick, J. K. Pearce, & J. Giordano (Eds.), *Ethnicity and family therapy* (pp. 108–122). New York: Guilford Press.

Rohter, L. (1997, August 10). In U.S. deportation policy, a Pandora's box. *The New York Times*, pp. A1, A6.

Rubin, V., & Comitas, L. (1975). *Ganja in society*. The Hague, Netherlands: Mouton.

Sowell, T. (1982). *Ethnic America*. New York: Basic Books.

Sue, D. W., & Sue, D. (1990). *Counseling the culturally different: Theory and practice* (2nd ed.). New York: Wiley.

Taussig, C. W. (1928). *Rum, romance and rebellion*. New York: Milton Balch.

U.S. Bureau of the Census. (1993). *Statistical Abstract of the United States*. Washington, DC: Author.

Warner-Lewis, M. (1991). *Guinea's other suns: The African dynamic in Trinidad culture*. Dover, MA: Majority.

Williams, E. (1976). *The Negro in the Caribbean*. Westport, CT: Greenwood.

III

Working with Clients of Native American and Latino Backgrounds

Typically, those people classified as "Hispanics" or more recently as "Latinos" are seen as a totally separate group from "Native Americans." Yet both groups have a common indigenous heritage underlying their unique cultures. As pointed out by the authors of the following four chapters, vestiges of this indigenous heritage are still reflected, in varying degrees, in the cultural norms and values of all these ethnocultural groups. Moreover, all these groups differ not only in their historical and cultural backgrounds but also, and even more important, in their assimilation and acceptance by the mainstream American society, thereby affecting the rate of substance abuse and their treatment options.

Nonetheless, the differences among these populations are great. As pointed out by Weaver (Chapter 4), despite our common stereotype of the "drunken Indian," the hundreds of Native American nations and tribes vary greatly in their use and abuse of alcohol and other drugs. Therefore, familiarity with the cultural norms and unique cultural treatment approaches, as well as with the level of assimilation to the mainstream culture, is essential when working with individuals of Native background.

Each of the three Latino groups discussed in this book, originating in Puerto Rico, Mexico, and Cuba, has had a different political and cultural relationship with the United States and consequently a different process of integrating into the mainstream society. The interrelationship between these processes, the use of substances, and the impact of economic opportunities on substance abuse raises interesting questions for both substance abuse prevention and treatment efforts. These questions are explored in the following section.

4

Native Americans
and Substance Abuse

Hilary N. Weaver

Virtually everyone is familiar with the stereotype of the drunken Indian—a once-noble warrior who has turned to drink because of cultural decimation, who became addicted to firewater through exploitive interactions with traders and frontiersmen, or who perhaps was genetically predisposed to alcoholism. Beliefs about Native Americans and substance abuse, primarily alcoholism, have been so widely discussed over the past few centuries that few people have stopped to critically examine what is actually known and empirically supported.

It is unwise to assume that widespread substance abuse exists among all Native populations. Some Native groups, such as the Lakota, have been studied extensively, whereas virtually no information is available for other groups, such as the Cayuga. Inconsistencies in the literature, for example, the differing statistics on whether men or women drink more, may be attributed to such factors as different populations having been sampled. In addition, existing literature on Native Americans has focused primarily on negative factors and social problems, which lends credibility to stereotypes (Fleming, 1992; Mail, 1992). Little attention has been given to strengths or positive factors within Native cultures and communities. Native Americans who are social drinkers are virtually never discussed in the literature, nor are they studied empirically.

Reliable data on extent and patterns of substance abuse among Native people are scarce due to problems in reporting and distrust of researchers

(Gurnee, Vigil, Krill-Smith, & Crowley, 1990). The literature on Native substance abuse is usually descriptive, with little empirical support and minimal guidance for clinicians interested in implementing appropriate interventions.

The fact that so much has been written about substance abuse and Native Americans suggests a belief that something about substance abuse in this population is qualitatively different than it is in other populations. Some authors have written about a distinctive style of "Indian drinking" (Escalante, 1980; Hamer, 1980; Weisner, 1984), and others have pointed to historical and cultural factors unique to Native people that may be related to substance abuse (Brown, 1980; Jilek, 1981; Waddell, 1980); however, it is stereotypical to rigidly apply any singular explanatory model or treatment philosophy to all Native people. Like people of other backgrounds, Native people use and abuse substances for a variety of reasons. Myths surrounding Native Americans and substance abuse must be critically examined before successful prevention and intervention efforts can be developed (May, 1994).

This chapter explores what is known and believed about substance abuse among Native Americans, including a brief history of Native people in North America, a discussion of which substances are most subject to abuse, and an analysis of the major theories that seek to explain substance abuse in this population. Implications for treatment are reviewed.

A BRIEF HISTORY OF NATIVE AMERICANS

Many different groups of indigenous people lived in the Americas at the time of the first European contact. Population estimates of indigenous people living north of the Rio Grande at the time of contact vary widely, ranging from approximately 1 million to 17 million. Such estimates are often politically and emotionally charged, as low estimates have been used to justify European expansion into indigenous territories (Stiffarm & Lane, 1992). It was easier to rationalize taking possession of a sparsely populated wilderness inhabited by a few backward savages than it was to morally justify colonizing, displacing, and destroying millions of human beings.

The history of the relationship between the European colonists and the indigenous people of the Americas is fraught with violence. The United States government often used military force to eliminate or move Native people who were in the way of White expansion. The Europeans brought with them diseases that decimated Native populations (Stiffarm & Lane, 1992). In speaking of the old days, one Native person interviewed on the subject of alcohol stated, "They first tried to get rid of us through disease like smallpox, diphtheria and all that and they couldn't, so they introduced us to this alcohol" (Maracle, 1993, p. 17).

Alcohol was frequently used as a trade item in exchange for natural resources such as furs (Maracle, 1993; Stiffarm & Lane, 1992). Alcohol was also used to deliberately trick Native people into relinquishing land. Clearly people who were under the influence of alcohol were at a disadvantage when entering into any sort of bargain, trade, or agreement. Many Native leaders recognized the danger of alcohol. Around the year 1800 Skenado, an Oneida leader, stated: "Drink no firewater of the white man. It makes you mice for the white men who are cats. Many a meal they have eaten of you" (Maracle, 1993, p. 1).

The genocide that was practiced against Native people was manifested in both physical and cultural forms. As indicated, warfare, disease, and alcohol were all used to physically destroy Native people. Other policies had assimilation as a goal. Many Native children were forcibly removed from their families and taken to English-speaking boarding schools run by the federal government and various churches, schools that were often thousands of miles away from their homes. Children were not allowed to speak their languages, practice their religions, or participate in any aspect of their cultures. Government-sponsored boarding schools were common until the mid-1970s, and many religious boarding schools are still in operation. Nearly 20% of Native American youth are still educated in boarding schools (Dick, Manson, & Beals, 1993).

CURRENT DEMOGRAPHICS

According to the 1990 census, almost 2 million Native people live in what is currently the United States (U.S. Bureau of the Census, 1993). Census data tend to undercount the population because many Native people identify primarily as citizens of Native nations and therefore resist being counted by what is essentially a foreign government, the United States (Kuhlmann, 1992; Native American Leadership Commission on Health and AIDS, 1994; Stiffarm & Lane, 1992). Although the United States officially bestowed citizenship on Native Americans in 1924, many Native people neither wanted nor accepted it and prefer to identify primarily or exclusively as members of their Native nations (Native American Leadership Commission on Health and AIDS, 1994; Stiffarm & Lane, 1992).

The United States government currently acknowledges the existence of more than 500 Native nations or tribes within its borders. The four largest of these nations, the Cherokee, Navajo, Chippewa/Ojibway, and Sioux (Lakota/Dakota/Nakota) each have populations of over 100,000. The terms "tribe" and "nation" both refer to groups of Native people that share a common ancestry, language, and culture; however, use of the word "nation" communicates a stronger belief in the inherent sovereignty of indigenous people. Other groups of Native people, such as the Homa in the Southeast and the Shinnecock of the northeastern United States, continue to exist without recognition by the federal government. The land base of Native people has been greatly reduced since initial contact with Europeans. Although many Native nations have retained some part of their original holdings, others have been moved to reservations outside their traditional areas (Stiffarm & Lane, 1992).

Native nations retain a sovereignty that in most cases includes more independence and self-governance than that held by the states. For example, many Native nations have their own social welfare systems, legal systems, and political systems. In addition, treaties between Native nations and the federal government (and, in a few cases, state governments) have established specific moral and legal relationships between these governments. The Indian Health Service is an example of one program provided to Native people by the federal government as part of its legal responsibilities. Some substance abuse treatment facilities that serve Natives are operated under the auspices of federal agencies such as the Indian Health Service. Others are run by Native nations or private organizations.

Although the label Native American has been applied to the indigenous groups in what is now the United States, it is important to remember that, in fact, there are hundreds of Native groups with no common language, culture, religion, or form of government. A Creek is likely to have as much in common with an Inuit as an Italian with a German. Although all Native groups have experienced colonization and oppression, the time of their first contact with Europeans varies greatly, as does the European group that they encountered. Some Native people have accepted assimilation into the values, norms, and beliefs of the dominant society, whereas others maintain their own languages, ways of life, and strong belief in their inherent sovereignty.

SUBSTANCES USED

Unlike people in most parts of the world, the people indigenous to most of what is now the United States and Canada did not have alcoholic beverages prior to contact with Europeans in the 15th and 16th centuries (Maracle,

1993). Although intoxicating substances such as peyote were used by some southwestern Native groups in ceremonial contexts, these substances were not used in a recreational or abusive manner. Today, these substances continue to be used in sacred contexts.

Although Native Americans have a higher consumption rate of alcohol than other ethnic groups in the United States, many Indians do not drink alcohol at all (Weisner, 1984). According to Weisner's comparative study of drinking styles, 52% of Native Americans abstain from alcohol, and 23% drink moderately. Although rapid consumption of alcohol with intent to achieve intoxication does seem to be a common pattern in Indian drinking (Moran & May, 1995), drinking norms vary considerably among nations (Beauvais & Trimble, 1992; Fleming, 1992; Young, 1992).

Native Americans who abuse substances are more likely than non-Natives to abuse only alcohol. In a study of urban Native Americans receiving outpatient substance abuse treatment, alcohol was the primary or secondary drug of choice for 90% of the sample, with marijuana as the other drug of choice (62%; Westermeyer & Neider, 1994). Young (1993) estimates that 75% of all Native American deaths can be directly or indirectly linked to alcohol. In spite of these statistics, our knowledge of substance abuse issues among Native Americans is limited.

> We simply do not know how serious a problem alcohol poses generally for Native Americans and their cultures. We do not even have a reliable notion of the incidence of alcoholism—in part because of logistical difficulties, but also because of the difficulty of defining *alcoholism* for objective study, across the cultural chasm. Even if we accept the evidence that a relatively high proportion of Native Americans use alcohol heavily, we have a paucity of information to help us evaluate whether or not the motivations for such behavior are pathological. (Brod, 1975, p. 1385)

Brod's statement, although made over two decades ago, is equally true today. Clinicians must keep in mind the limitations of our knowledge when reviewing any statistics or information about Native substance abuse.

Existing studies indicate that substance abuse is more prevalent among youth and young adults than among those over age 30, and many of the patterns visible in Native American adults were established during adolescence (Beauvais, 1992a; Young, 1987). Alcohol is the drug of choice for Native youth, although marijuana and inhalants are also used more than in the general population (Cole, Timmreck, Page, & Woods, 1992). Native Americans often decrease use of marijuana in early adulthood (Mitchell, Novins, & Holmes, 1999). Although use of inhalants varies considerably among nations (Young, 1987), inhalants are primarily used during early adolescence, and their use tapers off after age 13. Former inhalant users may continue to use other substances, such as alcohol. In general, Native adolescents use drugs and alcohol earlier, more heavily, and with more severe consequences, such as permanent disabilities and death, than is true for other adolescents (Beauvais, 1992a; Moncher, Holden, & Trimble, 1990). Many Native youth die in alcohol-related violence, car accidents, or suicide (Fleming, 1992; Young, 1992).

SUBSTANCE ABUSE AND NATIVE WOMEN

The different drinking norms that exist for men and women in Native cultures need more attention from both researchers and clinicians. The research on substance abuse for Native women is so sparse and poor that it is not possible to draw any reliable conclusions about substances used, patterns of use, or issues such as dual diagnosis. Only recently have helping professionals examined special issues of Native American women in recovery. Lowery (1999) provides a culturally based treatment model that shows promise with Native women.

By far most studies discuss drinking among Native American males. May and Smith (1988) and Topper (1985) point to drinking as being male oriented and male dominated, with men much more likely to be drinkers and to be problem drinkers than women. However, a more recent study of a Northwest coastal Native village found that women had a higher rate of problem drinking than men (8.4% for women vs. 3.6% for men) and a higher remission rate (82% vs. 52%; Leung, Kinzie, Boehnlein, & Shore, 1993). Among Indian Health Service patients, alcohol-related disorders for men have been found to consistently exceed those for women by a ratio of 2:1 in all age groups except for 14- to 19-year olds (Hisnanick, 1992). It is unclear if these findings reflect changing trends in substance abuse among women.

Fetal alcohol syndrome (FAS) is more prevalent among Native Americans than among the U.S. population as a whole, with approximately 1 in 99 Native Americans born with FAS (Committee on Interior and Insular Affairs, 1992). Nonetheless, disagreement exists about the prevalence of FAS in the Native population, with figures ranging from 6 times (Torres, 1995) to 30 times (Committee on Interior and Insular Affairs, 1992) the rate in the non-Indian community. This discrepancy may be due to variations between Native groups. For example, in some Native communities, such as the Pine Ridge and Rosebud Reservations in South Dakota, one in four children is born with FAS (Committee on Interior and Insular Affairs, 1992).

Few substance abuse treatment options are available for pregnant women (Committee on Interior and Insular Affairs, 1992). Many of the approaches used to prevent FAS work through the criminal justice system. Some nations have tried putting pregnant alcoholics in jail, but this policy may violate women's civil rights and place them in an environment without access to prenatal care (Torres, 1995). What is needed instead of a criminal justice approach is emphasizing prevention through public awareness, accessible treatment for women, better research on prevalence and treatment of FAS, and better diagnostic, medical, and social services for children with FAS (Committee on Interior and Insular Affairs, 1992).

THEORIES AND DYNAMICS OF SUBSTANCE ABUSE AMONG NATIVE AMERICANS

Although intertribal and regional differences limit the generalizability and applicability of any one causal model of Native American substance abuse, theories that seek to explain substance abuse among Native Americans have focused on various causes such as physiological susceptibility, cultural loss, and social and historical factors. Other explanations of substance abuse problems point to factors in the social environment of Native people, such as poverty and political oppression, and their psychological impact on people (Weisner, 1984; Wright & Watts, 1988).

Physiological Theories

It is a commonly held belief, even among Native people, that Native Americans possess a physiological predisposition to problem drinking (May & Smith, 1988; Moran & May, 1995). Yet the evidence for a biological predisposition is sketchy (Hill, 1989; Moran & May, 1995). The substantial genetic variability that exists within rather than between ethnic groups makes genetic models problematic (Reed, 1985). Genetic explanations of Indian drinking would need to take into account differences between full-blooded Indians and varying degrees of mixed heritage. Although some evidence indicates differential rates of metabolism (both slower and faster), metabolism rates have not been clearly linked to consumption rates or to problematic drinking (Reed, 1985).

Cultural Theories

A number of different theoretical views rely on culture as a primary explanatory factor in substance abuse. One points to particular factors within Native cultures that make intoxication desirable, whereas another points to substance abuse as a form of in-group behavior that promotes a sense of ethnic identity. Other related theories point to loss of culture and its psychological implications, rather than cultural factors per se, as the root cause of substance abuse.

Writings that espouse the first view identify a distinct style of Indian drinking and discuss the relationship of cultural attributes to alcohol consumption. For example, in many Native cultures communication with the spirit world through vision quests is highly valued. Alcohol may be seen as an easy and quick method to attain a state of altered consciousness (Hamer, 1980; Weibel-Orlando, 1985). However, Oetting and Beauvais (1991) point out that although ceremonial use of substances played a role in some Native cultures, particularly those in the Southwest, such substances were not used recreationally. Therefore, theories that point to substance abuse as an outgrowth of cultural practices do not stand up under scrutiny. Additionally, the diverse cultural practices of the hundreds of Native groups make such monolithic theories inappropriate.

Some authors interpret a tendency for Native Americans to drink to an extreme drunken state, or until the supply of alcohol is gone as a replication of traditional feast patterns in which rapid overindulgence was expected (Hamer, 1980). Indian drinking has been noted for being competitive, with the goal being rapid and complete intoxication rather than relaxation (Weibel-Orlando, 1985). This type of excessive consumption pattern could inadvertently lead to problem drinking or physical addiction.

Proponents of the second type of culturally based theory of substance abuse note that Indian drinking is almost always a group activity and that this characteristic reinforces social obligations and norms of reciprocity (Topper, 1985). During drinking gatherings, the subject of conversations is often related to Indian issues and topics that promote ethnic solidarity (Weibel-Orlando, 1985).

Many other theories that seek to explain Native drinking rely heavily on notions of the psychological response to deculturation or loss of cultural traditions (Hill, 1989; Jones-Saumpty, Hochaus, Dru, & Zeiner, 1983; Schinke et al., 1986; Segal, 1998; Topper, 1985). In particular, Native people of the Plains, such as the Lakota, who previously led lifestyles as hunters and warriors, are seen as more prone to problem drinking than Natives from more agricultural societies, such as the Hopi (Cooley, 1980).

Not all Indian cultures experienced the same level of deculturation; therefore, if deculturation does explain problem drinking, then according to theories that focus on cultural loss Indian groups should vary in their levels of problem drinking. And indeed some researchers have found this to be true (Weibel-Orlando, 1987). Topper (1985) cites the more recent increases in problem drinking among the Navajo as a result of increasing loss of culture. Brody (1980), however, points out that the disintegration of tribal society is of long standing and therefore is not an adequate explanation for contemporary problems. According to Brody, it is the conflict between Native norms and those of the dominant society that precipitate substance abuse rather than the loss of culture.

Substance abuse has also been related to acculturation issues such as cultural transition, cultural marginality, and identity conflicts (Nofz, 1988; Terrell, 1993). Oetting and Beauvais (1991), who have studied substance abuse among Native American adolescents, challenge the theories that cultural transition leads to substance abuse. They believe that a complex relationship exists between cultural identification and drug use, mediated by many variables such as peer relationships and family factors.

Psychological Theories

Some researchers consider psychological factors such as depression, external control orientation, and cognitive deficits to be important risk factors for Native Americans (Jones-Saumpty et al., 1983). However, it is important to note that all the theories that depict drinking as psychologically motivated seem to refer to external social phenomena such as loss of culture as the cause of psychological discomfort.

Social Theories

Some researchers trace the problems that contemporary Native people have with alcohol to historical antecedents. Alcohol was one of the major items of trade between Europeans on the frontier and Native Americans (Weibel-Orlando, 1985). Consequently, Indian styles of drinking may be patterned after the drinking styles of the Whites on the frontier who first came into contact with many groups of Native people (Lemert, 1980).

Some people believe that prohibiting the sale of alcohol to Native people (originally mandated by the federal government and later continued by many Native governments) encouraged rapid consumption that led to problem drinking (May & Smith, 1988). Additionally, prohibiting alcohol use on reservations has led to a lack of role models of responsible drinking.

According to Topper (1985), many Native people consume the alcohol quickly to avoid getting caught. This practice leads to rapid intoxication. In spite of these assertions, many reservations choose to maintain policies of prohibition, and 81% of Navajos surveyed by May and Smith (1988) favored prohibition.

PREVENTION AND TREATMENT ISSUES

The following cases illustrate some common dynamics and treatment issues for Native people who abuse substances. They also point out implications for prevention.

> Jeremy, a 40-year-old Choctaw, has been sober for 8 years. He began drinking heavily at age 14 while in boarding school. At school, he associated with a group of peers that valued heavy, competitive drinking. At age 25 he married a woman he met at a drinking party. He quit drinking "cold turkey" shortly after the birth of their third child. He began preaching the value of sobriety to many people in his community with much frustration and little success. Jeremy became involved in tribal politics in an effort to rescue his people from their problems. He worked long hours, which kept him away from his family. Within a year he put on more than 100 pounds. His only activity other than work was going to bingo games, often long distances from his home. Although at first he was resistant, friends convinced him that he still had a problem with addiction. He entered a Native-run treatment center based on a 12-step model that helped him recognize that his fanatical preaching of sobriety, overworking, overeating, and gambling were all symptoms of a continuing addiction.

> Sue is a 23-year-old Cree woman with a family history of substance abuse going back three generations. The home she was raised in was filled with alcohol and violence. She was moved repeatedly in the foster care system. As a child, she also experienced sexual abuse and was expelled from school for uncontrollable behavior. Her father died of exposure while intoxicated. Three cousins, a sister, two uncles, and her grandfather all died alcohol-related deaths. Sue used inhalants beginning at age 9 and used alcohol regularly as her drug of choice since age 11. She had three children, one of whom had fetal alcohol syndrome; the others had fetal alcohol effect (FAE). The children were in foster care at the time she came to treatment. She participated in five treatment programs over the past 8 years but was not able to remain sober for more than 6 weeks at a time. Most of these programs were court mandated and based on a 12-step model. One of the tribal elders be-

gan to involve her in the sweat lodge in the hopes of cleansing the alcohol from her system and bringing her back into the community through traditional activities.

Common Dynamics and Treatment Issues

The cases of Jeremy and Sue illustrate some common patterns and issues for Native people who abuse substances. The heavy, competitive drinking of young men followed by sobriety in middle age, evident in Jeremy's case, is not unusual. Drinking is a major problem in boarding schools, and for many Native youth, this is where their substance abuse problems start. Some possible reasons for substance abuse in the boarding schools include alienation from family and community support, peer pressure, and the historical association of boarding schools with traumatic and brutal policy designed to break Native cultures and socialize students into the dominant society.

It is not unusual for someone like Jeremy to stop drinking without the assistance of a formal treatment program. Native people often stop using substances when they reach an age at which they are expected to fulfill more community responsibilities. A 19-year follow-up of Native people with drinking problems found a 60–63% remission rate regardless of whether or not treatment was received (Leung et al., 1993).

Many community leaders have a history of substance abuse. Such a past does not necessarily carry stigma. People who are able to stop abusing substances and fulfill their responsibilities in the community are valued for their current roles and for their willingness to tell stories of their recovery as a means of reaching out to others.

The other addictive behaviors displayed by Jeremy (overwork, overeating, excessive involvement with bingo) can also be found among non-Indian clients; however, in this case the behaviors were manifested within an Indian context. Just as Indian drinking often takes place among Indian peers with Indian topics of discussion, bingo often takes place in an Indian setting with predominantly Indian participants. In Jeremy's case, overwork also occurred in an Indian context of tribal politics. The fact that many of his behaviors were manifested in an Indian context suggested that a successful intervention could be built on his connections to the community.

Sue's case illustrates the common pattern of multigenerational substance abuse and loss of many family members in alcohol-related deaths. Substance abuse is often just one of many problems—sexual abuse, foster care experiences, children with FAE, poverty, and other issues—that are facing such families. Intervening in this type of long-term, multiproblem situation can be very challenging. Multiple treatment programs and multiple relapses are common, as is court involvement and loss of children. In some cases, a desire to be reunited with her children can provide motivation for a woman's treatment.

There is no single intervention that is effective for all Native clients. Some can benefit from traditional healing practices, others from mainstream interventions, and some from a blend of the two. Still others may be difficult to reach through any of these methods. Service providers must begin with a comprehensive assessment to determine what intervention is likely to be most effective for any given client.

Assessment

Within most Native American cultures, quantity and frequency of alcohol consumption are not the primary guidelines for defining problem drinking. Instead, drinking is seen as a problem when it interferes with social roles, norms, and expectations. Jeremy's addictive behavior, although manifested within an Indian context, became problematic when it began to violate community norms. It was at that time that community members pressured him to get help. There was no indication that the heavy drinking he participated in as a youth was ever identified as a problem. As part of the assessment, the context for Jeremy's drinking, the consequences of his drinking, and his level of cultural connection had to be considered.

From what was known about Jeremy's case, he accepted some of the values of the dominant society while staying connected to his native culture. Treatment that bridges these worlds may be more viable than treatment based on either an exclusively indigenous or an exclusively dominant model. For example, it may be best to refer clients like Jeremy to a Native-run treatment facility that blends traditional approaches with a 12-step model.

Sue's case clearly illustrates the need to do a comprehensive family history to understand the client. The counselor must look at her past treatment experiences, explore the reasons why they failed, and examine any successes that she had. It is important to consider the client's strengths, as well as her weaknesses.

Although it is too early to tell whether Sue can maintain sobriety through the use of Native healing practices, the trauma and alienation she experienced since childhood may call for the type of healing that comes with establishing a positive connection to her cultural heritage and developing self-esteem and pride in her cultural identity. Because nonindigenous approaches failed in the past, indigenous approaches may hold hope for Sue's recovery.

Interventions with Individuals and Families

One critical premise that is echoed throughout the social work profession but is apparently forgotten when it comes to substance abuse treatment for Native people is, "start where the client is." The assumption is often made that culturally grounded programs are the most effective for Native clients. Many programs aimed at Native clients incorporate Native traditions, yet many of the clients in need of substance abuse services have been alienated from their traditions (Gurnee et al., 1990). Reconnection to culture may well be a powerful intervention for some, yet blindly offering culturally based programs without determining whether these fit the client's needs is likely to be ineffective. An assessment of the client must include looking at cultural dimensions, such as the meaning and role of culture in the client's life and the level and nature of the client's connection to culture.

Westermeyer and Neider (1994) reported lower success rates for treatment of Native Americans with substance abuse disorders than for non-Native American patients. The disease model of alcoholism, fairly prevalent in the United States, incorporates a focus on the individual that may not be appropriate for Native populations. One tenet of Alcoholics Anonymous (AA) and many treatment approaches is that it is important to accept the label of "alcoholic." Edwards and Edwards (1988) argue that this is counterproductive with Native clients, who are often sensitive to stereotypical labeling. Instead, they recommend treating drinking as an ordinary subject and focusing on responsible decision making in the context of drinking behavior.

Some Native people feel strongly that formal substance abuse treatment centers should not be allowed on Indian territory. Social agencies can be seen as the "White way," a way that prolongs problems for Native people. Solutions are seen as needing to come from within, as Natives help each other through telling their stories (Maracle, 1993).

Many Canadian Natives with substance abuse problems have benefited from Native treatment centers that combine the 12-step philosophy of Alcoholics Anonymous (AA) with elements from local Native cultures. Some of these centers operate using local Native languages (Maracle, 1993). Attneave (1982) suggests that some Native drinking practices, such as those that occur at bingos and celebrations, can be managed in a controlled way through contracting with clients to limit their drinking. For chronic substance abusers, she recommends referral to a treatment center with Indian staff that incorporates work with family members.

Alcoholics Anonymous groups have worked for some Native people, but such programs are less accessible to those who have limited literacy or speak little English. In order to reach these populations, AA and 12-step oriented programs may need to rely more on oral materials in the clients' native languages rather than using only written materials.

Some Native people have found help for their substance abuse problems through traditional teachings and ceremonies. The sweat lodge is a means of purification in many Native cultures that has been successfully used in the treatment of substance abuse.

In order to recruit and retain Native clients, agencies must be willing to do long-term outreach that leads to high visibility and respect within the Native community. The personal and professional characteristics of the counselors doing outreach are critical. If they are viewed as outsiders or people who do not care about the community, recruitment efforts may have minimal success. In order to retain and help clients, agencies must be able to recognize and incorporate cultural dynamics in the helping process and must be able to relinquish stereotypical ideas about various Native cultures and culturally based interventions. Clients who are successfully helped and who return to their communities are likely to encourage more people to seek help.

Interventions with Communities

If Native American drinking can be seen as a form of protest against White domination, then policies that are developed and treatment approaches that are administered by non-Indians are likely to be ineffective. Policy development and treatment interventions by Native Americans for Native Americans would be indicated. To eliminate the need for protest drinking, the conditions being protested against must change. Intervention and change at the societal level are necessary. For example, if alcohol is used to validate a sense of Indian identity, then providing other mechanisms to validate identity would be an appropriate prevention and treatment strategy. In fact, Native American religious and revitalization movements such as the Native American Church, the Indian Shaker Church, traditional Native spirituality, and Christian sects of Native Americans have proved to be effective means of offering a strong sense of Indian identity and reinforcing abstinence among their members (Slagel & Weibel-Orlando, 1986).

If problem drinking among Native Americans can be attributed, at least in part, to factors such as prohibition, poverty, and political oppression, then clearly a large-scale policy effort is more appropriate than individualized therapy. Topper (1985) believes that, due to the severity and nature of underlying social problems, treatment has no hope of solving the problem of alcoholism without dealing with the larger social picture. Community action and development approaches to deal with poverty and unemployment must be taken. For example, the pervasiveness of substance abuse and other problems in Sue's family may lead the counselor to explore the influences of her social environment, such as decisions about leaving or removing her children, on her recovery. In the long run, societal change may provide the most hope for cases such as this.

If problem drinking is caused by cultural loss, marginality, and feelings of powerlessness, then solutions must be found in cultural revitalization. This goal cannot be accomplished from the outside. For some Native people, acculturation into the dominant society may be realistic, whereas others may find hope in a return to their old traditions as adapted for today's world.

PREVENTION OF SUBSTANCE ABUSE

Beauvais (1992b) identified the primary factors related to substance abuse among Native youth as social structure, family socialization, low self-esteem, and peer associations, with the first two factors being most distantly and the last two being most closely linked to drug use. Therefore, prevention efforts must begin by considering factors such as social structure and then move forward, whereas treatment efforts must begin with peer associations and then work backward.

The issues of problem drinking as a learned behavior and of the lack of role models for moderate drinking cannot be resolved by legislation. However, if problematic behaviors are learned, then the possibility of learning new, less problematic, behaviors is always there. Consequently, strengthening competencies through educational approaches would be an effective preventive measure. Social support and recreation would also be appropriate prevention and treatment mechanisms (Schinke et al., 1986). Programs with a skill-building focus have been used with youth to help them learn healthy behaviors and to develop the ability to resist peer pressure. Youth who have the skills to function well in both Indian and non-Indian contexts are less likely to get involved with alcohol or other drugs (Moran & May, 1995). Prevention models such as the one developed by Moran (1999) for urban youth demonstrate important, ethnoculturally grounded approaches.

It is important that human service professionals be familiar with the history and contemporary context of social problems among Native people (Beauvais, 1992b). In a study of Native youth in a boarding school, family support was found to be correlated with lower alcohol use, indicating that preventive work must incorporate the family for maximum success (Dick et al., 1993). In Jeremy's case, prevention efforts incorporated within the boarding school could have counteracted the high-risk environment. In

Sue's case, prevention would have meant finding some way to break a multigenerational cycle. Growing up in such a heavily dysfunctional context put Sue at high risk. Although removal from the home might have been one option, it could have created problems in and of itself. Given the wide range of problems affecting Sue, addressing the issues on a community level with full participation of community members is required.

Edwards and Edwards (1988) emphasize that prevention efforts must be community specific and community based. Native community members should be involved in all aspects of developing appropriate services. Additionally, prevention efforts should be age specific and should address risk factors such as peer pressure, the influences of adult drinking behavior, stressful family environments, and acceptance of alcohol use in the community (Ma, Toubbeh, Cline, & Chisholm, 1998). Primary prevention efforts should provide opportunities for youth to increase their self-esteem, strengthen their sense of identity, develop educational and social skills, and contribute to the community. Groups for those who already drink or have developed substance abuse problems should include educational components, encourage responsible decision making, and reinforce Native values, cultures, and traditions.

CONCLUSION

Although much has been written about Native people and substance abuse, we are still left with the question, What do we really know? A critical review of the literature reveals that we may know less than we think. Further studies are required to really gain an understanding of the extent and nature of the problem. Culturally competent research that considers the diversity within Native people, including tribal, regional, gender, and age differences, and that explores the causes, extent, and potential solutions to substance abuse problems is essential. Without this foundation it is difficult to develop appropriate and effective intervention strategies.

Moreover, choices about prevention and intervention strategies and policies must come from within, not outside, Native communities. Such strategies must be tailored to the needs of specific Native groups and communities, and societal-level changes may be required to address the root sociocultural causes of substance abuse.

The high prevalence of substance abuse in Native communities is a reflection of other problems. A combination of clinical, spiritual, cultural, social, economic, and political action is needed to fully address the substance abuse problem. There is no one way that works for all Native people. Alcoholics Anonymous, Native spirituality, developing norms of social drinking, and quitting "cold turkey" have each worked for various people (Maracle, 1993). One of the most important factors for clinicians to keep in mind is to start where the client is. Theories and research may give some indication of what to look for and how to work with clients, but only the client has fully experienced his or her situation. It is imperative that clinicians critically examine the interventions they choose in order to ensure that these interventions are based on clients' needs and empirical findings rather than on stereotypical assumptions.

REFERENCES

Attneave, C. (1982). American Indians and Alaska Native families: Emigrants in their own homeland. In M. McGoldrick, J. K. Pearce, & J. Giordano (Eds.), *Ethnicity and family therapy* (pp. 55–83). New York: Guilford Press.

Beauvais, F. (1992a). The consequences of drug and alcohol use for Indian youth. *American Indian and Alaska Native Mental Health Research, 5*(1), 32–37.

Beauvais, F. (1992b). An integrated model for prevention and treatment of drug abuse among American Indian youth. *Journal of Addictive Diseases, 11*(3), 63–80.

Beauvais, F., & Trimble, J. E. (1992). The role of the researcher in evaluating American-Indian alcohol and other drug abuse. In M. A. Orlandi, R. Weston, & L. G. Epstein (Eds.), *Cultural competence for evaluators: A guide for alcohol and other drug abuse prevention practitioners working with ethnic/racial communities* (pp. 173–201). Rockville, MD: U.S. Department of Health and Human Services, Public Health Service, Alcohol, Drug Abuse, and Mental Health Administration, Office for Substance Abuse Prevention, Division of Community Prevention and Training.

Brod, T. M. (1975). Alcoholism as a mental health problem of Native Americans. *Archives of General Psychiatry, 32*, 1385–1391.

Brody, H. (1980). Indians on skid row: Alcohol in the life of urban migrants. In J. Hamer & J. Steinbring (Eds.), *Alcohol and native peoples of the North* (pp. 209–266). Lanham, MD: University Press of America.

Brown, D. N. (1980). Drinking as an indicator of community disharmony: The people of Taos pueblo. In J. O. Waddell & M. Everett (Eds.), *Drinking behavior among Southwest Indians* (pp. 83–102). Tucson: University of Arizona Press.

Cole, G., Timmreck, T. C., Page, R., & Woods, S. (1992). Patterns and prevalence of substance abuse among Navajo youth. *Health Values, 16*(3), 50–57.

Committee on Interior and Insular Affairs. (1992). *Indian Fetal Alcohol Syndrome Prevention and Treatment Act* (Serial No. 102-52). Washington, DC: U.S. Government Printing Office.

Cooley, R. (1980). Alcoholism programs. In J. O. Waddell & M. Everett (Eds.), *Drinking behavior among Southwest Indians* (pp. 205–213). Tucson: University of Arizona Press.

Dick, R. W., Manson, S. M., & Beals, J. (1993). Alcohol use among male and female

Native American adolescents: Patterns and correlates of student drinking in a boarding school. *Journal of Studies on Alcohol, 54*(2), 172–177.

Edwards, E. D., & Edwards, M. E. (1988). Alcoholism prevention/treatment and Native American youth: A community approach. *Journal of Drug Issues, 18*, 103–114.

Escalante, F. (1980). Group pressure and excessive drinking among Indians. In J. O. Waddell & M. Everett (Eds.), *Drinking behavior among Southwest Indians* (pp. 183–204). Tucson: University of Arizona Press.

Fleming, C. (1992). American Indians and Alaska Natives: Changing societies past and present. In M. A. Orlandi, R. Weston, & L. G. Epstein (Eds.), *Cultural competence for evaluators: A guide for alcohol and other drug abuse prevention practitioners working with ethnic/racial communities* (pp. 147–171). Rockville, MD: U.S. Department of Health and Human Services, Public Health Service, Alcohol, Drug Abuse, and Mental Health Administration, Office for Substance Abuse Prevention, Division of Community Prevention and Training.

Gurnee, C. G., Vigil, D. E., Krill-Smith, S., & Crowley, T. J. (1990). Substance abuse among American Indians in an urban treatment program. *American Indian and Alaska Native Mental Health Research, 3*(3), 17–26.

Hamer, J. (1980). Drinking as a way of life. In J. Hamer & J. Steinbring (Eds.), *Alcohol and native peoples of the North* (pp. 107–153). Lanham, MD: University Press of America.

Hill, A. (1989). Treatment and prevention of alcoholism in the Native American family. In G. W. Lawson & A. W. Lawson (Eds.), *Alcoholism and substance abuse in special populations* (pp. 247–272). Rockville, MD: Aspen.

Hisnanick, J. J. (1992). The prevalence of alcohol abuse among American Indians and Alaska Natives. *Health Values, 16*(5), 32–37.

Jilek, W. (1981). Anomic depression, alcoholism and a culture- congenial Indian response. *Journal of Studies on Alcohol* (Suppl. 9), 159–170.

Jones-Saumpty, D., Hochaus, L., Dru, R., & Zeiner, A. (1983). Psychological factors of familial alcoholism in American Indians and Caucasians. *Journal of Clinical Psychology, 39*, 783–790.

Kuhlmann, A. (1992). American Indian women of the Plains and Northern Woodlands. *Mid-American Review of Sociology, 16*(1), 1–28.

Lemert, E. (1980). Alcohol in the life of the Northwest Coast Indians. In J. Hamer & J. Steinbring (Eds.), *Alcohol and native peoples of the North* (pp. 49–71). Lanham, MD: University Press of America.

Leung, P. K., Kinzie, J. D., Boehnlein, J. K., & Shore, J. H. (1993). A prospective study of the natural course of alcoholism in a Native American village. *Journal of Studies on Alcohol, 54*(6), 733–738.

Lowery, C. T. (1999). A qualitative model of long-term recovery for American Indian women. In H. N. Weaver (Ed.), *Voices of First Nations people: Human services considerations* (pp. 35–50). New York: Haworth Press.

Ma, G. X., Toubbeh, J., Cline, J., & Chisholm, A. (1998). The use of a qualitative approach in fetal alcohol syndrome prevention among American Indian youth. *Journal of Alcohol and Drug Education, 43*(3), 53–65.

Mail, P. D. (1992). Do we care enough to attempt change in American Indian alcohol policy? *American Indian and Alaska Native Mental Health Research, 4*(3), 105–111.

Maracle, B. (1993). *Crazywater: Native voices on addiction and recovery.* Toronto: Penguin Books.

May, P. A. (1994). The epidemiology of alcohol abuse among American Indians: The mythical and real properties. *American Indian Culture and Research Journal, 18*(2), 121–144.

May, P. A., & Smith, M. B. (1988). Some Navajo Indian opinions about alcohol abuse and prohibition: A survey and recommendations for policy. *Journal of Studies on Alcohol, 49,* 324–334.

Mitchell, C. M., Novins, D. K., & Holmes, T. (1999). Marijuana use among American Indian adolescents: A growth curve analysis from ages 14 through 20 years. *Journal of American Academy of Child and Adolescent Psychiatry, 38*(1), 72–79.

Moncher, M. S., Holden, G. W., & Trimble, J. E. (1990). Substance abuse among Native-American youth. *Journal of Consulting and Clinical Psychology, 58*(4), 408–415.

Moran, J. R. (1999). Preventing alcohol use among urban American Indian youth: The seventh generation program. In H. N. Weaver (Ed.), *Voices of First Nations people: Human services considerations* (pp. 51–67). New York: Haworth Press.

Moran, J. R., & May, P. A. (1995). American Indians. In J. Philleo, F. L. Brisbane, & L. G. Epstein (Eds.), *Cultural competence for social workers: A guide for alcohol and other drug abuse prevention professionals working with ethnic/racial communities* (pp. 3–39). Rockville, MD: U.S. Department of Health and Human Services, Public Health Service, Substance Abuse and Mental Health Services Administration, Center for Substance Abuse Prevention.

Native American Leadership Commission on Health and AIDS. (1994). *A Native American leadership response to HIV and AIDS.* New York: American Indian Community House.

Nofz, M. P. (1988). Alcohol abuse and culturally marginal American Indians. *Social Casework, 69,* 67–73.

Oetting, E. R., & Beauvais, F. (1991). Orthogonal cultural identification theory: The cultural identification of minority adolescents. *International Journal of the Addictions, 25*(5/6), 655–685.

Reed, T. E. (1985). Ethnic differences in alcohol use. *Social Biology, 32,* 195–209.

Robbins, R. (1980). Alcohol and the sub-Arctic cultures: A hypothesis. In J. Hamer & J. Steinbring (Eds.), *Alcohol and native peoples of the North* (pp. 155–207). Lanham, MD: University Press of America.

Schinke, S. P., Gilchrist, L. D., Schilling, R. F. II, Walker, R. D., Loyclear, V. S., Bobo, J. K., Maxwell, J. S., Trimble, J. E., & Cvetkovich, G. T. (1986). Preventing substance abuse among American Indian and Alaska native youth: Research issues and strategies. *Journal of Social Service Research, 9*(4), 53–67.

Segal, B. (1998). Drinking and drinking-related problems among Alaska natives. *Alcohol Health and Research World, 22*(4), 276–280.

Slagel, A. L., & Weibel-Orlando, J. (1986). The Indian Shaker church and Alcoholics Anonymous: Revitalistic curing cults. *Human Organization, 45*, 310–319.

Stiffarm, L. A., & Lane, P., Jr. (1992). The demography of Native North America: A question of American Indian survival. In M. A. Jaimes (Ed.), *The state of Native America: Genocide, colonization, and resistance* (pp. 23–53). Boston: South End Press.

Terrell, M. D. (1993). Ethnocultural factors and substance abuse: Toward culturally sensitive treatment models. *Psychology of Addictive Behaviors, 7*(3), 162–167.

Topper, M. D. (1985). Navajo "alcoholism": Drinking, alcohol abuse, and treatment in a changing cultural environment. In L. A. Bennett & G. M. Ames (Eds.), *The American experience with alcohol: Contrasting cultural perspectives* (pp. 227–251). New York: Plenum Press.

Torres, C. (1995). *Another broken promise: Budget cuts and Native American health* [Online]. Available: http://hcs.harvard.edu/~perspy/dec95/fetal. html

U.S. Bureau of the Census. (1993). *We the . . . First Americans*. Washington, DC: U.S. Government Printing Office.

Waddell, J. O. (1980). Drinking as a means of articulating social and cultural values: Papagos in an urban setting. In J. O. Waddell & M. Everett (Eds.), *Drinking behavior among Southwest Indians* (pp. 37–82). Tucson: University of Arizona Press.

Weibel-Orlando, J. (1985). Indians, ethnicity, and alcohol: Contrasting perceptions of the ethnic self and alcohol use. In L. A. Bennett & G. M. Ames (Eds.), *The American experience with alcohol: Contrasting cultural perspectives* (pp. 201–226). New York: Plenum Press.

Weibel-Orlando, J. (1987). Drinking patterns of urban and rural American Indians. *Alcohol Health and Research World, 11*(2), 8–13, 54–55.

Weisner, T. S. (1984). Serious drinking, White man's drinking and teetotaling: Drinking levels and styles in an urban Indian population. *Journal of Studies on Alcohol, 45*, 237–249.

Westermeyer, J., & Neider J. (1994). Substance disorder among 100 American Indian versus 200 other patients. *Alcoholism: Clinical and Experimental Research, 18*(3), 692–694.

Wright, R. W., & Watts, T. D. (1988). Alcohol and minority youth. *Journal of Drug Issues, 18*, 1–6.

Young, T. J. (1987). Inhalant use among American Indian youth. *Child Psychiatry and Human Development, 18*, 36–45.

Young, T. J. (1992). Substance abuse among Native American youth. In G. W. Lawson & A. W. Lawson (Eds.), *Adolescent substance abuse: Etiology, treatment, and prevention* (pp. 381–390). Gaithersburg, MD: Aspen.

Young, T. J. (1993). Alcohol prevention among Native-American youth. *Child Psychiatry and Human Development, 24*(1), 41–47.

5

Substance Abuse
among Cuban Americans

Eugenio M. Rothe
Pedro Ruiz

Addiction to drugs and alcohol has been identified as a major problem among the different subgroups of Hispanics who live in the United States. Among these groups, Cuban Americans number more than 1 million and constitute the third largest Hispanic subgroup, following the Mexican Americans and the Puerto Ricans (U.S. Bureau of the Census, 1990). For all Hispanic subgroups, our knowledge and understanding of the intimate link between addiction and its sociocultural context is seriously lacking (Ruiz & Langrod, 1997).

In the past, attempts at understanding the link between addiction and its sociocultural context have been complicated by the individual differences encountered among each of the various Hispanic subgroups. Even though they share a common Iberian heritage, Spanish language, and Catholic religion, Hispanics in the United States differ markedly in terms of ethnic background, socioeconomic status, political ideology, type of migration, and cultural heritage. These differences may explain why Hispanics choose to settle in particular geographical locations within the United States (usually those in which there are a sizable number of compatriots who can validate the individual's social values and cultural identity). These differences also help to explain why the stereotype of the "typical Hispanic" is an erroneous oversimplification. Marked differences in the patterns of alcohol and drug abuse also exist among the various Hispanic subgroups who reside in the United States. Some of these differences appear to be related to specific factors characteristic of a particular subgroup and are not necessarily shared by the majority of Hispanics. For example, substance abuse was found to be higher among Mexican American and Puerto Rican adolescents living in female-headed households; however, this factor did not appear to be of importance among Cuban American adolescents (Sokol-Katz & Ulbrich, 1992).

Cultural changes associated with migration, life stress, and socioeconomic and demographic factors have also been implicated in the genesis of substance abuse. Marked differences in these factors appear among the various Hispanic subgroups (Pumariega, Swanson, Holzer, Linskey, & Quintero-Salinas, 1992; Ruiz & Langrod, 1997). These various causative factors require individualized treatment approaches. Failure to recognize these differences can lead to a negative impact on the treatment process and may account for the tendency of U. S. Hispanics to underutilize treatment services (Langrod, Alksne, Lowinson, & Ruiz, 1981; Ruiz & Langrod, 1997; Ruiz, Langrod, Lowinson, & Marcus, 1977). Improvement in treatment outcomes and increased effectiveness of national health policies will depend on achieving a better understanding of the peculiarities of the Hispanic population in question and in tailoring the treatment to the needs of each subgroup (Ruiz, 1996).

In order to promote better understanding of the problem of substance abuse among Cuban Americans, this chapter focuses on the following topics: the history and the characteristics of the Cuban migration; the demographic profile of Cuban Americans in the United States; the changes in the values and identity of the Cuban American family; the importance of acculturation and biculturalism among Cuban Americans and its impact on their mental health; the impact of alcohol, drugs, and HIV among Cuban Americans; and appropriate treatment approaches.

CUBAN AMERICANS IN THE UNITED STATES

The 1990 census showed that there were 1,014,000 Cubans residing in the United States at the end of the 1980s, composing 0.4% of the total U.S. population. Approximately 87% reside in the south Florida area (Jorge, Suchlicki, & Leyva de Varona, 1991; U.S. Bureau of the Census, 1990), but considerable numbers of Cubans have also settled in New York, New Jersey, Illinois, Texas, and California (Boswell, Rivero, & Diaz, 1984).

An estimated 200,000 Cubans lived in the United States prior to 1959, and almost 700,000 additional Cubans arrived in the United States following

Castro's takeover in 1959. The early pre-Castro immigrants were largely divided into three social classes. The largest group was composed of unskilled rural laborers who had immigrated to the United States looking for financial improvement. The second group consisted of professionals, especially those in health care, who found it difficult to move up economically and socially in Cuba due to the saturation of health professionals in the urban areas. The third group consisted of workers, mainly from the tobacco industry, who settled in the United States at the turn of the century during the War of Independence against Spain (Jorge et al., 1991; Ruiz, 1982).

The Cuban Migration

January 1, 1959, signaled the beginning of the political events in Cuba that culminated with the ascension to power of the government led by Fidel Castro, which later turned to Communism. This situation led to a massive exodus of Cubans from the island. It is estimated that between 1959 and 1970, Cuba lost more than 10% of its 1959 population of approximately 6 million people (Jorge et al., 1991).

Several distinct phases of Cuban migration to the United States have been identified, each phase comprising different socioeconomic, racial, and age groups. These groups experienced different levels of social support, economic achievements, and adaptation problems, including substance abuse and mental health problems (Jorge et al., 1991; Rothe, 1992).

The first migration took place between 1959 and 1962 and was primarily composed of members of the upper classes and of those connected to the previous political regime of Fulgencia Batista. The second wave occurred between 1962 and 1965 as a consequence of Castro's proclamation of a Communist government in Cuba. It consisted primarily of the upper and upper middle classes who did not wish to live under Communism.

The third migration phase took place between 1965 and 1973, after the government announced the collectivization of all privately owned land. This group of immigrants consisted mostly of middle-class Cubans who lived in small towns and in rural areas. These three migration phases were overrepresented by the White descendants of European colonizers who made up the Cuban elite.

The Cubans who migrated during these years saw their relocation to the United States as a "temporary phenomenon" and regarded their migratory status as "political exile." However, the intensification of the cold war between 1959 and 1980 led to the realization that a return to the island was highly unlikely (Bernal, 1982; Rothe, 1995). As a consequence, these immigrants began investing their energies into forming a cohesive community and achieving economic growth and upward mobility: In only three decades many of these Cuban Americans have made significant local, regional, and national contributions in key areas such as politics, the judicial system, the economy, education, medicine, sports, architecture, and the arts—achievements that led them to be labeled "the Cuban miracle" or "the golden exile" ("Cuban Success Story," 1967; "Flight from Cuba," 1971). Their success was facilitated by the massive financial aid ($56 million by 1967) that was provided through federal and nonfederal agencies such as the Cuban Refugee Center (Jorge et al., 1991). Such help was not available to later Cuban, or any other Hispanic, immigrants.

The fourth migration phase was mostly composed of more than 15,000 unaccompanied Cuban children and adolescents who were allowed into the United States on visa waivers while their parents waited for U.S. visa permits in order to travel to the United States. The children were scattered over 40 states, and many spent their entire adolescent years in foster homes while awaiting reunification with their parents.

The fifth migration phase primarily consisted of an assortment of political prisoners released by Castro and of individuals escaping the island in small boats between 1959 and 1980. The sixth phase came with the Mariel boatlift of 1980. This new phase of migration of about 125,000 Cubans, mostly young males (Bernal, 1982), was more representative of the ethnocultural and socioeconomic composition of Cuba as a whole and included Blacks and individuals of mixed Spanish and African heritage (mulattos).

In 1994, another massive exodus took place in which Cubans took to sea in homemade seacrafts and small boats. Approximately 32,000 Cubans (including 2,500 children and adolescents) were rescued at sea by the U.S. Coast Guard and eventually were able to enter the United States. This last Cuban migration resulted in a U.S. government decree on May 4, 1995, that stated that all future Cuban immigrants would no longer be considered political exiles but illegal aliens and would, therefore, be repatriated to Cuba (Ackerman & Clark, 1995).

Ethnocultural Characteristics

As we stated, Whites were overrepresented among the earlier Cuban immigrants. These immigrants tended to have middle-class aspirations and a capitalistic orientation (Queralt, 1984; Rumbaut & Rumbaut, 1976) and did not experience many problems with discrimination. Later Cuban migrations, however, were more representative of the racial and ethnocultural composition of Cuba, which is estimated to be 73% White (direct descendants of the Spanish colonizers) and 27% Black or mulatto (descendants of African slaves), and were more likely to experience prejudice and discrimination—dynamics that may have increased their vulnerability to substance abuse.

Thus, despite their overall success in terms of socioeconomic variables, Cuban Americans have slightly lower incomes, educational levels, and rates of home ownership than non-Hispanic Whites. However, when compared with African Americans and other Hispanics in the United States, Cuban Americans have higher incomes and lower rates of unemployment and of female-headed households and are better educated (U.S. Bureau of the Census, 1991). As a group, Cuban Americans in the United States are achievement oriented and highly individualistic in their work goals. At times, their attitude of elitism, along with their often staunch political conservatism, has alienated Cuban Americans from other Hispanics, who tend to perceive Cuban Americans as arrogant.

Family Dynamics

The traditional Cuban view of the family is dependent on *machismo* and *marianismo*. The male is at the top of the family hierarchy; he is expected to be the main provider and is responsible for discipline and financial decisions. The mother is the moral authority, providing affection and keeping the family together; she is venerated for her kindness, tolerance, and purity. Children are taught to value respect, love, and dignity; this triad, representing the core of Hispanic cultural values, is considered to foster mental health (Ruiz, 1982).

In Cuba, it is not uncommon to have grandparents, uncles, and even neighbors participate in the raising of the children (Bernal, 1982; Rumbaut & Rumbaut, 1976). Moreover, sons and daughters are expected to live with their parents until they marry, and grandparents are kept with the family until their deaths. The transition from the model of the extended family with traditional Cuban values to the two-income nuclear-family model typical in the United States has had a profound impact on traditional gender roles and family dynamics among Cuban Americans. Currently, the tradition of "obedience to the parents and loyalty to the family" is still strong among many Cuban Americans and may sometimes come into conflict with the Anglo-Saxon values of independence and self-reliance.

Like other Hispanics, Cuban Americans place great value on personal trust and kinship and tend to value the judgment and approval of family and friends over those of professionals. They tend to develop strong affiliations with individuals rather than with institutions, a characteristic that permeates clinical transactions and is referred to as *personalismo* (Queralt, 1984; Rothe, 1992, 1995).

Role of Religion

Prior to the rise of Communism, the majority of Cubans were Catholic, and many Cuban Americans still turn to the Catholic Church for help with social and emotional problems (Clark, 1992). Others practice the Afro-Cuban religions of *santería* and *brujería*, which were initially brought to Cuba by slaves from West Africa, particularly from Congo and Nigeria. Santería resulted from the ban by the Catholic Spanish colonizers on the worship of African deities. Consequently, the African deities were transposed onto the effigies of the Catholic saints (*santos*) and the various representations of the Virgin Mary (Sandoval, 1977).

ACCULTURATION OR BICULTURALISM: THE CUBAN AMERICAN DILEMMA

Immigrants who are uprooted from their native culture and who lose their social network support without the ability to redevelop it in the host country are confronted with major stressors. Without the benefit of a social support system that values and validates their cultural and ethnic identity, immigrants may internalize potential negative images of themselves, leading to ethnic self-hate (Vega, Zimmerman, Gil, Warheit, & Apospori, 1993). This social phenomenon has been found to be responsible for alcohol and drug abuse among certain ethnic minority groups the United States (Ruiz, 1996; Vega et al., 1993).

According to studies by Szapocznik and colleagues (1978; 1988), the well-acculturated Cuban American adolescent who moves away from his or her heritage, who does not speak Spanish, and who is separated by a cultural gap from his or her parents and their community may experience the same degree of alienation as the poorly acculturated Cuban American adult who cannot speak English and who remains marginal to the culture of the host country. It is biculturalism that enables the immigrant to negotiate the demands of the host culture without losing connection and a sense of belonging to his or her own ethnocultural group. Such process allows for a validation and reaffirmation of the immigrant's identity by both the new and the old culture, thus allowing the immigrant to consolidate his or her sense of self. It is this model of biculturality, as reflected in South Florida where English and Spanish are spoken interchangeably and transactions can be conducted in either language (Bernal & Gutierrez, 1984; Botifoll, 1988), that has been held as one of the major factors in the success of many Cuban Americans. Such biculturality may also serve as a protective factor against mental illness and substance abuse (Rumbaut & Rumbaut, 1976;

Ruiz, 1997). For example, a study conducted in Miami by Szapocznik, Scopetta, and King (1978) revealed that out of the 50 Hispanic heroin addicts who were interviewed, 48 had developed their addiction while living in other, larger metropolitan areas in the United States. This finding supports the belief that cities like Miami provide a "cultural enclave" that validates the individual's sense of cultural and ethnic identity and minimizes risks for substance abuse (Botifoll, 1988; Grenier & Perez, 1996).

Rogler, Cortes, and Malgody (1991) have addressed the relationship between the socioeconomic variables of migration and the onset of psychopathology, including substance abuse. The best predictor of problems was high unemployment rates, whereas a higher level of education on the part of the immigrant, as well as having immigrated at an earlier age, facilitated positive acculturation. Rumbaut and Rumbaut (1976) suggest that among Cuban Americans who arrived in the United States prior to 1980, their high level of education and occupational skills, their motivation for success, and their strong sense of Cuban identity and ethnic consciousness facilitated their adaptation. Moreover, the strong sense of family cohesion among the Cuban American community allowed the Cuban immigrants to retain their culture and tradition while engaging in positive interactions with the host culture (Szapocznik & Hernandez, 1988).

ALCOHOL, DRUG ABUSE, AND HIV

Despite many commonalities, Cuban Americans in the United States are a heterogeneous group, and what may be true for the majority may not necessarily apply to a given individual. The stresses of migration and the disruption of the traditional family ties have produced "psychological casualties" among some Cuban Americans, resulting in alcohol and drug abuse, depression, and other emotional and mental disorders.

Alcohol and Drug Use among Cuban Americans

There is a sparsity in the literature with regard to epidemiological studies on alcohol and drug abuse among Cuban Americans. In general, the use and abuse of alcohol and drugs has been correlated with degree of acculturation, income, and educational levels. In regard to education and income levels, as discussed earlier, Cuban Americans tend to fare better than African Americans and other Hispanic and to follow closely behind non-Hispanic Whites. Thus it is not surprising that Cuban Americans seem to fare better than other Hispanic subgroups in terms of substance abuse. According to the 1991–1993 National Survey on Drug Abuse

(Substance Abuse & Mental Health Services Administration [SAMHSA], 1998), the "prevalence of a need for drug abuse treatment" among Cuban Americans was only 2.6% (compared with 3.7% among Puerto Ricans, 3.6% for Mexican Americans, and 2.5% for Caucasians), and their rate of alcohol dependence was the lowest (less than 1%) among all Hispanic subgroups. However, the rate of "heavy alcohol use" among Cuban Americans was 2.8%—lower than that for Mexican Americans (6.9%) or Puerto Ricans (4.0%), but higher than those for groups of other Caribbean or Central American origin (2.5% and 2.2%, respectively). Accordingly, "the results of this report suggest that relatively acculturated Hispanics, such as those who have lived in the United States long enough to become fluent in English, are in greater need of illicit drug abuse prevention and treatment services than less acculturated Hispanics" (SAMHSA, 1998, p. 12).

A study by Szapocznik and colleagues (1978) has identified an increase in substance abuse and antisocial behaviors among well-acculturated Cuban American male adolescents who lived with their poorly acculturated parents. It has been postulated that "gaps" in the cultural orientation between the generations or between the individual and the majority culture of the host society could lead to intrapsychic conflicts that could result in dysphoric feelings that might lead to acting out behaviors, including substance abuse.

Recent data regarding substance abuse among Cuban American women are lacking; however, past studies have reported that Cuban American women, particularly those who were "poorly acculturated" and struggling with intergenerational and sex-role conflicts, tend to abuse benzodiazepines, which are easily obtained over the counter in Cuban-owned and -operated pharmacies in South Florida (Allgulander, 1978; Gonzalez & Page, 1979). The changing family values have been particularly stressful for the traditional Cuban American female who is not employed outside the house and is considered the keeper of the family values. It is not uncommon for mental health professionals to encounter a middle-aged Cuban American woman who, after her exposure to a more permissive American culture, comes to the realization that she has spent her life with a husband whom she does not love and whose sexual interactions she rejects. A profound sense of loss ensues, often complicated by an agitated depression, as the woman realizes that she does not have the resources to make any changes in her life and that she is trapped in her predicament (Rothe, 1992).

HIV/AIDS among Cuban Americans

Despite the fact that Miami, the American city in which most Cubans reside, ranks second in the nation among metropolitan areas with the most

AIDS cases among Hispanics (104 per 100,000; Diaz, Buehler, Castro, & Ward, 1993), the risk factor for Cuban Americans is more likely to be homosexual transmission of HIV than the use of intravenous drugs. However, the social stigma of homosexuality resulting from the Hispanic cultural value of *machismo* and the frequent family ostracism contribute to the marginalization of homosexuals in the Cuban American community. Such marginalization, in turn, may lead to social isolation, depression, and risk of substance abuse, as well as more risk-taking sexual behaviors, completing a vicious cycle that increases the risk of contracting HIV infection.

Substance Abuse in Cuba

Official statistics of alcohol and drug consumption in Cuba have been unavailable in traditional literature for more than three decades (Rothe, 1994). However, a 1997 newspaper article ("Alcoholismo bate," 1997, p. 2-B) reported that during that year, alcohol consumption in Cuba "broke historical records." According to this article, a survey conducted by the Cuban National Institute of Hygiene, Epidemiology, and Microbiology among 14,300 Cubans living on the island showed that 45.2% of Cubans were "regular drinkers" and that 7.8% were classified as "alcoholics," with individuals between 40 and 59 years old being the most affected, followed by those between the ages of 20 and 29. Alcohol abuse was also found to be related to an increase in the number of motor vehicle accidents, revocation of driver's licenses, incidents of domestic violence, and a decrease in labor productivity ("Alcoholismo bate," 1997). This article did not venture any information regarding any possible precipitating factors that could be responsible for these increases, although the dire financial situation that has affected Cuba since 1992 is a likely contributing factor (Rothe, 1994).

There are no known data regarding drug use or drug-related HIV/AIDS cases in Cuba.

TREATMENT

The treatment of alcohol and other drug abuse need not vary for Cuban Americans. However, once the appropriate medical treatment protocol is selected (detoxification, relapse prevention, methadone maintenance, or others), important sociocultural considerations should be taken into account when designing the patient's individual treatment plan. The degree of cultural sensitivity employed in the treatment design may result in the success or failure of the particular intervention.

Traditionally, in pre-Castro Cuba, the middle class subscribed to "mutualistic clinics" that were similar, in some respects, to American health maintenance organizations (HMOs) at which for a fixed monthly fee the entire family received medical care. These mutualistic clinics have mushroomed in Miami (Ruiz, 1985) and provide a familiar "entry point" into treatment for many Cuban American substance abusers. However, although offering culturally sensitive treatment, some of these clinics may lack the knowledge to diagnose and treat substance abuse, and thus some individuals may be misdiagnosed and untreated for their substance abuse.

Language sometimes represents an important barrier in the accessibility of mainstream mental health and substance abuse treatment and accounts for the underutilization of all mental health services by Hispanics in the United States (Ruiz & Langrod, 1997). The availability of bicultural and bilingual professional staff, Spanish-speaking Alcoholics Anonymous (AA) and Narcotics Anonymous (NA) groups, and methadone clinics represent a key element in the success of treating the Cuban American substance abuser (Langrod et al., 1981; Ruiz, 1996; Ruiz & Langrod, 1997).

The values of *machismo* can also occasionally present an obstacle to the treatment of substance-abusing Cuban American men (Bernal, 1982; Queralt, 1984; Ruiz, 1996; Ruiz & Langrod, 1997). Although belief systems are difficult to change and education sometimes takes a long time to produce results, one way to address this problem is by confronting the substance abuser and reframing his behavior as a neglect of his role as head of the family, thereby appealing to his sense of responsibility, which requires that he command dignity and respect in exercising this role (Rothe, 1992).

In general, Cuban Americans tend to seek concrete and practical solutions to their problems and tend to be present oriented, and they are not usually inclined to seek long-term psychotherapies for the purpose of achieving insight or personal growth. They value a personal relationship with the treating professional and clinical staff and expect a mutual recognition of dignity and respect, as well as the open mutual expression of affection and care (Ruiz, 1982).

Szapocznik and his colleagues (1978) found that Cuban Americans view their doctors and other professionals in a linear hierarchical relationship. They expect their doctors to assume a position of authority and to provide clear and concise instructions for treatment. They also expect praise from their doctors if instructions are followed correctly.

Like other Hispanics, Cuban Americans place great value on the extended family. The failure to include key figures in the family hierarchy may result in resistance to treatment. This is particularly true when working with substance-abusing Cuban American women and adolescents.

Treatment of Adolescents

Most of the research in the treatment of Cuban American substance abusers has been done on male adolescents, who have been found to have higher rates of behavioral problems and substance abuse because they acculturate faster than other members of the family. Consequently, they find themselves alienated from their families of origin (Szapocznik et al., 1988).

Researchers found that using a combination of structural and strategic family therapy in the treatment of these adolescents has provided very successful results. They found that the core symptoms of family dysfunction that contribute to the adolescents' acting out behavior, including substance abuse, present themselves as a resistance in the initial phase of treatment, thus demarcating diagnostically what needs to be changed. The structural–strategic family approach seeks, among other things, to restore parents to their traditional hierarchical role in the family constellation and to facilitate the development of a cultural continuum between the generations. Such an approach leads to a decrease of alienation in the substance-abusing adolescent (Santiesteban & Szapocznik, 1994; Santiesteban et al., 1996).

Treatment of Women

The Cuban women who abuse benzodiazepines (Gonzalez & Page, 1979) frequently resist any attempts at tapering down the dose of the particular antianxiety agent. Because benzodiazepines are easily obtained over the counter in pharmacies in many Cuban communities, any treatment attempt of this kind is likely to fail. Rothe (1992) has suggested that rather than addressing benzodiazepine abuse directly, the clinician employ a combination of supportive and cognitive–behavioral individual and group therapy in which unresolved grief and pathological mourning are addressed. Such an approach is likely to decrease use and dosage of drugs. Accomplishments, such as having overcome the many difficulties of exile, having raised a family under difficult circumstances, and having "started a new life from scratch" are highlighted and validated, thus restoring the patient's self-esteem, dignity, and respect. It is not uncommon for the clinician to be showered by gifts from an elderly Cuban American who will say to his or her therapist, on the first visit, "You could be my son (daughter)." This immediate transferential reaction signals the beginning of the painful mourning process that will follow (Rothe, 1992).

Some Cuban elderly have found support in community organizations such as Cuban Municipalities in Exile, in which every small Cuban town and village is represented and in which its members reconnect and socialize with their former childhood acquaintances and their descendants. Such activities allow them to maintain their cultural and family traditions and minimize the loneliness and isolation that may lead to substance abuse.

CONCLUSIONS

Cuban Americans continue to adhere to their cultural heritage and traditions, although this practice may vary among second- and third-generation Cuban Americans. They also continue to face the challenges of adaptation and acculturation, and, even though they appear to fare better than other Hispanic subgroups, many psychological casualties continue to occur.

Cuban Americans present particular migration characteristics, modes of acculturation, and sociodemographic variables that differ from those found among other Hispanic subgroups in the United States. These characteristics are important in understanding the genesis of psychopathology and substance abuse problems and have a major impact on the effectiveness, delivery, and accessibility of health services and treatment of substance abusers.

Substance abuse and HIV infection have been identified as devastating problems for Hispanics in the United States. In spite of this concern, very little epidemiological and treatment outcome research has been conducted, especially with Cuban Americans. Such research, however, should be culturally sensitive, employing an ethnographic methodology and instrumentation that can better help to conceptualize the particular research paradigm for this population. Research findings, in turn, can then be applied to improve treatment interventions. Additionally, there is a strong need for education in order to address issues such as *machismo* and homosexuality within the Cuban American culture. These are the clinical and programmatic challenges that must be faced as we enter into the 21st century.

REFERENCES

Ackerman, H., & Clark, J. (1995). *The Cuban Balseros: Voyage of uncertainty* (Monograph of the Policy Center of the Cuban National Council). Miami, FL: Cuban National Council.

Alcoholismo bate record historico ["Alcoholism breaks historical records"]. (1997, November). *El Nuevo Herald, 4,* 2-B.

Allgulander, C. (1978). Dependence on sedatives and hypnotic drugs: A comparative clinical and social study. *Acta Psychiatria Scandinavica, 705*(Suppl.), 7–101.

Bernal, G. (1982). Cuban families. In M. McGoldrick, J. K. Pearce, & J. Giordano (Eds.), *Ethnicity and family therapy* (pp. 187–208). New York: Guilford Press.

Bernal, G., & Gutierrez, M. (1984). Cubans. In L. Comas-Díaz & E. E. H. Griffith (Eds.), *Clinical guidelines in cross cultural mental health* (pp. 131–154). New York: Wiley.

Boswell, T., Rivero, M., & Diaz G. (1984). *Demographic characteristics of pre-Mariel Cubans living in the United States* (Monograph of the Research Institute of Cuban Studies). Miami, FL: University of Miami, Graduate School of International Studies.

Botifoll, L. (1988). *How Miami's image was created* (Monograph of the Research Institute of Cuban Studies). Miami, FL: University of Miami, Graduate School of International Studies.

Clark, J. (1992). *Documento de Consulta* (Monograph of the Encuentro Internacional de Comunidades de Reflexión Eclesial Cubana en la Diaspora). Miami, FL: Catholic Archdiocese of Miami.

Cuban success story in the United States. (1967). *U.S. News & World Report, 62,* 104–106.

Diaz, T., Buehler, J. W., Castro, K. G., & Ward, J. W. (1993). AIDS trends among Hispanics in the United States. *American Journal of Public Health, 83*(4), 504–509.

Flight from Cuba: Castro's loss, U.S. Gain. (1971). *U.S. News & World Report, 70,* 74–77.

Gonzalez, D., & Page, J. B. (1979, November). *Cuban women, sex role conflicts and use of prescription drugs.* Paper presented at the annual meeting of the American Anthropological Association, Miami, FL.

Grenier, G., & Perez, L. (1996). Miami spice: The ethnic cauldron simmers. In S. Pedraza & R. G. Rumbaut (Eds.), *Origins and destinies: Immigration, race, and ethnicity in America.* Belmont, CA: Wadsworth.

Jorge, A., Suchlicki, J., & Leyva de Varona, A. (1991). *Cuban exiles in South Florida: Their presence and contributions* (Monograph of the Research Institute of Cuban Studies). Miami, FL: University of Miami Press.

Langrod, J., Alksne, L., Lowinson, J., & Ruiz, P. (1981). Rehabilitation of the Puerto Rican addict: A cultural perspective. *International Journal of the Addictions, 16*(5), 841–847.

Pumariega, A., Swanson, J. W., Holzer, C., Linskey, A. O., & Quintero-Salinas, R. (1992). Cultural context and substance abuse in Hispanic adolescents. *Journal of Child and Family Studies, 1*(1), 75–92.

Queralt, M. (1984) Understanding Cuban immigrants: A cultural perspective. *Social Work, 29,* 115–121.

Rogler, L. H., Cortes, D. E., & Malgady, R. G. (1991). Acculturation and mental health status among Hispanics. *American Psychologist, 46*(6), 585–597.

Rothe, E. (1992, May). *The Cuban American: Mental health after three decades of exile.* Paper presented at the annual meeting of the American Psychiatric Association, Washington, DC.

Rothe, E. (1994, August). *The Cuban American medical system: Myths and realities.* Paper presented at the University of Miami/Jackson Memorial Hospital, Department of Family Medicine, Grand Rounds, Miami.

Rothe, E. (1995, May). *The Miami Cubans: Immigrants or new Americans?* Paper presented at the annual meeting of the American Psychiatric Association, Miami Beach, FL.

Ruiz, P. (1982). Cuban Americans: Migration, acculturation and mental health. In A. Gaw (Ed.), *Cross-cultural psychiatry* (pp. 69–89). Boston: John Wright, PSG.

Ruiz, P. (1985). Cultural barriers to effective medical care among Hispanic-American patients. *Annual Review of Medicine, 36,* 63–71.

Ruiz, P. (1996). Alcohol and Hispanic Americans. In Group for the Advancement of Psychiatry (Ed.), *Alcoholism in the United States: Racial and ethnic considerations* (Report No. 141). Washington, DC: American Psychiatric Press.

Ruiz, P., & Langrod J. G. (1997). Hispanic Americans. In J. H. Lowinson, P. Ruiz, R. B. Millman, & J. G. Langrod (Eds.), *Substance abuse: A comprehensive textbook* (3rd ed., pp. 705–711). Baltimore: Williams & Wilkins.

Ruiz, P., Langrod, J., Lowinson J., & Marcus N. (1977). Social rehabilitation of addicts: A two-year evaluation. *International Journal of the Addictions, 12*(1), 173–181.

Rumbaut, R., & Rumbaut, R. (1976). The family in exile: Cuban families in the United States. *American Journal of Psychiatry, 133*(4), 395–399.

Sandoval, M. (1977). Santería: Afro-Cuban concepts of disease and its treatment in Miami. *Journal of Operational Psychiatry, 8*(1), 52–63.

Santiesteban, D. A., & Szapocznik, J. (1994). Bridging theory, research and practice to more successfully engage substance abusing youth and their families into therapy. *Journal of Child and Adolescent Substance Abuse, 3*(2), 9–24.

Santiesteban, D. A., Szapocznik, J., Perez-Vidal, A., Murray, E. H., Kurtines, W. M., & LaPerriere, A. (1996). Efficacy and intervention for engaging youth and families into treatment and some variable that may contribute to differential effectiveness. *Journal of Family Psychology, 10*(1), 35–44.

Sokol-Katz, J. S., & Ulbrich, P. M. (1992). Family structure and risk taking behavior: A comparison of Mexican, Cuban and Puerto Rican Americans. *International Journal of the Addictions, 27*(10), 1197–1209.

Substance Abuse and Mental Health Service Administration. (1998, April). *Disparity seen in substance use among racial/ethnic subgroups.*

Szapocznik, J., & Hernandez, J. R. (1988). The Cuban American family. In C. Mindez, R. W. Haberstein, & R. Wright (Eds.), *Ethnic families in America: Patterns and variations* (3rd ed.). New York: Elsevier.

Szapocznik, J., Scopetta, M. A., & King, O. E. (1978). Therapy and practice in matching treatment to the special characteristics and problems of Cuban immigrants. *Journal of Community Psychology, 6,* 112–122.

Szapocznik, J., Perez-Vidal, A., Brickman, A. L., Foote, F. H., Santiesteban, D., & Hervis, O. (1988). Engaging adolescent drug abusers and their families in treatment: A strategic structural system approach. *Journal of Consulting and Clinical Psychology, 56,* 552–557.

U.S. Bureau of the Census. (1990). *Current population reports* (Series P-20, No. 449 (3).

Vega, W. A., Zimmerman, R., Gil, A., Warheit, G. J., & Apospori, E. (1993). Acculteration strain theory: Its application in explaining drug use behavior among Cuban and other Hispanic youth. *American Journal of Public Health, 83(2),* 185–189.

6

Substance Abuse in the Mexican American Population

Louis R. Alvarez
Pedro Ruiz

Substance abuse is an enormous health problem among the Mexican American population in the United States (Substance Abuse and Mental Health Services Administration, 1997). The 13.4 million Mexican Americans, that is, people of Mexican birth or ancestry, are the second largest ethnic minority in the United States and constitute the largest Hispanic subgroup, composing 63% of the U.S. Hispanic population (U.S. Bureau of the Census, 1992). It has been estimated that by the year 2000, Mexican Americans will account for the majority of the individuals under the age of 30 living in the southwestern United States (Western Interstate Commission on Higher Education, 1987).

For many Mexican Americans, drugs and alcohol are a major means of coping with the hardships of poverty, discrimination, and minority status. The reemerging anti-immigrant sentiment in the United States, reduced entitlements, inadequate health insurance coverage, and disproportionately lower federal spending on treatment than on law enforcement are fueling the substance abuse crisis among Mexican Americans. This chapter is a practical guide for both public health and mental health professionals working with Mexican American clients affected by substance abuse. It seeks to advance an understanding of important sociocultural and demographic variables in evaluating and treating the Mexican American substance abuser and in establishing effective substance abuse prevention programs. It addresses the (1) historical background and cultural heritage of Mexican Americans, (2) epidemiology of substance abuse among Mexican nationals in Mexico and Mexican Americans in the United States, (3) etiology of substance abuse among Mexican Americans, (4) cultural issues in the substance abuse treatment of Mexican Americans, (5) principles of substance abuse treatment of Mexican Americans, and (6) implications for prevention and public policy.

HISTORICAL BACKGROUND
AND CULTURAL HERITAGE

The histories of Mexico and of the United States are closely intertwined. Unlike other Hispanics, most of whom arrived in the second half of the 20th century, the ancestors of Mexicans, who were indigenous Indians, inhabited much of what constitutes the United States almost 6 centuries ago (Novas, 1994). The history of Mexico is distinguished by a long line of advanced Indian civilizations that included the Olmec, the Maya, and the Aztec. It is understandable that Mexican Americans resent being told that Columbus "discovered" America when their ancestors developed highly sophisticated cultures and built wondrous cities centuries before the arrival of Columbus. Mexicans are often offended when the term "Americans" is used to refer to only U.S. citizens (Kennedy Center for International Studies, 1990), as this does not acknowledge that Mexico is part of North America and that its citizens have an equal right to be called Americans.

The history of Mexico and its people is characterized by a recurring theme of domination and exploitation by foreign powers, including the United States. After Mexico was defeated by the United States in the Mexican War (1846–1848), it was coerced into signing the Treaty of Guadalupe Hidalgo, which forced it to cede Texas, New Mexico, California, Arizona, Nevada, Utah, and half of Colorado to the United States—thereby losing two-fifths of its national territory (Novas, 1994). The present quasi-democratic, single-dominant-party system that first evolved in Mexico in the 1930s has had only limited success in effective land distribution or fair economic development. The great inequality of wealth and opportunity that has persisted has further stimulated migration to the United States.

Mexican Culture

Mexico's rich culture is characterized by an exuberant vitality that is reflected in its magnificent music, literature, and art. Religion greatly affects the lives of most Mexicans, and it is a predominantly Roman Catholic nation. The Virgin of Guadalupe, the patron saint of Mexico and the symbol of its national identity, is a ubiquitous presence in Mexican life (Toor, 1985). In Mexican culture, an individual's family and personal interests are ascribed more value than his or her occupation, so that a person's job does not define him or her as much as it tends to do in mainstream U.S. culture (Shorris, 1992).

The mind-set of the traditional Mexican woman is often associated with the cultural construct of *marianismo*, focusing on the Virgin Mary as an ideal of duty, self-sacrifice, passivity, and chastity. Today, women in Mexico are still not able to fully participate in society because institutionalized sexism sometimes relegates them to a secondary status.

MEXICAN AMERICANS

Mexican Americans are a heterogeneous group, with approximately 80% of the population concentrated in California, Texas, Arizona, and New Mexico, and the remainder located mostly in Colorado and Illinois (U.S. Bureau of the Census, 1992). The majority of Mexican Americans live in large cities, with Los Angeles having the largest concentration of people of Mexican descent outside of Mexico City. The typical Mexican American household tends to be larger and younger than other households in the United States: Mexican Americans have a median age of 23, compared with a median of 32 for White non-Hispanics (Chavez, 1993), and live in households of 3.8 persons, compared with 2.6 persons in non-Hispanic households (U.S. Bureau of the Census, 1992). Most Mexican Americans speak English and Spanish with varying degrees of fluency.

Mexican Americans have been described as a decent, generous, and honorable people (Toor, 1985). They are known for their strong work ethic and are imbued with an indomitable will to provide for their families (Toor, 1985). The labor force participation rate of Mexican American men (80.5%) is higher than that of non-Hispanic men (74.3%; U.S. Bureau of the Census, 1992). The high regard that Mexican culture has for working is illustrated in one of the more common Mexican *dichos* (folk sayings): "*El flojo trabaja doble*," translated as "He who is lazy ends up working twice as much."

Despite their high labor force participation, studies of Mexican Americans show that they are least likely to be covered by health insurance. This is often a significant impediment to receiving adequate substance abuse treatment. According to the National Council of La Raza (NCLR, 1992),

36% of people of Mexican origin were uninsured in 1990 compared with 21% of other Hispanics and 13% of Whites.

In spite of their sacrifices and numerous contributions to American society, Mexicans and Mexican Americans have encountered prejudice in the United States for much of its history. In the 1930s the Federal Bureau of Narcotics fabricated information about the "epidemic" of marijuana use by "reefer mad" Mexicans in order to further the agency's own growth and power (Glick & Moore, 1990). This led to a long-standing label of deviance being placed on Mexicans and Mexican Americans in the United States. During the Depression years of the 1930s approximately one-half million people of Mexican descent, including many Mexican Americans whose families had lived in the United States for generations, were deported from the United States without the slightest regard for their civil rights (Novas, 1994). Mexican farmworkers in the United States have historically been subjected to rampant prejudice, physical mistreatment, and deadly pesticide exposure, even though they have been the backbone of U.S. agricultural prosperity in California and in the Southwest. The history of great injustices perpetrated on Mexican laborers in the United States has been seared into the minds of present-day Mexican Americans and fuels the mistrust that many Mexicans and Mexican Americans have toward Anglos today. Perhaps no one has embodied the finest qualities of Mexican Americans and represented the worker's struggle for justice and equality better than César Chávez. Facing incredible odds and experiencing countless setbacks, he persevered to form the first successful farmworker's union. Mexican American women have additional struggles. Whereas in Mexico *marianismo* affords women protection and respect, in the United States the value system it perpetuates is at odds with their adopted American culture. Moreover, the Chicana may have to struggle against "triple oppression"— poverty, racism, and sexism—in the United States while still being expected to fulfill all her traditional duties to her family (National Association for Chicano Studies, 1993).

Since the 1960s, many Mexican Americans have chosen to call themselves Chicanos as a symbol of their pride and solidarity. The term "Chicano" has gone through several transformations, but it most commonly refers to people of Mexican descent born in either the United States or Mexico and raised in the United States (Hurtado & Gurin, 1995). In addition to containing qualities characteristically found both in so-called American and Mexican cultures, Chicano culture also contains many unique hybrid characteristics not typical of either parent culture (Garza & Gallegos, 1995).

EPIDEMIOLOGY OF SUBSTANCE
ABUSE IN MEXICANS

For thousands of years indigenous peoples in Mexico used native hallucinogens such as peyote and sacred mushrooms in religious rites. According
to the Mexican government, drug abuse among the general population of
Mexico has remained low over the years except in the area near the Mexico–United States border (U.S. Department of State, 1996). Recent drug
surveys in Mexico are not very comprehensive because they are carried out
in metropolitan areas, not in the numerous rural communities. Since 1970,
several studies have reported that inhalants were the most commonly
abused substances, followed by amphetamines, cannabis, and tranquilizers.
Heroin, LSD, and cocaine were reportedly used by a smaller percentage of
the Mexican population (U.S. Department of State, 1996).

Unlike illicit drug use, the use of alcohol has increased in recent years.
In Mexico, a male drinking companion is often called a *cuate,* meaning a
"twin brother," and the festive gathering at which drinking takes place is
sometimes called a *pachanga* (Gilbert & Gonsalves, 1985). Mexico's annual alcohol consumption increased from 1.9 liters per person in 1970 to
2.9 liters in 1993. In particular, consumption of beer has risen steadily,
from 29.1 liters per person in 1970 to 47.0 liters in 1993 (U.S. Department
of State, 1996).

EPIDEMIOLOGY OF SUBSTANCE
ABUSE IN MEXICAN AMERICANS

Alcohol Use

Alcohol is by far the drug of greatest abuse among Mexican Americans
(Caetano, 1985). Alcohol is woven into the social fabric of family life of Mexican Americans, and its traditional convivial use is well accepted (Gilbert,
1985). To a significant extent, drinking is also accepted for its utilitarian use
as a method of reducing anxiety (Caetano, 1987). Studies (Cervantes,
Gilbert, Salgado de Snyder, & Padilla, 1990) have also suggested that Mexican American men have a greater tendency than Whites to self-medicate with
alcohol out of the expectation that it will relieve depressive symptoms.
Studies indicate that Mexican Americans hold more permissive attitudes toward alcohol intoxication than other Hispanic subgroups (National Institute
on Drug Abuse, 1987). Data from the Substance Abuse and Mental Health
Services Administration's (SAMHSA; 1993) National Household Survey on

Drug Abuse on past-month prevalence of drug use indicates that persons of Mexican ancestry report the highest prevalence of heavy alcohol use compared with other Hispanics (6.9% vs. 5.5%). Heavy alcohol use is defined as consuming five or more drinks on the same occasion on 5 or more days in the past month. Caetano (1985) found that among Hispanic men, Mexican Americans also drink more frequently.

The correlation between alcohol intake and acculturation among Mexican Americans has been noted by many researchers (Caetano, 1987). In studying Mexicans who migrate to the United States, Caetano and Medina-Mora (1988) found that changes in drinking patterns among men seem to occur shortly after they arrive in the United States. Gilbert and Cervantes (1986) have hypothesized that the pattern of frequent heavy drinking among Mexican American men results from both native culture and acculturation. In other words, the heavy drinking more typical in Mexican culture combines with the more frequent drinking typical of American culture, leading to both heavy and frequent drinking. Whereas in the general population, heavy drinking, alcohol dependency, and alcohol-related social problems are at their highest in the years between ages 18 and 29 and decrease from that point with age, such a drop does not take place among Mexican American men (Gilbert & Cervantes, 1986). This is troubling because heavy drinking is occurring when these men are older and generally have increased responsibilities and increased health problems (Aguirre-Molina & Caetano, 1994). The impact of drinking is consequently more severe at this point in their lives.

Mexican Americans are disproportionately struck by alcohol-related diseases, and they are overrepresented among those experiencing alcohol-related deaths (National Center for Health Statistics, 1990). A study by Rosenwaike (1987) found that Mexican American men have a 40% higher risk of death from cirrhosis than White men. Data from the National Center for Health Statistics in 1990 ranked chronic liver disease and cirrhosis as the seventh most frequent cause of death in Mexican Americans, whereas they ranked tenth among Whites and African Americans (National Center for Health Statistics, 1990).

According to the 1993 National Household Survey on Drug Abuse, Mexican American women report the highest prevalence of heavy alcohol use when compared with other Hispanic women (SAMHSA, 1993). Caetano (1985) also found that Mexican American women accounted for a greater proportion of frequent high maximum drinkers compared with other Hispanic women (Herd & Caetano, 1987). Studies also demonstrate that adolescent Mexican American females clearly represent an emerging risk group (Mora & Gilbert, 1991). Mexican American girls are beginning

to experiment with alcohol at approximately 13 years of age and have abstention rates only slightly higher than Mexican American boys (Gilbert &
Alcocer, 1988). Despite these findings, research on drinking patterns
among Mexican American men and women supports the existence of a
double standard in that drinking is an accepted activity for males but not
for females (Gilbert, 1985).

The association between acculturation and drinking is stronger among
Mexican women than among Mexican men (Mora & Gilbert, 1991). Mora
and Gilbert (1991) observe that among first-generation Mexican American
women, abstinence rates are as high as for women in Mexico, but for second-generation women abstinence rates fall dramatically, and light to moderate drinking greatly increases. Alcohol ingestion increases in frequency
and quantity, especially among highly acculturated, educated, employed,
and middle-class Mexican American women (Gilbert, 1987), among whom
traditional sanctions against female drinking appear to break down.

Drug Use

Patterns of drug use by Mexican Americans vary by age group and region of the country. The Substance Abuse and Mental Health Services
Administration's (1993) National Household Survey on Drug Abuse
found that the rate of illicit drug use for Mexican Americans (6.2%) was
higher than for Hispanics overall (5.9%). However, because national
studies usually collect and clump together data for Mexican Americans
with those for other Latino subgroups under the category "Hispanics,"
the true extent of the problem of drug use among Mexican Americans is
probably underestimated (Rouse, 1987). Such clumping of data also pre-
vents a distinct understanding of the ethnocultural, socioeconomic, and
biological characteristics of Mexican Americans, which is vital in compre-
hending and treating their drug use. Moreover, many Mexican Americans
are reluctant to disclose illicit drug use for fear of prosecution and possible deportation.

Heroin

Increased heroin trafficking in the 1990s and the greater supply of heroin in
inner-city barrios is in large measure responsible for the recent resurgence
of heroin use among Mexican Americans (Castro, 1994). Mexican American heroin addicts are often referred to as *tecatos* (addicts) and those with a
long-term heroin addiction are also known as *veteranos* (Mata & Jorquez,
1988). Rouse examined the percentage of hospital admissions for Mexican

Americans and Whites in Texas, stratified by age groups. He found that among the oldest group, those aged 26 and over, 70% of Mexican American admissions were for heroin abuse, compared with only 28% of White admissions (Rouse, 1987).

Studies of heroin addicts on methadone maintenance found that Mexican Americans were generally older at their first admission for methadone, had been addicted for longer periods of time, had lower levels of educational attainment and lower socioeconomic status, and displayed a higher proportion of school problems than White addicts (Hser, Anglin, & Liu, 1990). In addition, those Mexican American men who were not involved in treatment early in their addictions took the longest time to end their use of narcotics and to find employment (Hser, Anglin, & Liu, 1990).

Inhalants

The bulk of the inhalant abuse research related to Mexican Americans consists of local community- or school-based studies (Texas Commission on Alcohol and Drug Abuse, 1990). Much of this literature reflects sample sizes that are inadequate for making reliable estimates of those affected by these substances (Mata, Rodriguez-Andrew, & Rouse, 1993). Although some studies have not found Mexican Americans to be more likely than non-Hispanic Whites to use inhalants, there appear to be circumscribed areas, such as the United States–Mexico border region, in which epidemics of inhalant abuse are common (Mata & Rodriguez-Andrew, 1988). Moreover, several studies indicate that Mexican Americans use inhalants at earlier ages than Whites, with some finding inhalant use among children as young as 7 years old (De Barona & Simpson, 1984). Rouse (1987) found that treatment admissions of adolescents for inhalant abuse were more likely among Mexican Americans than among Whites, with 33% of Mexican American 12- to 17-year-olds admitted for inhalant use compared with 5% of Whites.

Rodriguez-Andrew (1985) found that Mexican Americans aged 12 to 14 did not perceive inhalant use as dangerous. As a result, these youths are probably less aware of the fact that inhalants can be as lethal as cocaine or heroin and may cause irreversible brain, kidney, and liver damage following chronic exposure (Hecht, 1980). Most experts agree that fatalities are underreported, especially among the Mexican American children who are truant and homeless (Dyer, 1984). The cognitive deficits arising from chronic inhalant abuse further mitigate against the future participation of these youth in the educational process. Although inhalant abuse among Mexican Americans cuts across socioeconomic lines, low-income individuals are overinvolved because of the availability and minimal cost of inhalants (Dyer, 1984). The leading types of inhalants abused by Mexican Americans are gasoline or lighter fluid (36%), shoe polish, glue, or toluene (33%), and spray paint (33%; National Institute on Drug Abuse, 1987).

A serious concern related to those Mexican Americans who abuse inhalants is that, like alcohol and marijuana, inhalants are a so-called gateway drug and frequently part of a polydrug pattern of use among Mexican Americans (De Barona & Simpson, 1984). Rodriguez-Andrew's (1985) pilot study of Mexican American children in housing projects found that 68% of chronic inhalant users and 82% of recreational users reported also using marijuana once a day. Almost half (47%) of the chronic users and 27% of the recreational users reported drinking alcohol once a day. The multiple-drug-use phenomenon is especially alarming when one considers that the average age of the respondents was approximately 14 years and that the effects of multiple drug use may have an adverse impact on their cognitive and emotional development (Rodriguez-Andrew, 1985).

Marijuana

The Substance Abuse and Mental Health Services Administration's (1993) survey on past-month prevalence of drug use indicates that Mexican American men report less marijuana use (5.7%) than other Hispanic men, whereas Mexican American women report less use (2.7%) than some but not all Hispanic women. Amaro, Whitaker, Coffman, and Heeven (1990) found that acculturation is more strongly associated with marijuana use among Mexican American women than among men. Moreover, the most acculturated and least educated women were most likely to report the greatest marijuana use (Amaro et al., 1990).

Although analysis of data from the Client Oriented Data Acquisition Process (Rouse, 1987) found that the percentages of admissions for marijuana abuse among Mexican American and White clients were comparable across all age groups, there is cause for concern because marijuana is also a gateway drug, often leading to polysubstance abuse among Mexican Americans.

Cocaine

Mexican Americans report a slightly higher prevalence of cocaine use (1.5%) compared with other Hispanics (1.3%; SAMHSA, 1993). Among Hispanic females, Mexican American women report the highest prevalence of cocaine use (1.1%), whereas Mexican American men were second only to Puerto Rican men (1.9% vs. 2.4%) in prevalence of cocaine use (SAMHSA, 1993). Little data is available on the specific use of crack cocaine by Mexican Americans. It is striking that in the Hispanic Health and Nutrition Examination Survey conducted between 1982 and 1984 (Amaro et al., 1990), Mexicans who spoke English were found to be 25 times more likely than those who spoke only Spanish to have used cocaine during the previous year—once again reflecting the association of acculturation with substance use.

HIV/AIDS among Mexican Americans

Perhaps nowhere else is the effect of substance abuse on the Mexican American population potentially more devastating than in the transmission of the human immunodeficiency virus (HIV). The HIV/AIDS Surveillance Report of HIV and AIDS cases reported in the United States through December 1997 by the Centers for Disease Control and Prevention (CDC) indicate that, among individuals born in Mexico and living in the United States, there were 1,117 AIDS cases, with 7% of these cases being attributed to injecting drug use (CDC, 1997). It should not be lost upon clinicians that the use of any drug by Mexican Americans, whether injected or not, can lead to other high-risk behaviors and result in HIV infection.

SOCIOECONOMIC AND ETHNOCULTURAL FACTORS IN SUBSTANCE USE

Although an in-depth discussion of economic and social policies lies outside of the purview of this chapter, they are of paramount importance in any attempt to discern the etiology of substance abuse in the Mexican American population (Ruiz & Langrod, 1997).

Impact of Poverty

In analyzing the various conditions that predispose Mexican Americans to substance abuse, we find impressive evidence that poverty is among the most significant of all risk factors (Booth, Castro, & Anglin, 1990). Mexican Americans are clearly overrepresented among the poor in the United States (U.S. Bureau of the Census, 1992). Mexican American families are almost three times as likely as non-Hispanic families to be poor: 1 in 4 Mexican American families (27.4%) compared with 1 in 10 non-Hispanic families (10.2%) lived below the poverty level in 1991 (U.S. Bureau of the Census, 1992).

According to 1992 census data, the median earnings of Mexican men in the United States were $12,959, compared with $14,503 for all Hispanic men and $22,628 for non-Hispanic men. More than one third (35.3%) of Mexican men earned less than $10,000, compared with less than one fourth of non-Hispanic men (23.6%; U.S. Bureau of the Census, 1992). The median earnings of Mexican women were also lower compared with all Hispanic women ($9,260 vs. $10,399) and significantly less than the median of $13,216 for non-Hispanic women (U.S. Bureau of the Census, 1992).

The condition of poverty provides few opportunities to buffer the inordinate stress and economic hardship experienced by Mexican American families, often leaving them devoid of hope and with little capacity to cope. Alcohol and other drugs thus become one of the few ways of dealing with destitute circumstances. Poverty itself can also intensify the adversity and suffering experienced by the Mexican American substance abuser by amplifying the harmful social and health-related consequences of alcohol and other drug use. When poverty is added to the inequality, discrimination, and economic insecurity in their lives, Mexican American youths may be more vulnerable to peer pressure and negative influences. Moore (1990) reports that, among young people, a friend's use of a drug may be the greatest single factor influencing initiation and continued drug use. Because many of these youths are unable to see a meaningful purpose to their lives, they engage in living for the moment and have little to empower them to resist the allure of drugs.

Educational Status

The strong relationship between dropping out of school and the use of drugs has been well documented (Fagan & Pabon, 1990). The general finding in the 1996 National Household Survey on Drug Abuse that illicit drug use rates remain inversely correlated with educational status is dramatically evident among Mexican Americans (SAMHSA, 1997). The Mexican American Drug Use and Dropout study begun in 1987 has shown that Mexican American dropouts have the highest rates of drug use (Chavez, Edwards, & Oetting, 1989). According to the U.S. Bureau of the Census (1992), Mexican Americans are the least educated of all Hispanic subgroups and the most undereducated of all ethnocultural groups in the United States, with dropout rates reaching as high as 58% in some communities (National Center for Education Statistics, 1989). Of all Mexicans 25 years old and older in 1993, less than half completed high school (45.2%), compared with 81.5% of non-Hispanics (U.S. Bureau of the Census, 1992). These trends are especially disheartening because dropouts are more difficult to reach with school-based preventive and rehabilitative efforts. In particular, after dropping out, these Mexican American students may no longer have access to reliable information about the harmful consequences of drugs. This situation may translate to a decrease in the perceived risk of using these substances and lead eventually to heightened alcohol and drug use.

Acculturation

One of the most extensively studied of all cultural constructs among Hispanics is acculturation, which refers to the social and psychological process whereby immigrants and their offspring adopt the values, attitudes, and behaviors of the host culture (Padilla, 1980). The relationship of acculturation to substance abuse among Mexican Americans has at times been unclear and dependent on the theoretical perspective used by researchers to define acculturation. Nevertheless, the weight of the research indicates that higher levels of acculturation into U.S. society, as reflected mainly by English-language use, are associated with higher levels of drug use among Mexican Americans (Amaro et al., 1990). Pumariega, Swanson, Holzer, Linskey, and Quintero-Salinas (1992) report in their study of 4,157 Mexican American and Mexican youths living along the United States–Mexico border that the Mexican youths had significantly lower rates of both recent and problematic drug use than their Mexican American counterparts on the U.S. side of the border. It has been postulated that Mexican American youth who are more acculturated than their parents may bond less to them, resulting in a less cohesive family unit (Cervantes, 1993). Given the important role of the family as a social support network for Mexican Americans, the consequences of a disruption in these ties can be severe (Cervantes, 1993). However, it is important to emphasize that, regardless of their level of acculturation, the realities of discrimination, entrapment in poverty, and disillusionment with their inability to achieve upward socioeconomic mobility can alienate Mexican Americans from mainstream U.S. society and galvanize them to use drugs.

Marketing by the Alcohol and Tobacco Industries

Aggressive marketing by the alcohol and tobacco industries frequently targets Mexican Americans because the youth and growth of this population make it a very profitable market (Moore, Williams, & Qualls, 1996). One of the more popular methods employed has been to sponsor cultural events such as El Cinco de Mayo celebrations in order to create an environment conducive to the use of alcohol. Such marketing is very disconcerting because it represents an additional risk factor for drug use to Mexican American youth and because studies suggest that with increasing numbers of risk factors the student's vulnerability to substance abuse markedly rises (Yin, Zapata, & Katims, 1995).

ASSESSMENT AND TREATMENT ISSUES WITH MEXICAN AMERICANS

A central tenet in the substance abuse treatment of Mexican Americans is that the clinician be knowledgeable about some of the more significant cultural values and beliefs of their Mexican American clients. It is imperative that treatment agencies have Spanish-speaking and, if possible, culturally competent staff who can enhance the therapeutic alliance with the client. The celebrated Mexican poet Octavio Paz once wrote: "What sets the world in motion is the interplay of differences." A given Mexican American patient can fall anywhere along the continua of acculturation and language preference. A clinician should guard against making assumptions about the client's needs and possible response to treatment on the basis of blanket cultural generalizations. To avoid this reductionistic tendency will require taking into consideration the personal characteristics of the patient, as well as those particular cultural values from the client's Mexican American background that apply to the individual. Although the following discussion offers descriptions of cultural characteristics that capture the flavor of traditional Mexican family values, descriptions such as these do not always do justice to generational, geographic, economic, and social class differences among Mexican Americans. It must be understood, for instance, that a growing percentage of Mexican Americans are well educated, belong to the middle class, speak mostly English, and do not ascribe to traditional values. Nonetheless, because sociocultural factors do play a prominent role in initiating and maintaining drug use among Mexican Americans (Ruiz & Langrod, 1997), they must be taken into account during treatment. Such factors include *familismo,* fatalism, *machismo, personalismo,* dignity, and religion.

Familismo

A distinctive characteristic of Mexican culture is the importance of the family. *Familismo* is the cultural trait that refers to the significance of the family to the individual and that characterizes it as a source of solidarity, cohesiveness, harmony, and emotional closeness (Marin & Marin, 1991). Family members are imbued with a strong sense of responsibility to each other within the family unit. For this reason the family has been seen as a critically important target in substance abuse prevention and treatment with Mexican Americans (Cervantes, 1993). It is noteworthy that although a strength of the Mexican American is support from the family, over-reliance on the family can also at times discourage the individual from seeking professional help (Sanchez Mayers & Kail, 1993).

Fatalism and Motivation for Treatment

The trait of fatalism is one that has been well described in the Mexican American population (Soriano, 1994). Fatalism is the belief that life's misfortunes are "meant to be" or inevitable and that one should accept his or her fate. The construct of fatalism may be more common among Mexican Americans because of their disproportionate level of socioeconomic hardship. The experience of being a beleaguered minority with limited access to the opportunity structure in the United States may engender feelings of hopelessness and contribute to their fatalistic attitude.

Some scholars postulate that an exaggerated ascription of the cultural value of fatalism, with its implied sense of passivity and resignation, to Mexican Americans has played a role in advancing certain pejorative views of Mexican Americans (Soriano, 1994). A particularly egregious misconception is that Mexican Americans are not as motivated as other groups to seek treatment. A careful analysis of such so-called unmotivated cases may reveal that the client experienced an erosion of confidence in a specific treatment because of a bad fit with the intervention or the clinician. A clinician can use fatalism to overcome the Mexican American client's resistance to entering treatment and to assist him or her to remain in treatment. For example, the clinician might say: "You are here for a reason. You were meant to be helped." Another challenge faced by the clinician related to fatalism is educating the Mexican American client about the disease model of addiction. If the client has a strong degree of fatalism in his or her belief system, the danger exists that he or she may feel predestined to continue with the use of alcohol or drugs. The clinician must inform the client that though he or she may have a predisposition or heightened vulnerability toward substance abuse, he or she is certainly not predestined to become an addict. This therapeutic approach empowers Mexican American clients to assume a strong measure of responsibility for their substance use and not abdicate their role as active participants in their treatment and recovery.

Role of *Machismo*

The ethnocultural value that demarcates gender identity in Hispanic and Mexican men is known as *machismo*. A common definition of *machismo* is that it is a set of traits possessed by the male that include bravery, strength, and, most important, being a good provider to his family (Lara-Cantu & Navarro-Arias, 1986). However, considerable individual variance exists in the degree to which the Mexican American male relates to *machismo*. *Machismo* may contribute significantly to the denial of alcohol and other drug-related problems in the Mexican American community because of the individual's reluctance to admit that he has a problem. It is fairly common for the Mexican American male to avoid presenting for substance abuse treatment because it is perceived as an admission of weakness and may result in considerable humiliation.

Drinking alcohol without displaying intoxication or loss of self-control is considerably influenced by *machismo*, as a man's supposed strength is often measured by the quantity he consumes. A growing body of evidence (Schuckit, 1994) now indicates that a low level of response or reduced sensitivity to alcohol, especially among the sons of alcoholics, is a potent predictor of future alcoholism. Consequently, it is crucial that clinicians educate their Mexican American clients about the increased risk of developing alcohol problems should they have a family history of alcoholism or an ability to "drink people under the table." Because drinking has such deeply ingrained associations with *machismo,* clinicians must frequently remind their male clients that outdrinking others should not be viewed as a positive attribute because it might indicate a predisposition toward alcohol dependency.

Personalismo and Dignity

The cultural construct of *personalismo* is an especially prominent characteristic of Mexican and Mexican American populations (Martinez, 1993). It describes a proclivity toward informality in social situations, enjoying the company of others and engaging in pleasant conversation, referred to as *la plática*. This construct helps explain why Mexican Americans have a distaste for the impersonal or business-like aspects of situations (Soriano, 1994). *Personalismo* may influence the Mexican American individual to be more likely to trust and cooperate with a clinician whom they feel is personable.

Mexican Americans generally ascribe considerable importance to their sense of dignity. Clinicians should be highly sensitive to comments or actions that may transgress the substance abuser's sense of honor and dignity, which is already probably diminished from living in a society that holds drug users in contempt. The failure of substance abuse programs to retain Mexican Americans is sometimes due to the confrontational style employed by clinicians. The clinician may find it useful to explain the rationale for certain procedures to clients beforehand to avoid the appearance of impugning their character, especially with the thorny issue of compulsory urine testing for drugs. It is beneficial to relay to the patient that the primary purpose of urine testing is to gauge the effectiveness of substance abuse treatment, not to catch the client in a lie. The clinician can explain to the client that the nature of an addictive illness is such that it may preclude the client's being truthful on certain occasions, regardless of the client's well-intentioned efforts or inherently honest character.

It is strongly suggested that clinicians make special efforts to allow Mexican American patients to express disagreement with them. This suggestion is based on the observation that some Mexican Americans adhere strictly to traditional values that may deem it disrespectful to question authority outwardly (Martinez, 1993). If not given the opportunity to oppose a particular policy or treatment, the Mexican American client may become quietly noncompliant.

Religion

Religion and/or a sense of spirituality are often major influences in the lives of Mexican Americans and sources of comfort in times of stress (Toor, 1985). Catholicism can serve a particularly supportive function for those who have dissolved ties with their families as a consequence of their drug use. The local Catholic Church can also play an important role by empowering Mexican American drug users to seek treatment. However, it cannot be assumed that all Mexican Americans will find a religious approach helpful.

ISSUES IN ASSESSMENT

A possibly contentious issue when a Mexican American client presents for an evaluation of his or her substance abuse is addressing whether or not an actual alcohol or drug problem exists. Building on the traditional Mexican value of respect for authority figures, the clinician should thoroughly review with the client the criteria for making a diagnosis of substance abuse or dependence. Although clinicians in the addiction field have realized that they cannot rely solely on measures of quantity and frequency of drug use to make a diagnosis, many Mexican Americans tend to ascribe much importance to these criteria in deciding whether they have a substance abuse problem. Therefore, the clinician needs to emphasize that the most salient factor for diagnosing a drug use problem is a "loss of control" that is best demonstrated by the client's continuing to take a drug even though it is causing significant problems in his or her life. The clinician must educate the Mexican American client that the pattern of curtailing or intermittently discontinuing the use of a drug only to eventually start again simply represents the chronic, relapsing nature of the addiction process. This approach will prevent the client from minimizing or denying that he or she truly has a substance abuse problem that requires treatment.

Assessing for Dual Diagnosis

Significant numbers of Mexican Americans suffer from posttraumatic stress disorder and major depressive disorder. Many of these individuals may self-medicate with drugs. Many medications that have significant abuse potential, such as Valium, can be obtained without a prescription in some parts of Mexico, a situation that can lead to unsupervised and indiscriminant use in the United States. Moreover, sharing one's own supply of medications to relieve the distress of a family member or a friend is a culturally sanctioned practice among many Mexican Americans. Therefore, as part of the assessment process, it is important for the clinician to inquire as to whether the client is using any medication, whether prescribed or given to them by friends or relatives.

Assessing the Degree of Acculturation

The clinician must become aware of differences among Mexican Americans by assessing for the degree of acculturation. Inquiring whether the individual was raised in the United States or in Mexico serves to demonstrate respect for the uniqueness of the client's heritage and enhances rapport. Assessing for acculturation helps in developing appropriate treatment approaches. For example, it might not be appropriate to treat an overly shy, English-dominant, well-acculturated Mexican American with too much *personalismo,* whereas a more recent Mexican immigrant may be offended by a clinician who is too formal in his or her approach. Any general guidelines that purport to represent all Mexican Americans must be used judiciously and selectively, if at all.

TREATMENT STRATEGIES

Establishment of a Therapeutic Alliance

When the Mexican American client first presents to the treatment provider, the clinician should explain the issue of confidentiality to the client's full satisfaction. The objective is to engender as much trust as possible in the clinical setting and to promote therapeutic disclosure. Many Mexican Americans have been exposed to anti-immigrant legislation, which has led them to have a pronounced mistrust of all institutions. Moreover, in order to foster the honest communication of sensitive material, it is imperative that the therapist be nonjudgmental about the client's substance use and convey respect, warmth, and empathy at all times. This nonjudgmental approach by the clinician is immensely important because it is often the most influential of all the factors affecting the Mexican American's decision to remain in treatment (Sanchez & Mohl, 1992). Research (Delgado & Humm-Delgado, 1993) indicates that many Hispanics, including Mexican Americans, often ascribe to a nondisease or moral model of addiction wherein the drug abuser is stigmatized because he or she is said to lack moral fortitude or to possess a "weak character." Also, because Mexican Americans may have less precise concepts of time than other populations (Brigham Young University, 1990), the clinician may need to be more flexibile in scheduling appointments when working with the Mexican American client.

Use of Cognitive Approach

In working with the Mexican American substance abuser, the clinician may find it helpful to engage the client in therapy that is practical, active, and problem solving in its orientation. Such a treatment approach is more consistent with cultural expectations and with the realities of living in deprived socioeconomic circumstances. Organista, Dwyer, and Azocar (1993) found it beneficial to explore and challenge forms of prayer that seem to lessen the probability of active problem solving. For example, patients can be instructed to shift their prayers in a more active direction by discussing the saying, "God helps those who help themselves." Cognitive–behavioral strategies can also be used in prevention programs aimed at teaching Mexican American adolescents to effectively cope with peer pressure. For example, through behavioral rehearsal and role playing, adolescents can learn communication skills that enable them to gain confidence and resist pressures to use alcohol and drugs.

Use of 12-Step Programs

Clinicians need to be sensitive to the possibility that certain treatment options may be less appropriate for some Mexican American clients than for others. For example, some men who identify strongly with *machismo* may be uncomfortable with the 12-step approach of Alcoholics Anonymous (AA). The notion of admitting to being powerless over alcohol, as is stated in the first step of the AA creed, may strike a painful chord in those clients who for most of their lives have felt the powerlessness and diminished sense of self-worth created by discrimination. The religious appeal to a "higher power" that AA prescribes may not be enough to compensate for feeling disempowered. For thousands of other Mexican Americans, however, AA and other 12-step programs have been a valuable resource and, when appropriate, should be considered as part of a treatment plan.

CASE REPORT

The following is a brief case report that demonstrates some of the more salient issues in treating the substance-abusing Mexican American patient.

> Miguel, a 35-year-old, bilingual, unemployed, Mexican American civil engineer came to the Family Treatment Center with his wife, Maria. According to his wife, Miguel had become increasingly irritable and depressed and had begun to drink alcohol frequently and in large amounts in the weeks following the loss of his job. It was agreed that Miguel would be seen individually for a couple of sessions so that the clinician would have a better understanding of Miguel before seeing the couple. The clinician suggested that Maria consider going to an Al-Anon meeting in the interim. At the outset of therapy, Miguel was reluctant to discuss the difficulties at home, stating often that "anyone else out of work would also be having a rough time" and that he was entitled to drink when he felt like it. Miguel downplayed his drinking as something "I can take or leave anytime." The therapist empathized with the problems Miguel was facing but was clear that in order to derive any benefit from therapy it would be necessary for Miguel to refrain from all alcohol use. The therapist acknowledged the challenging nature of this task and stated that he would wholeheartedly support Miguel in his struggle to achieve abstinence. He impressed upon Miguel that his problem with alcohol was not a sign of weakness but that it impeded his effectiveness as the head of the family. This view allowed Miguel to maintain his dignity and fostered a continuing investment in treatment.

In the initial sessions the therapist allowed Miguel wide latitude and considerable time to describe his expectations of treatment. The therapist obtained a detailed accounting of Miguel's alcohol use and its impact on his daily functioning. Miguel was agreeable to pursuing additional treatment for his alcohol abuse but rejected a referral to either a Spanish- or English-speaking AA group because a friend had told him that AA was a "religious" organization, which did not appeal to him. Miguel stated that his preference was to learn how he could help himself and not feel dependent on others to maintain his sobriety. After further discussion it was felt that a referral to a Rational Recovery group might be a better match for Miguel's belief system. The therapist also referred Miguel to a seminar that focused on dealing with unemployment and searching for a new job. Soon after attending the seminar, Miguel was able to discuss some of his other stressors. He admitted feeling that he had "let down" his family because of not being able to contribute financially and expressed particular shame after friends joked that his wife, was "supporting" him. He was also upset at being unable to continue sending money to his parents in Mexico, which had always been a great source of pride for him. As therapy progressed, Miguel became less resistant to admitting that he had lost control of his drinking. The therapist used reframing to help Miguel see that, in admitting his problems and seeking assistance, he was also helping his family to get through this difficult period. He successfully appealed to Miguel's sense of *machismo*, as Miguel was able to appreciate that by abstaining from alcohol he was actually reinforcing his position as the head of the family. In the later stages of treatment the therapist was able to assist Miguel in challenging some of his distorted cognitions relating to his drinking, including his grossly exaggerated estimate of the number of men who drank in order to cope with stress. Miguel came to realize that there were actually several individuals in his neighborhood who were experiencing economic hardship but had not resorted to using alcohol. A few days later, Miguel enrolled in a class to improve his computer skills. Near the termination of therapy and with Miguel's consent, the therapist invited his wife to come in order to educate her about alcohol abuse. Maria felt much more positive about their relationship and was eager to learn about ways that she could support her husband in his sobriety.

This case illustrates some key points that are useful in understanding specific dynamics in working with substance-abusing Mexican American clients. It demonstrates the tremendous importance ascribed to employment in the Mexican American culture and how the therapist's sensitivity to this issue laid the foundation for a trusting alliance and allowed him to effectively engage the client in discussing his alcohol abuse. A major task for the therapist was addressing Miguel's view that his alcohol use was simply an adaptive response to being unemployed. The key to the therapist's success was eventually leading Miguel to recognize and deal with his alcohol use as an issue independent of the loss of his job. The therapist was able to advance the process by which Miguel assumed responsibility for his drinking and took the necessary steps toward his recovery. The empathic, nonjudgmental, and flexible approach utilized by the therapist greatly enhanced communication with his client and led to a satisfactory outcome.

CONCLUSION

Although Mexican Americans are a heterogeneous population and although the etiology of substance abuse is complex and multifactorial, it is important to underscore the role of socioeconomic and ethnocultural conditions in the evolution and persistence of alcohol and drug abuse in this population. In the context of these conditions clinicians can better comprehend the tremendous toll that substance abuse has taken on Mexican Americans. We have incontrovertible evidence that the solution to the drug problem must involve solutions to the draconian problems of poverty, undereducation, discrimination, and inadequate health insurance coverage that face Mexican Americans.

The presently ineffective and misinformed U.S. drug policy, based disproportionately on law enforcement and ignorant of relevant socioeconomic variables, has done little to ameliorate the plague of alcohol and drug use in Mexican American communities. We cannot expect to eradicate drugs from Mexican American communities by using prisons to serve as the major repository of our hopes for success.

Future research on the Mexican American population must target polysubstance abuse and undertake controlled treatment outcome studies to determine which treatments are most effective. It is through well-planned research that we can best reduce the surfeit of misinformation that tends to "criminalize" Mexican American drug users and obfuscates society's recognition of the need to prioritize treatment and rehabilitation.

A public health approach that treats addiction as a chronic illness and utilizes harm-reduction strategies has considerable merit in helping Mexican Americans afflicted with the pernicious problem of drug abuse. The most effective model of treatment would involve comprehensive integrated human service programs that emphasize prevention and early intervention and target high-risk Mexican Americans. Public health officials must be indefatigable in replacing moralistic, vitriolic, and specious arguments with a policy predicated on reason and scientific study.

Treatment programs should seek partnerships with schools, churches, and law enforcement agencies to reduce the availability and demand for alcohol and drugs in the Mexican American community. There is an unprecedented need for more school-based interventions that have a long-term commitment to preventing dropouts. Because education is one of the most effective strategies available to deter thousands of Mexican American youth from starting down the road to addiction, the educational messages must be culturally relevant and should be delivered considerably earlier in the educational process, prior to first drug exposure.

In conclusion, clinicians must help their Mexican American clients recognize that their struggles with substance abuse are not insurmountable but are possible to overcome with a commitment to education and an unwavering participation in treatment. The treatment approaches outlined in this chapter can bring dignity and meaning back to the lives of those Mexican Americans grappling with the scourge of substance abuse.

REFERENCES

Aguirre-Molina, M., & Caetano, R. (1994). Alcohol use and alcohol-related issues. In C. W. Molina & M. Aguirre-Molina (Eds.), *Latino health in the U.S.: A growing challenge* (pp. 393–417). Washington, DC: American Public Health Association.

Amaro, H., Whitaker, R., Coffman, G., & Heeren, T. (1990). Acculturation and marijuana and cocaine use: Findings from HHANES 1982–84. *American Journal of Public Health, 80*(Suppl.), 54–60.

Booth, M. W., Castro, F. G., & Anglin, M. D. (1990). What do we know about Hispanic substance abuse? A review of the literature. In R. Glick & J. Moore (Eds.), *Drugs in Hispanic communities* (pp. 21–43). New Brunswick, NJ: Rutgers University Press.

Brigham Young University. (1990). *Culturegram for the 90's: Mexico* (Publication Services No. 280 HRCB). Provo, UT: Kennedy Center for International Studies.

Caetano, R. (1985, November). *Drinking patterns and alcohol problems in a national sample of U.S. Hispanics.* Paper presented at the National Institute of Alcohol Abuse and Alcoholism Conference, Bethesda, MD.

Caetano, R. (1987). Acculturation and drinking patterns among U.S. Hispanics. *British Journal of Addiction, 82,* 789–799.

Caetano, R., & Medina-Mora, M. E. (1988). Acculturation and drinking among people of Mexican descent in Mexico and the United States. *Journal of Studies on Alcohol, 49,* 462–471.

Castro, F. G. (1994). Drug use and drug-related issues. In C. W. Molina & M. Aguirre-Molina (Eds.), *Latino health in the U.S.: A growing challenge* (pp. 425–441). Washington, DC: American Public Health Association.

Cervantes, R. C. (1993). The Hispanic family intervention program: An empirical approach to substance abuse prevention. In R. S. Mayers, B. L. Kail, & T. D. Watts (Eds.), *Hispanic substance abuse* (pp. 101–114). Springfield, IL: Thomas.

Cervantes, R. C., Gilbert, M. J., Salgado de Snyder, N., & Padilla, A. M. (1990). Psychosocial and cognitive correlates of alcohol use in young adult immigrant and U.S. born Hispanics. *International Journal of the Addictions, 25*(3), 1990–1991.

Chavez, E. L. (1993). Hispanic dropouts and drug use: A review of the literature and methodological considerations. In M. R. De La Rosa & J. L. Recio Adrados (Eds.), *Drug abuse among minority youth: Advances in research and methodology* (NIDA Research Monograph No. 130, NIH Publication No. 93-3479, pp. 224–232). Washington, DC: U.S. Government Printing Office.

Chavez, E. L., Edwards, R., & Oetting, E. (1989). Mexican American and White American school dropouts' drug use, health status, and involvement in violence. *Public Health Reports, 104*(6), 595–604.

De Barona, M., & Simpson, D. (1984). Inhalant users in drug abuse prevention programs. *American Journal of Drug and Alcohol Abuse, 10*(4), 503–518.

Delgado, M., & Humm-Delgado, D. (1993). Chemical dependence, self-help groups, and the Hispanic community. In R. S. Mayers, B. L. Kail, & T. D. Watts (Eds.), *Hispanic substance abuse* (pp. 145–156). Springfield, IL: Thomas.

Dyer, M. (1984). Inhalant abusers: A neglected aspect in substance abuse treatment. *Grassroots,* 1–2.

Fagan, J., & Pabon, E. (1990). Delinquency and school dropout. *Youth and Society, 20*(3), 305–354.

Garza, R. T., & Gallegos, P. I. (1995). Environmental influences and personal choice. A humanistic perspective on acculturation. In A. M. Padilla (Ed.), *Hispanic psychology: Critical issues in theory and research* (pp. 3–14). Thousand Oaks, CA: Sage.

Gilbert, M. J. (1985). Alcohol-related practices, problems, and norms among Mexican Americans: An overview. In National Institute on Alcohol Abuse and Alcoholism (Ed.), *Alcohol use among ethnic minorities* (pp. 115–134). Rockville, MD: U.S. Department of Health and Human Services.

Gilbert, M. J. (1987). Alcohol consumption patterns in immigrant and later generation Mexican American women. *Hispanic Journal of Behavioral Sciences, 9,* 299–313.

Gilbert, M. J., & Alcocer, A. (1988). Alcohol use and Hispanic youth: An overview. *Journal of Drug Issues, 18,* 33–48.

Gilbert, M. J., & Cervantes R. (1986). Patterns and practices of alcohol use among Mexican Americans: A comprehensive review. *Hispanic Journal of Behavioral Sciences, 8,* 1–60.

Gilbert, M. J., & Gonsalves, R. (1985). *The social context of Mexican and Mexican American male drinking patterns.* Paper presented at the annual meeting of the American Anthropological Association, Washington, DC.

Glick, R., & Moore, J. (1990). Introduction. In R. Glick & J. Moore (Eds.), *Drugs in Hispanic communities* (pp. 1–17). New Brunswick, NJ: Rutgers University Press.

Hecht, A. (1980). Quick route to danger. In *FDA Consumer* [Newsletter]. Rockville, MD: U.S. Department of Health and Human Services.

Herd, D., & Caetano, R. (1987). *Drinking patterns and problems among White, Black, and Hispanic women in the U.S.: Results from a national survey.* Berkeley, CA: Pacific Medical Center Research Institute, Alcohol Research Group.

Hser, Y., Anglin, M. D., & Liu, Y. (1990). A survival analysis of gender and ethnic differences in responsiveness to methadone maintenance treatment. *International Journal of the Addictions, 25,* 1295–1315.

Hurtado, A., & Gurin, P. (1995). Ethnic identity and bilingualism attitudes. In A. Padilla (Ed.), *Hispanic psychology: Critical issues in theory and research* (pp. 89–103). Thousand Oaks, CA: Sage.

Lara-Cantu, M. A., & Navarro-Arias, R. (1986). Positive and negative factors in the measurement of sex roles: Findings from a Mexican sample. *Hispanic Journal of Behavioral Sciences, 8,* 143–155.

Marin, G., & Marin, B. V. (1991). Hispanics: Who are they? In G. Marin & B. V. Marin (Eds.), *Research with Hispanic populations* (Vol. 23, pp. 13–17). Newbury Park, CA: Sage.

Martinez, C. (1993). Psychiatric care of Mexican Americans. In A. C. Gaw (Ed.), *Culture, ethnicity, and mental illness* (pp. 431–462). Washington, DC: American Psychiatric Press.

Mata, A., & Jorquez, J. S. (1988). Mexican American intravenous drug users' needle-sharing practices: Implications for AIDS prevention. In R. J. Battjes & R. W. Pickens (Eds.), *Needle sharing among intravenous drug abusers: National and international perspectives* (NIDA Research Monograph No. 80, pp. 40–58). Rockville, MD: U.S. Government Printing Office.

Mata, A., & Rodriguez-Andrew, S. (1988). Inhalant abuse in a small rural South Texas community. In R. A. Crider & B. A. Rouse (Eds.), *Epidemiology of inhalant abuse: Update* (NIDA Research Monograph No. 85). Rockville, MD: U.S. Government Printing Office.

Mata, A., Rodriguez-Andrew, S., & Rouse, B. A. (1993). Inhalant abuse among Mexican Americans. In R. S. Mayers, B. L. Kail, & T. D. Watts (Eds.), *Hispanic substance abuse* (pp. 65–80). Springfield, IL: Thomas.

Moore, D. J., Williams, J. D., & Qualls, W. J. (1996). Target marketing of tobacco and alcohol-related products to ethnic minority groups in the United States. *Ethnicity and Disability, 6,* 83–98.

Moore, J. W. (1990). Gangs, drugs and violence. In M. R. De La Rosa, E. Lambert, & B. Gropper (Eds.), *Drugs and violence: Causes, correlates, and consequences* (NIDA Research Monograph No. 103, pp. 160–176). Rockville, MD: U.S. Government Printing Office.

Mora, J., Gilbert, J. (1991). Issues for Latinas: Mexican American women. In P. Roth (Ed.), *Alcohol and drugs are women's issues* (pp. 43–47). Metuchen, NJ: Women's Action Alliance and Scarecrow Press.

National Association for Chicano Studies. (1993). *Chicana voices: Intersections of class, race, and gender* (pp. 47–61). Albuquerque: University of New Mexico Press.

National Center for Education Statistics. (1989). *Dropout rates in the United States: 1988.* Washington, DC: U.S. Government Printing Office.

National Center for Health Statistics. (1990). *Vital Statistics of the United States, 1987: Vol. 2. Mortality. Part A* (DHHS Publication No. 90-1101). Washington, DC: U.S. Public Health Service.

National Council of La Raza. (1992). *Hispanics and health insurance. Vol. 1. Status.* Washington, DC: Labor Council for Latin American Advancement, National Council of La Raza.

National Institute on Drug Abuse. (1987). *Use of selected drugs among Hispanics: Mexican Americans, Puerto Ricans, and Cuban Americans.* Washington, DC: U.S. Government Printing Office.

Novas, H. (1994). *Everything you need to know about Latino history.* New York: Plume.

Organista, K. C., Dwyer, E., & Azocar, F. (1993, October). Cognitive behavioral therapy with Latino outpatients. *Behavior Therapist, 16*(9), 229–233.

Padilla, A. (1980). The role of cultural awareness and ethnic loyalty in acculturation. In A. Padilla (Ed.), *Acculturation: Theory, models, and some new findings* (pp. 47–84). Boulder, CO: Westview Press.

Pumariega, A. J., Swanson, J. W., Holzer, C. E., Linskey, A. O., & Quintero-Salinas, R. (1992). Cultural context and substance abuse in Hispanic adolescents. *Journal of Child and Family Studies, 1*(1), 75–92.

Rodriguez-Andrew, S. (1985). Inhalant abuse: An emerging problem among Mexican American adolescents. *Children Today, 14*(4), 23–25.

Rosenwaike, I. (1987). Mortality differentials among persons born in Cuba, Mexico, and Puerto Rico residing in the U.S., 1979–81. *American Journal of Public Health, 77,* 603–606.

Rouse, B. A. (1987). Substance abuse in Mexican Americans. In R. Rodriguez & M. T. Coleman (Eds.), *Proceedings of the Fifth Robert Lee Sutherland Seminar: Mental health issues of the Mexican origin population in Texas* (pp. 135–151). Austin, TX: Hogg Foundation for Mental Health.

Ruiz, P., & Langrod, J. G. (1997). Hispanic Americans. In J. H. Lowinson, P. Ruiz, R. B. Millman, & J. G. Langrod (Eds.), *Substance abuse: A comprehensive textbook* (3rd ed., 705–711). Baltimore: Williams & Wilkins.

Sanchez, E. G., & Mohl, P. C. (1992). Psychotherapy with Mexican American patients. *American Journal of Psychiatry, 149*(5), 626–630.

Sanchez Mayers, R., & Kail, B. L. (1993). Hispanic substance abuse: An overview. In R. S. Mayers, B. L. Kail, & T. D. Watts (Eds.), *Hispanic substance abuse* (pp. 5–16). Springfield, IL: Thomas.

Schuckit, M. A. (1994). Low level of response to alcohol as a predictor of future alcoholism. *American Journal of Psychiatry, 151,* 184–189.

Shorris, E. (1992). *Latinos: A biography of the people.* New York: Norton.

Soriano, F. I. (1994). The Latino perspective. A sociocultural portrait. In J. U. Gordon (Ed.), *Managing multiculturalism in substance abuse services* (pp. 117–144). Thousand Oaks, CA: Sage.

Substance Abuse and Mental Health Services Administration. (1993). *1991–1993*

National Household Survey on Drug Abuse. Washington, DC: U.S. Government Printing Office.

Substance Abuse and Mental Health Services Administration. (1997). *Preliminary results from 1996 National Household Survey on Drug Abuse* (DHHS Publication No. SMA 97-3149). Rockville, MD: Author.

Texas Commission on Alcohol and Drug Abuse. (1990). *The 1990 Texas School Survey of Substance Abuse.* Austin, TX: Author.

Toor, F. (1985). *A treasury of Mexican folkways.* New York: Crown.

U.S. Bureau of the Census. (1992). *The Hispanic population in the United States: March 1990. Current Population Reports* (Series P-20, No. 449). Washington, DC: U.S. Government Printing Office.

U.S. Department of State. (1996). *International Narcotics Control Strategy Report.* Washington, DC: Bureau for International Narcotics and Law Enforcement Affairs.

Western Interstate Commission on Higher Education. (1987). *From minority to majority.* Boulder, CO: WICHE.

Yin, Z., Zapata, J. T., & Katims, D. S. (1995). Risk factors for substance abuse among Mexican American school-age youth. *Hispanic Journal of Behavioral Sciences, 17*(1), 61–76.

7

Toward an Understanding of Puerto Rican Ethnicity and Substance Abuse

Catherine Medina

The problem of alcohol and other drug (AOD) abuse is one that affects all segments of society in the United States; however, its impact has been particularly severe on the social and health status of people of color (Substance Abuse and Mental Health Services Administration, 1995). AOD abuse has had a devastating effect on the Puerto Rican community, especially on the family and on the social networks that traditionally have served as stabilizing structures protecting the Puerto Rican people from daily negative economic, social, health, and educational stressors.

The literature on substance abuse and treatment approaches regarding Puerto Ricans is not extensive, and findings are often conflicting. Moreover, the use of the term "Hispanic" has not allowed for a differential analysis of substance use by each ethnocultural subgroup within this category. What seems significant in the literature is not the prevalence of substances used by different groups but the type of substance and method of use and the health and social impact on a community. Research findings indicate that substance abuse treatment programs that are not culturally sensitive promote a perception of inaccessibility and have high dropout rates (De La Rosa, 1987; Delgado, 1980; Marin, 1993; Moore & Mata, 1981; Obeso & Bordatto, 1979). Some of the culturally sensitive factors that may be significant in working with Puerto Rican clients are: an understanding of Puerto

Rico's historical background and cultural heritage and its political relationship to the United States, the socioeconomic profile of Puerto Ricans in the United States, the client's ethnic and racial identity, migration patterns, the impact of acculturation, the influence of language, and perception of gender roles.

This chapter focuses on the relationship between ethnocultural issues, substance abuse, and clinical interventions with Puerto Rican clients. It provides the clinician with some knowledge regarding Puerto Ricans, their social situation in the larger American society, and the cultural and sociopolitical contexts that place an individual at risk for AOD problems.

PUERTO RICAN HISTORICAL BACKGROUND AND ITS RELATIONSHIP TO THE UNITED STATES

On the island of Puerto Rico, the constant easterly trade winds have been waving both the U.S. and the Puerto Rican flags from government buildings and the airport since 1952, when Puerto Rico first became a commonwealth. Puerto Ricans refer to this status as *Estado Libre Asociado* (Associated Free State). Both Spanish and English are spoken, although the majority of the islanders prefer their native tongue. The island's post offices, radio, television licensing, custom services, and trade are all under U.S. federal control, and Puerto Rico receives federal subsidies for education, public housing, highway construction, and social programs. The currency used on the island is the U.S. dollar, and industry is primarily U.S. owned. Puerto Rico is a major producer and exporter of manufactured goods and high technology equipment. It produces 7% of the world's total supply of pharmaceuticals, including all of the birth control pills used in the United States. The island is also the world's largest producer of rum and liquor, which can be purchased in the supermarkets 7 days a week (Pariser, 1997).

Strategically, Puerto Rico is the site of an immense U.S. naval base, which shields America's southern coast; approximately 13% of the land is occupied by the U.S. military (Wagenheim, 1975). Puerto Ricans on the island do not participate in U.S. elections and do not have a voting voice in the U.S. Congress, yet as U.S. citizens they serve in the U.S. Army during wartime. The island's government is divided into executive, legislative, and judicial branches similar to those of the mainland. The governor is the island's highest ranking elected official. Puerto Rico has it own supreme court; contested decisions are heard by the U.S. Supreme Court. Spanish is the language used by both its legislature and courts. Politics is viewed by many natives as Puerto Rico's national sport, with many heated debates focusing on health, education, law enforcement, and particularly on its confusing political status of a commonwealth.

The United States–Puerto Rico Relationship

Using Eriksonian theory and the works of Memmi (1968) and Fanon (1965), Bird (1982) shows how Puerto Rico's long-standing colonial experience negatively affects individual self-definition, self-esteem, and dependency. Its colonial status deprives its people of self-determination and self-efficacy. Its dependency on the U.S. Congress to decide Puerto Ricans' social, political, and economic status reinforces its marginal existence. This political situation parallels the themes many Puerto Rican clients bring into treatment—self-doubt, low self-esteem, and dependency. These affective states reflect cultural, sociopolitical, and economic identities that have transferential meanings in the therapeutic relationship. Therefore, it is important for clinicians to have some understanding of Puerto Rico's political history and its unique relationship to the United States, because they will be significant in understanding the client's view in relationship to addiction and dependency issues.

The United States influence on the island was first felt in 1898 when Puerto Rico became its colony after the Spanish American War, only 7 months after having won home rule from Spain (Wagenheim, 1975). After 4 centuries of colonial rule, Spain granted Puerto Rico political autonomy in 1897 through a royal decree, giving Puerto Rico more political power than ever before in its history. The Puerto Rican people could elect voting delegates to Spain's legislative bodies and vote on insular matters, such as budget, tariffs, and taxes, and could undertake commercial treaties. However, Puerto Rico's political freedom was short-lived. The Spanish American War of 1898 changed the history of the Puerto Rican people.

Puerto Rico was once again a colony, but this time under U.S. military rule. Its status as a U.S. territory had both economic and political implications. In a *New York Times* editorial dated July 11, 1898, at that time, Puerto Rico was described as "the real gem of the Antilles" because of its rich soil and its "commanding position between the two continents" (cited in Wagenheim, 1975, p. 61). In 1900, the U.S. Congress passed the Foraker Act that created a political body called "We the People of Puerto Rico," whose members were identified as neither U.S. citizens nor citizens of an independent nation. However, this act gave President William McKinley the authority to appoint a governor from the United States and an 11-man executive council, the majority of whom were from the United States, to lead a civil government of 35 island residents elected to the Puerto Rico House of Delegates. An elected resident commissioner with no voting power would represent Puerto Rico in the U.S. House of Representatives. This law regulated Puerto Rico's commerce and judicial matters and was the beginning of formalizing Puerto Rico's colonial relationship to the United States. The United States maintained absolute power to veto any local law and mandated English as the official language of instruction in the public schools, even though very few of the residents spoke English. Whereas in the past Puerto Rico was able to share a cultural heritage and language with the ruling Spaniards, now the Puerto Rican leaders had to communicate their political and civil needs in a foreign tongue or through translators. Much of the struggle between Puerto Rico and the United States then and now stems from differences in culture and language and disagreement over the right to self-determination. These issues often arise within the culture of the agency and/or within the therapeutic process and become a source of conflict. It is important to know how the political status of Puerto Rico influences its people in daily life, especially in its relationship to self-identity.

The Jones Act of 1917 imposed United States citizenship on Puerto Ricans against their will (Montilla, 1997). U.S. citizenship obligated all eligible Puerto Rican males to serve in the U.S. Armed Forces during World War I. The sole legislative body in Puerto Rico at the time, the House of Delegates, elected by Puerto Rican voters in 1914, responded with a memorandum to the U.S. Congress insisting on retaining Puerto Rican citizenship and rejecting U.S. citizenship. Although this petition went unheard, to this date Puerto Ricans have the distinctive peculiarity of having both Puerto Rican and U.S. citizenship (Montilla, 1997). It was not until 1948 that the people of Puerto Rico elected their first governor, and in 1952 it gained the status of an United States commonwealth. Under this unique political status, Puerto Rico obtained some local autonomy and was able to restore Spanish as its official language. English became the second language, and it continues to be required for all students in the public elementary schools. As a commonwealth, Puerto Rico elects its own governor, local legislators, and a commissioner who represents it in the U.S. Congress but who has no vote on any legislation, even those affecting the island (Pariser, 1997). Although island Puerto Ricans are U.S. citizens, they cannot vote in U.S. elections; yet much of their fate is determined by the U.S. Congress through the House Committee on Insular Affairs and the Senate Committee on Territorial and Insular Affairs. Puerto Ricans' contradictory political status—dual citizenship and commonwealth—is an area of continuous political debate both in Puerto Rico and in the United States. Recently, this duality was challenged in the case of Ramìrez versus Brás, and on November 18, 1997, the Supreme Court of Puerto Rico upheld the constitutional basis of Puerto Rican citizenship (Garcia-Passalacqua, 1997).

Puerto Ricans have two languages, two citizenships, two basic philosophies of life, two flags, two anthems, and two loyalties. Within this duality there is a sense of nationalism, or ethnocultural identity, that permeates every corner of the Puerto Rican consciousness (Navarro, 1998). It is based not on an opposition to the United States, but rather on a Puerto Rican sense of pride developed out of its history as a distinct people with a complex and diverse cultural spirit. It is exemplified by Puerto Rico's own fine arts, folklore, national symbol (*el coquí*), and social and cultural institutions, and it is expressed in sending Puerto Rican teams and contestants to compete in the Olympics and in international beauty pageants, thereby maintaining a separate national identity from the United States.

THE PUERTO RICAN CULTURAL
HERITAGE AND ETHNIC IDENTITY

Puerto Rican identity has been influenced by different races and ethnic groups. The cultural ancestry is a mixture of Taíno Indian, African, and White European—mostly Spaniard. The island was inhabited by the Taíno Indians when Spain invaded and colonized it in the 16th century. The Taínos had named the island *Boriquen* ("Land of the Noble Lord") because they believed that their supreme creator, Yukiyu, lived there in the heights of the lush mountains. After the Spanish invasion, Columbus renamed the island San Juan in honor of Don Juan, the son of the king and queen of Spain. In 1508 the island had its first Spaniard governor, Ponce de León, and with the settling of Spaniards on the island it was renamed Puerto Rico ("Rich Port") in 1511.

The early Spanish military interests in Puerto Rico were replaced by its interest in gold mining (1508–1535) and later by the production of sugarcane (1535–1640). Authoritative estimates put the Taíno population at 30,000 when the Spaniards arrived; it is believed that most of the natives died by their own hands, from hunger, and from being overworked by the Spanish colonists on the island (Fernandez-Mendez, 1970). With the Taíno population in decline, the Spaniards began to transport African slaves to work in the sugarcane industry.

Puerto Ricans' ethnocultural identity is derived from a national pride in the blend of its three distinct cultures. The mixture of Taíno Indian, African, and Spanish cultural traditions is transmitted from one Puerto Rican generation to another through its values and language and through such specific characteristics as perception of time, sense of control, level of group centeredness, beliefs about social and personal space, and preferred behavioral patterns of interpersonal interactions. Ethnic identity is the extent to which an individual or group endorses and commits to distinct values, beliefs, and behaviors associated with an ethnocultural tradition, but more important is the response it elicits from others through social interaction (Marsella, 1990). The influences of these three distinct cultures are evident today in many of the attitudes, beliefs, and rituals of the Puerto Rican culture. For example, the cultural value that Puerto Ricans put on avoiding direct confrontation (*simpatía*) and on preserving a peaceable demeanor is reminiscent of Taíno tranquility (Garcia-Preto, 1996). Differences are settled in a "nice way" (*a la buena*), and resistance is expressed in a "relaxed fight" (*pelea monga*), a noncooperation rather than a direct counterattack, especially in relationship to someone in authority or a professional. A direct negative reply to a request is also avoided. The emphasis on kinship, familism, metaphysical forces, and the value of the group rather than the individual are also symbolic of the Taíno influence. The Spaniards brought their language, literature, food, the Catholic religion, and a patriarchal family structure to the island. The African influence is reflected in food, spirituality, medicine men, and music. The African sense of fatalism as an enslaved race is expressed today in Puerto Rican idioms such as "whatever God wills" (*lo que Dios quiera*) and in the belief that motivation or change is the result of a supernatural power rather than self-efficacy.

This blending of the Taíno, Spanish, and African cultures has resulted in the unique ethnocultural identity of the Puerto Rican. The pride in the richness and diversity of their cultural heritage is a significant part of the Puerto Rican identity. The cultural heritage is reinforced by most mainland Puerto Rican families through preservation of their language, music, and folk stories (*cuentos*) of the *jibarito* (folk hero) and through frequent visits to relatives on the island.

Racial Identity

Traditionally, social identification in Puerto Rico has been based on class, not color (Pariser, 1997). Unlike the dichotomous Black and White skin-color categorization commonly used in the United States, the Puerto Rican people acknowledge racial differences on a continuum between White and Black. The skin-color spectrum is expressed in words such as *blancos* (whites), *trigueños* (olive skinned), *prietos* (dark-skinned), and *negros/negritos* (black-skinned). *Negro/negra* is also used as a term of endearment meaning "dear" or "honey." Such classification of skin color on a continuum denotes the wide range of racial characteristics based on the historical mixture of races that make up the Puerto Rican identity. In the past, it also discouraged racism and allowed for more acceptance of different skin colors. Historically, Puerto Ricans have viewed skin color as unimportant, but over the years the U.S. presence on the island has enhanced the awareness of racial differences among Puerto Ricans (Bonilla-Silva, 1997; Wagenheim, 1975). Because most American immigrants to the island are White and wealthier than the average islander, success has increasingly become equated with Whiteness. Moreover, the racial dichotomy and prejudice experienced by the Puerto Rican people in the United States has lead to increasing feelings of low self-esteem, rejection, and family conflict for many. For example, in his acclaimed autobiography, Piri Thomas (1967) describes his descent into drug addiction and his own and his family's struggle with his Black skin color on the mainland. Although within his family he was viewed as Puerto Rican and *trigueño*, outside his home he was considered Black (*negrieto*). This conflict led to a major identity crisis. Thomas (1997) notes that after a heated argument with his younger brother, he told his father: "you and James think you're White, and I'm the only one that found out that I am not. I tried hard not to find out. But I did. . . . What's wrong with not being White? I'm proud to be a Puerto Rican, but being Puerto Rican does not make the color" (p. 68). As Thomas found out, in the United States skin color defines identity and serves as the basis for racism and discrimination against many Puerto Ricans.

PUERTO RICANS IN THE UNITED STATES

Puerto Ricans are the second largest Hispanic group in the United States, with approximately 2.7 million living on the U.S. mainland (U.S. Bureau of the Census, 1995). Growing up Puerto Rican in the United States is a unique experience in self-definition. Vega (1997) notes that of all the groups in the United States, Puerto Ricans present the greatest problem in being categorized as ethnic citizens of the United States. Most groups will refer to their all-inclusive ethnic diversity and absorption into the U.S. culture by stating they are Mexican American, Cuban American, African American, and so forth. There are no Puerto Rican Americans. For the Puerto Rican, such ethnic categorization is redundant because of the interrelationship between the United States and Puerto Rico. The majority of Puerto Ricans on the mainland and on the island value both their ethnocultural heritage and their U.S. connection and citizenship. The unique cultural identity of the Puerto Ricans in the United States is reinforced by the back-and-forth migration pattern and strong family ties between the island and mainland relatives. As a result, many preserve a strong hold on ethnic identification and language. Others feel torn in their identity because of the emotional, social, and economic implications of belonging to a discriminated-against minority group in the United States.

Migration Patterns

Historically, migration patterns have been dependent on the economic and employment opportunities both in Puerto Rico and on the mainland. Large numbers of Puerto Ricans began arriving on the mainland in the late 1940s and early 1950s in pursuit of economic and educational success or adventure or to join relatives already living in the United States. They settled in the inner cities, mostly in the northeast part of the country. Since the 1980s, due to industrialization of the island and the impact of the global economy, many Puerto Ricans have lost their jobs, especially in the garment industry, leading to increased migration to the mainland (Melendez & Melendez, 1993). In addition, there also has been an increase in the number of professionals leaving the island in pursuit of greater economic opportunities in the United States (Garcia-Remis, 1993).

Although the majority of Puerto Ricans in the United States reside in New York City, the high rates of crime, unemployment, drugs, poverty, and school dropout and the history of discrimination have had a great impact on their social mobility in that city and influenced the more recent migration patterns (Garcia-Preto, 1996; Rodriquez, 1988). According to Novas (1994) only 6% of island Puerto Ricans with college degrees migrated to New York, whereas 24% migrated to Texas. Garcia-Preto (1996) found that Puerto Ricans who migrate to regions outside of New York City tend to do better than other Hispanic subgroups in the same area. For example, in Texas, Puerto Ricans graduate from college at a higher rate than Mexicans Americans and have a higher per capita income (Garcia-Preto, 1996). A study of Puerto Ricans in Lorain, Ohio, and in San Francisco found that in those cities Puerto Ricans also have fared better economically, with higher incomes per capita than other Hispanics (Novas, 1994).

Because Puerto Ricans do not need any special documentation to travel between the island and the U.S. mainland, their pattern of migration tends to be a back-and-forth movement between the two places. According to Garcia-Preto (1996), going back to the island represents freedom from the prejudice, discrimination, and isolation experienced by many in the United States. The migration experience—the preparation for separating from one's native land, the context of exit and entry into the mainland—

influences the Puerto Rican family's adaptation and adjustment (Vega & Gil, 1999). Even those who have been born in the United States are likely to be influenced by their families' past migration history and their experiences in seeking social and economic success in the United States.

Demographic Profile of Puerto Ricans in the United States

Ethnic minority group status in the United States is frequently correlated with socioeconomic status, access to life chances, and entry into the opportunity structure. Despite a growing number of upper-middle-class professionals, the majority of Puerto Ricans in the United States reflect a demographic profile characterized by poverty, poor and limited education, substandard housing, and limited political power. According to Cheung (1989), an ethnic group's socioeconomic position in relation to the larger society has been shown to play an explanatory role in substance abuse. The following data represent the social indexes that increase the likelihood for some Puerto Rican individuals to abuse substances:

- Puerto Ricans have the lowest socioeconomic status among all the Hispanics in the United States, who, as a group, have a poverty rate almost three times as high as their non-Hispanic White counterparts. Approximately 38% of all Puerto Ricans on the mainland live in poverty, with unemployment rates of 31% for males and 59% for females over the age of 16 (U.S. Bureau of the Census, 1991a). Household income patterns follow the poverty pattern, with Puerto Ricans having the lowest median income of $16,200, compared with $22,439 for Mexicans, $25,900 for Cubans, and $30,500 for non-Hispanic Whites (Russell, 1996).
- Twenty-four percent of Puerto Ricans on the mainland are without telephones in their homes versus 8% of households nationally (Russell, 1996).
- Puerto Ricans show the lowest percentage of married couples and the highest percentage of single-parent and female-headed families with 43% of families headed by a single parent compared with 30% for all Hispanic groups and 20% for non-Hispanics (U.S. Bureau of the Census, 1991).
- Puerto Ricans are believed to have the highest dropout rate among all Hispanics (Mizio, 1983), who as a group lag behind the total population in educational attainment. In 1994, only 53% of Hispanics received a high school diploma compared with 81% of the national population (Russell, 1996).

Impact of Acculturation

Acculturation is a dynamic and interactional process that reflects modifications and changes toward native cultural values that occur as a result of exposure to alternate culture. It refers to the psychosocial process whereby immigrants and their children change their behavior and attitudes toward members of the host society based on their contact and exposure to the new dominant culture (Berry, 1980; Padilla, 1980). Acculturation depends on the length of time spent in the different culture, on social context, on exposure to and intensity of the alternate culture, on level of education, and on language, socioeconomic, and psychological factors. The process of acculturation has been linked as a critical variable in the development of family dysfunction and higher levels of personal disorganization, such as the emergence of mental illness, teen pregnancy, delinquency, and alcohol and drug problems (Amaro, Whitaker, Coffman, & Heeren, 1990; Anderson & Rodriquez, 1984; Gill, Vega, & Dimas, 1994; Oetting & Beauvais, 1991; Rogler, Cortes, & Malgady, 1991; Szapocznik, Kurtines, & Fernandez, 1980; Vega & Amaro, 1994). Studies have shown that alcohol consumption and drug use patterns among Hispanics varies by acculturation level (Marin, Posner, & Kinyon, 1991; Vega & Amaro, 1994; Vega, Hough, & Romero, 1983).

The different levels of acculturation among family members creates familial and intergenerational conflicts and affects the Puerto Rican client and his or her family's capacity to function in the larger society. According to Rodriquez, Recio, and De La Rosa (1992), a survey of Puerto Rican adolescent males in the South Bronx found that family involvement had a significant negative effect on drug use but that acculturation also played an indirect yet an important role in drug use. For example, consistent with the importance of family in the Puerto Rican culture (*familismo*—having a sense of attachment, respect, duty, and obligation), the less acculturated the adolescent male was, the more actively involved he was with his family and the less likely to be involved in problem behavior. On the other hand, the acculturated adolescents were less involved with their families and more involved with deviant peer bonding, often leading to drug use.

A comparative study between Puerto Rican adolescents in New York City (including those born in New York and those born in Puerto Rico but living in New York) and island adolescents (including those who never lived outside of Puerto Rico, as well as those who were born in New York but whose families returned to the island) found that the longer island migrants lived in New York City, the greater their drug use (Velez & Ungemack, 1989). The National Institute on Drug Abuse (1992) also found that because of the broader acceptance of drugs in the United States, drug use by Puerto Rican youth on the mainland tends to be higher than on the island. The more permissive attitudes and acceptance of drugs as the mode in the United States gradually erode the traditional Puerto Rican cultural values that serve as protective mechanisms against drugs—*familismo* (familism), *personalismo* (personalism), *dignidad* (dignity), *respeto* (respect), and *vergüenza* (shame).

However, participation in more than one culture is not necessarily a negative experience. Oetting and Beauvais (1991) argue that increasing identification with one culture does not produce a decreasing identification with another culture. Because the process of acculturation in a pluralistic society is multidimensional, a differential pattern of acculturation occurs when the adaptation is bicultural. For example, second- and third-generation mainland Puerto Ricans share some cultural values with island relatives, emphasizing respect, dignity, and an interdependent, humanistic view toward spirituality, hierarchy of parents, family, and community; at the same time they are adapting to a distinct mainland culture with its emphasis on individualism, self-reliance, and anonymity. Therefore, an individual does not live in a cultural dichotomy but in a multidimensional world with many "cultural selves." However, in order to navigate multiple cultures successfully, social interactions with the host society must be nonthreatening. As indicated previously, the environment in the United States has not been positive in the overall experience of many Puerto Ricans.

It is important to keep in mind that the acculturation process is an interactional one and includes elements of individual choice within different cultural and social contexts. Additionally, because the environment does not affect individuals uniformly but scatters its effects differentially, we cannot realistically conclude that particular cultural environments will automatically produce certain behaviors, such as AOD abuse. In most cases, individuals have the capacity to adjust, adapt, and change both their internal and external environments. It is only within this psychosocial context that the clinician can understand the intrinsic relationship of ethnicity and drug use patterns.

Language

Puerto Ricans in the United States display different levels of proficiency in both English and Spanish. Some are bilingual and have mastered both languages artfully; some do not speak Spanish; some do not speak English. The substance abuse clinician needs to have an understanding of the client's language dominance, because it is through the use of language that experiences, events, memories, and perceptions are coded and organized. Language conveys representations of intrapsychic forces, and words are powerful symbols that give voice to expression. Language is symbolic of affective development, ethnocultural identity, and perceptual affinity. It is through language that clients share their deepest thoughts, ideas, and feelings and organize an action plan. The native tongue holds the fullest complement of sensorial, affective, and cognitive elements related to early experiences (Amahti-Mehler, Argentieri, & Canestri, 1993; Buxbaum, 1949; Greenson, 1950; Loewald, 1980). A second language can be used frequently to intellectualize emotional content and thus be devoid of affect. The bilingual client has more than one linguistic code to process and organize experiences and may have to shift languages to express an affective state. Studies indicate that the memory of an event in the language in which it occurred is more descriptive and affective for the bilingual client (Javier & Munoz, 1993). An event that is translated into the language of the clinician rather than being expressed in the language in which the client experienced and processed it may be altered in its meaning.

Gender Roles

In the Latino culture, *machismo* is referred to as the traditional role of the man, which is to be strong, dominant, and the provider and protector of the family. It is the man's responsibility to control his own and his family's fate and destiny. *Machismo* signifies male dominance and has been linked to sexual potency and physical courage. This cultural construct affects the whole pattern of family relations: It plays an important role in defining power and privilege, in setting the emotional climate for decision making, and in structuring communication patterns within the Puerto Rican family. Traditionally, the Puerto Rican family has been patriarchal, and *machismo* gives men authority over women.

The traditional female role of the Puerto Rican woman, *marianismo*, is to be nurturing, to be deferential to the male partner, and to be self-sacrificing (Sue & Sue, 1990). The woman is expected to remain morally, spiritually, and sexually pure, loyal and respectful of her partner in order to maintain his dignity (*dignidad*). This cultural construct is derived from the religious belief in the Virgin Mary and stresses that women are morally and spiritually superior to men and capable of enduring all suffering (Stevens, 1973).

These values are seen as complementary rather than opposing cultural forces in defining and organizing gender roles. They help maintain a social order that upholds the power of the *macho completo* (the complete man) and *respeto* (respect), *familismo* (family unity—saving face for each other), and the honor of the woman (*hembrismo*). Traditionally, many Puerto Rican women tend to reaffirm male role prerogatives because challenging male dominance would bring *vergüenza* (shame) to the family.

Although the traditional gender-role ascriptions of *machismo* and *marianismo* remain dominant, within the last decade these cultural constructs have undergone ongoing modifications. These changes reflect the changes in family structure, with an increasing number of single mothers heading families; the greater number of women in the labor market; the increase in educational level of Puerto Rican women; and increased exposure to the mainland culture and the feminist movement. These changes have affected the role of the Puerto Rican woman, especially on the mainland. The fact that an increasing number of Puerto Rican families are headed by women poses a direct challenge to the cultural male dominance and creates conflict and role strain among couples. Such role strain can make Puerto Rican couples and families more vulnerable to depression, domestic violence, and substance abuse problems.

ASSESSMENT AND TREATMENT INTERVENTIONS

Cultural norms and values can be found within the context of the client's therapeutic stories and in their patterns of substance use and abuse. If the web of culture is not explored in the client's stories, the clinician may be left with assumptions that can be stereotypic, and the client may feel misunderstood and drop out of treatment. In order to create motivation for change, the clinician must assess ethnocultural variations and develop treatment goals that are culturally sensitive. Using an intervention that has been created for non-Hispanic Whites and simply translating it into Spanish or incorporating certain Puerto Rican cultural traditions into a mainstream intervention may not be enough to produce behavior change strategies for the Puerto Rican client.

Treatment is culturally competent when interventions are based on an understanding of Puerto Rican cultural values, when they reflect the client's subjective culture (i.e., the client's individual cultural attitudes, expectancies, and norms), and when they respect the behavioral preferences and expectations of the Puerto Rican client. The clinician working with a Puerto Rican client can enhance the effectiveness of treatment by understanding and working with the sociopolitical background and cultural scripts and values that clients present in their stories and interpretation of events.

Ethnic labeling is a sociopolitical process, and in substance abuse counseling it is critical to assess the psychological implications that a given label such as racial or ethnocultural identity has on the individual. According to Phinney (1990), strong ethnic identity, when accompanied by a positive mainstream orientation, is related to high self-esteem. Conversely, individuals experience problems in self-esteem when they lack a sense of ethnic identity and have difficulty adapting to the mainstream group. An understanding of the Puerto Rican client's ethnocultural identity within a social context gives new or expanded meanings to presenting problems and effective interventions in treatment. Relevant to treatment is the client's description of "self" in relationship to ethnic attributes. For example, in the United States, a dark-skinned individual (*trigueño*) may be characterized as a Black Puerto Rican—a characterization that may be inconsistent with the individual's own ethnic self-identification but that may, nonetheless, increase the likelihood of discrimination in employment or housing. Therefore, exploring the client's ethnocultural identification also includes his or her unique sense of self, migration experience, level of acculturation, educational attainment and socioeconomic status, language proficiency, family structure and roles, attitude toward his or her own and other groups, gender roles, religious and friendship affiliations, music and food preferences, and participation in cultural activities. Understanding the uniqueness of the client's background helps move the practitioner toward a more complete assessment of the person, his or her stressors and behaviors, and his or her motivation for change.

It is within the therapeutic context that the client experiences the treatment program as a safe place to examine oneself and to change. The client's political consciousness influences ethnocultural identity and worldview, but more important it helps a clinician to understand how the client perceives experiences and interactions with the dominant culture group members and institutions, including the therapeutic relationship. For example, because *respeto* (respect) governs all positive reciprocal interpersonal relationship in the Puerto Rican culture, it also dictates appropriate behavior with authority figures (Diaz-Royo, 1976). The Puerto Rican client may not directly express disapproval of a treatment plan; but out of *respeto* for the dignity of the authority figure, the clinician, he or she may appear to be compliant yet fail to follow through with treatment recommendations. Occasionally, the client chooses to do the opposite of what was mutually agreed on in a contract. The clinician may experience this interaction as resistance, when in fact it is a *pelea monga* (a relaxed fight)—a passive noncooperation reflecting the client's sense of being misunderstood rather than an expression of anger, autonomy, or assertiveness toward the clinician. Or a clinician may feel that a Puerto Rican client's sense of fatalism impedes the treatment by putting the responsibility of change in the hands of fate or of a higher power rather than of oneself. The clinician therefore needs to explore the level of control the client feels (self-efficacy) and what social supports the client will need to effect change. For many Puerto Rican clients, because of the cultural emphasis on the other rather than on oneself, self-efficacy is contingent on other close-knit relationships.

A recurrent theme for many Puerto Rican clients in substance abuse treatment is *vergüenza* (shame), which is experienced in relationship to behaviors such as neglecting their children and families, prostitution, stealing, and other criminal behavior that support their addictions. This affect is deeply rooted in relationship to the family rather than in the individual. Each member is expected to protect the safety, interest, dignity, and honor of the family. Family orientation is so strong as a Puerto Rican core cultural value that it has been characterized in the literature by the term "familism" (Zayas, 1988). *Vergüenza* is most effectively worked through in relationship to other family members, such as the client's spouse or significant other, children, mother, father, and siblings. Puerto Rican clients may be more motivated into modifying their substance abuse for the sake of their families rather than themselves (familism rather than individualism). Among family members, loyalty, interdependence, and cooperation are stressed rather than confrontation, individualism, and competition. Spanish-speaking Alcoholics Anonymous (AA) groups and the *espiritista* (spiritist, which is a healer who has the gift of being able to communicate with the spirits of the dead regarding the problems of the living) can be helpful in providing additional support, as well as pressure and external controls to help the client maintain sobriety (Comas-Díaz, 1982).

Another consideration is that many Puerto Ricans on the mainland feel a sense of shame in not being able to communicate in English or in having an accent. Sometimes the clinician can facilitate communication and the client's use of the language by incorporating a few Spanish words. Such behavior promotes a person-to-person contact (*personalismo*), relates the belief in the innate worth and uniqueness of the individual, and reduces the client's skepticism of the treatment relationship.

Cultural exploration is an ongoing process because the cultural context is always changing. For the clinician, the challenge of cultural competency is the exploration of the different meanings that a narrative has for the client. The following case illustrations provide some understanding of the complexity of ethnocultural identity for Puerto Rican clients within their particular social context.

Ms. J is a 27-year-old New York–born woman who identified herself as Puerto Rican. She had a 12th-grade education, was unemployed, and lived with her parents, her 4-year-old daughter, and a nephew.

Ms. J had never married and was currently separated from her lover. The father of her daughter had died of AIDS 3 years previously. The presenting problem was feeling depressed after being physically assaulted by her lover after she refused to use heroin. She stated, "I want to be clean and take care of my family." At the time of intake, she had just been detoxified and had stopped using alcohol, crack, and heroin. Ms. J was self-referred to a community mental health center and was assigned to a clinician familiar with substance abuse problems and with Puerto Rican culture. Ms. J's substance abuse history is as follows:

- She started drinking at age 15 and using drugs at 26.
- She drank two to three times a week, averaging seven to nine alcoholic drinks each day.
- She used six to eight bags of heroin a month and crack twice a week.
- She used more than one drug at a time and was unable to control her use.
- She experienced withdrawal symptoms when she didn't use drugs, but had no blackouts or flashbacks.
- She had no reported medical problems and had previously been tested and found HIV negative.
- She had no psychiatric history.
- Her father and sister also have histories of substance abuse.

The client's longest period of "staying clean" was 10 months without any treatment intervention, at which time she worked as a cashier and was living with the father of her daughter. The client identified heroin as her main drug of choice and was spending an average of $3,000 monthly. Her drug use was financially supported by prostitution and stealing.

Ms. J. stated that she felt guilty about her drug use and felt that she had neglected her family because of it. She had been having serious problems with her mother, who had been critical of her substance use. She described her mother as insignificant in her substance abuse but important in her recovery process because of the structure she provided in the home and her role as a caregiver. Her father was described as a "very important" figure whom she enjoyed spending time with playing cards or dominos and watching baseball games. Her father had stopped drinking 9 years before and was very supportive of her abstinence. He was willing to help in any way he could but had been very sick lately, having been diagnosed with prostate cancer. He had never been treated for his alcoholism, but he stopped drinking because he lost several jobs and his wife threatened to leave him. Her mother believes that Ms. J should be able to stop just like her father did. As her situation was explored in treatment, Ms. J's *vergüenza* and her sense of hopelessness were so strong that she was viewed as a potential suicide risk. After exploring her familial relationships, it became clear that she feared her father's death, and her mother's subsequent rejection of her for not helping out. She felt worthless, "unlike my mother."

Treatment consisted of working with the client and her family on the positive restructuring of communication patterns, expectations, and roles. Treatment included both individual and family sessions in which either the mother or both parents participated, depending on her father's physical condition. Initially the parents showed a tendency to focus on the problems of the past; however, the clinician emphasized the present and the need to effect change that would be helpful to the client's present recovery. Past experiences were used only if they were helpful to promoting hope and effecting change and healing. For example, the clinician explored how Ms. J was able to remain clean for a period of 10 months just prior to and following the birth of her daughter. The clinician worked with the family to support their strengths and needs and to clarify perceptions, feelings, and behaviors that would help them function as a family unit. A written contract outlining their goals and behaviors was signed by family members each week for about 6 weeks. The contract was modified as needed, and Ms. J was responsible for holding the contract. The client was able to reassert herself in the role of daughter and mother and to maintain her recovery.

During individual sessions, the clinician provided information and practical advice about domestic violence, safe sex practices, and legal and health issues. From a traditional Anglo therapeutic perspective Ms. J's dependency on her family may have been an issue, but from a cross-cultural perspective it was clear that her family had to be used as a support system in this client's recovery process and that her dependence on her family was an important factor in maintaining her recovery. The individuation process was viewed as countertherapeutic to the cultural values of this Puerto Rican family system. The pervasive theme was how to maintain cooperation and empowerment among family members during the different phases of the client's recovery.

The second case shows the significance of broadening the clinician's therapeutic lens to include an understanding of the conflicts that stem from acculturation and gender adaptation while balancing and accepting differences in cultural values and treatment interventions. An understanding of the Puerto Rican client's ethnocultural identity within a social context gives new or expanded meanings to presenting problems and effective interventions in treatment.

Mrs. O is a 36-year-old Puerto Rican–born woman. She first came to the mainland when she was 10 years old and experienced a back-and-forth migration between the island and the mainland. Mrs. O was a professional, fluently bilingual and the only one among her family to graduate from college. In treatment with a Spanish-speaking clinician, she spoke both Spanish and English, depending on the affective material. Her use of language in sessions was symbolic of her back-and-forth migration between the island and the mainland and reflected how she perceived her situation. When the material was emotionally painful or pleasurable, she spoke in Spanish. When the material was factual and nonthreatening or when she wanted to avoid some emotion, she spoke in English. At times, she used both languages, and this behavior usually symbolized her feelings of lack of control or of uncertainty or confusion. When she referred to her job or to an experience in which she encountered racism or discrimination, she felt oppressed and powerless, feelings that she expressed in both languages. Both languages conveyed the urgency to do something about how she was feeling but also to remedy the structural racism.

Mrs. O was married to a man she had first met in Puerto Rico. He was *un negrito* who, although highly intelligent, had no formal education and limited job skills and who, upon migrating to the mainland, had difficulties earning enough money to financially support his wife and their 8-year-old son. She became the main financial and emotional provider. Her husband began to drink heavily and became physically and emotionally abusive toward her. Mrs. O was conflicted between leaving her husband, which was common behavior among her Anglo peers, and working on the relationship, as advised by her family, priest, and neighborhood friends. She became pregnant with a second child in the hope of cementing their relationship and increasing her sense of self-worth through her role of motherhood. Her husband became more distant and began to deal drugs to support his family. When she approached her mother and other family members regarding his criminal activity, they told her that she needed to stand by him and should accept his new employment because now he was the "provider." His mother stated that it was the will of God and that she should pray that he would change his ways.

Mrs. O told the clinician that she planned to seek an *espiritista* to get some advice as to what she should do and perhaps his help in changing the course of events. The *espiritista* acted as a medium, calling on the client's ancestors and giving her some herbs for her *nervios* (nerves). After a couple of visits, he advised her to talk to the *compadre*, the godfather who had acted as a witness during their marriage and had baptized their son. The *compadrazco* (godparenthood) is a kinship system with binding obligations and responsibilities in terms of emotional, financial, and personal support. The *compadre* was asked to talk to Mr. O about his responsibility to protect the family and to set an example for his son to be *un macho completo* (a real man). This cultural value implies that a real man accepts his destiny and affirms his dignity with moral standards.

With the encouragement of the clinician, Mrs. O followed the *espiritista*'s advice and also asked her priest to accompany the *compadre* in speaking to her husband. She would not be included in the dialogue among the men, nor would it be mentioned that she sought their help. The clinician gave Mrs. O the names of alcohol treatment facilities that she felt would be most sensitive to her husband's cultural values. Mrs. O then gave this list to the priest. Thus with the help of the *espiritista,* the *compadre,* the priest, and the clinician, her husband entered an intensive outpatient treatment program and began his recovery.

Following the completion of his substance abuse treatment program, Mr. O agreed to attend couples treatment with his wife. During the joint sessions he was able to explore the connection between his migration experience and his use of substances and how his expectations, dreams, and hopes were shattered by the stressors, isolation, and racism he experienced in the United States. The clinician explored Mr. O's expectations of his wife and helped the couple negotiate a plan that would work for both of them. Differences, including those in gender-role expectations, were discussed and validated. Both agreed that they had difficulties communicating with each other and decided to turn to their family members and their *compadrazgo* relationships for help when needed.

In working with Mrs. O. and in referring the husband to a treatment program, the clinician took into consideration the couple's cultural values and beliefs, as well as their level of acculturation. The clinician supported the family's network role in problem solving—a role that is common within the Puerto Rican community. She helped Mr. O to resume his dignity and his sense of *machismo* by exploring what could be negotiated in the couple's relationship to maintain his recovery, while valuing Mrs. O's acculturation level, her gender role, and the many differing ways to "help" in the Puerto Rican culture.

SUBSTANCE ABUSE IN PUERTO RICO

The use of alcohol and other drugs is a major problem affecting Puerto Rico's social welfare. Out of a total population of 3.8 million, it has been estimated that about 500,000 individuals suffer from an alcohol- or drug-related problem. Child and partner abuse, assault, rape, suicide, homicide, and school desertion have been linked with AOD. An estimated 65% to 70% of crimes committed in Puerto Rico are drug related (U.S. Department of Justice, 1997). This report notes that in 1995–1996, Puerto Rico's Mental Health and Anti-Addiction Services Administration (MHAASA) treated 38,524 clients, with the majority addicted to heroin (10,667), cocaine (7,000), and speedball (a combination of heroin and cocaine; 4,515). Of those serviced 88% were men, 12% women; 59% were inmates or on parole; 62% were between 18 and 44 years old; and 36% were under 18 years old. Forty-six percent had completed high school; 42% did not complete high school; 11% had some education beyond high school; and 54% were unemployed. MHAASA found a strong relationship between drug use and access to drugs, between drug use among peers and social acceptance among adolescents, and between drug use and criminal activity (U.S. Department of Justice, 1997).

It is difficult to examine the role of AOD in Puerto Rico isolated from the political economy associated with its sale and distribution. Drug smuggling and trafficking is a major concern for Puerto Rico because of its coastline and easy access to the U.S. market for sale and distribution. In 1996, the Drug Enforcement Administration estimated that 40% of all cocaine entering the mainland transits through the eastern Caribbean, specifically Puerto Rico (Ruiz-Guitierrez, 1996). The U.S. federal government reduced its drug interdiction funding by 40% in a 3-year period (1992–1995). Consequently, Puerto Rico experienced an unprecedented wave of drug trafficking at a time when the purity of drugs increased and the prices decreased. Cocaine kilogram prices are lower in Puerto Rico than in any city in the United States, and the purity level is very high, ranging from 80–90%. Crack is easily accessible, resulting in a growing rate of addiction. Similarly, the island's production of rum and its inexpensive cost greatly increases the use of alcohol, particularly among youth.

Puerto Rico's war on drugs policy is referred to as *mano dura* (hard hand) and calls for the militarization of *puntos* (drug distribution points), targeting public housing as a major distribution point. In 1993, the National Guard began occupying 20 public housing projects as a deterrent to drug sale and use. Fences, access controls, and bulletproof guard stations have been constructed around the housing projects, and the guardsmen hand out pens, pencils, and erasers with the slogan, "Say No To Drugs" (Pariser, 1997). This policy has been sharply criticized because of the unprecedented military presence and the fact that drug-related homicides have not decreased, nor have drug dealers been stopped. Instead the *puntos* have been dispersed.

Prevention and Treatment Approaches Used in Puerto Rico

During 1996–1997 Puerto Rico consolidated its drug, alcohol, and mental health services under the MHAASA to effect an integrated service delivery system. Puerto Rico's alcohol and drug intervention approaches include prevention, law enforcement, corrections, treatment, information systems, and technological improvements (U.S. Department of Justice, 1997). The focal points for drug prevention programs are the schools and public housing projects through on-site drug education programs for youth and parents, such as The Drug Abuse Resistance Education (D.A.R.E.) program, *Rescate a Tiempo* ("On Time Rescue"), and *Yo Sí Puedo* ("Yes, I Can"). These programs emphasize behavioral modification techniques, cognitive skills, and community-based efforts coordinated by multidisciplinary teams consisting of police, education, justice, and social service departments.

The major treatment modalities are methadone maintenance, residential treatment, and rehabilitation programs in correctional facilities. Treatment interventions are built around the patient's community and involve family members, peers, community-based programs, and work settings.

Alcohol Anonymous (AA) meetings are held throughout the island. AA's collective group consciousness and the belief in a higher power are seen as compatible with Puerto Rican value systems. The meetings are further modified to be culturally responsive by valuing the family and the community.

Much of the current emphasis in treating AOD abusers is on building support, strength, and resources within the neighborhood and lessening reliance on government programs. Such intervention strategies are dependent on the community's infrastructure, such as the priest or minister, the *espiritista* (spiritist), the *compadre* (godparent), the extended family, the neighbor, the grocery store owner, or a teacher. This philosophy extends to abstinence and recovery, in which the emphasis is on the need to protect and preserve the family and the community rather than the individual self. It is believed that the motivation to change will occur because of the attachment to and love for the family and community rather than because of any value attached to self-reliance.

SUBSTANCE ABUSE IN THE UNITED STATES

As indicated previously, data about Puerto Rican substance use on the mainland are limited because of the use of the catchall terms "Hispanics" or "Latinos." Morgan (1990) notes that drug use among ethnocultural minorities in the United States is best understood in terms of drug enforcement policies that promote oppression and social and class conflict. An example of this phenomenon is the easy availability of illegal drugs, coupled

with a lack of economic opportunity for uneducated youth in minority urban communities. This awareness of structural racism and poverty as antecedents for drug abuse is increasing. According to Rodriquez (1988), economic and sociopolitical conditions have led to the development of a peer
group orientation that emphasizes survival skills based on bending the law.
This has resulted in a street economy involving the active selling and buying
of illicit drugs and the acceptance of certain drugs, such as marijuana, as
the norm in some Puerto Ricans neighborhoods. Stressors associated with
unemployment, poverty, low educational achievement, high crime rates,
racism, and discrimination, combined with easy access to drugs, influence
AOD use and abuse among Puerto Ricans in poor neighborhoods (Bonilla-
Silva, in press; Cheung, 1989; Mayers & Kail, 1993; Vega & Miranda,
1985). It is not the environmental factors by themselves that contribute to
drug use behaviors but the internalization of membership in a marginalized
and vulnerable subgroup. AOD abuse is also linked to domestic violence
among Puerto Rican families and to their low educational achievement. Alcohol and illicit drug abuse are a major cause of incarcerations and deaths
among Puerto Rican males. One cannot refer to the devastating effects of
AOD use without mentioning its relationship to HIV/AIDS, especially on
communities of people of color. However, this is another area in which the
available information and research is classified under the categories of Hispanic or Latinos, not by subgroups. It is worth noting that AIDS is the leading cause of death for Hispanic women between 25 and 34 years of age
(Centers for Disease Control and Prevention, 1995). The majority of these
women have been exposed to HIV through a steady sexual partner who is
an intravenous drug abuser. Although no exact numbers for Puerto Rican
women are given, this statistical information notes that heterosexual HIV
transmission is an increasing risk for this subgroup.

When examining AOD use among the three major Hispanic subgroups
in the United States—Mexican, Cuban, and Puerto Rican—differences related to choice of substances, age, and gender are evident and at times contradictory. English-speaking Puerto Rican males between the ages of 18
and 24 have the highest prevalence of illegal drug use, with the exception of
inhalants (De La Rosa, Khalsa, & Rouse, 1990). Puerto Ricans reported
the highest prevalence of both marijuana (National Clearinghouse for Alcohol and Drug Information, 1993) and cocaine (National Institute on
Drug Abuse, 1989) use; the latter is particularly prevalent among Puerto
Rican youth (12–17 years). Additionally, both Puerto Rican men (28%)
and women (17%) have a higher rate of lifetime use of cocaine than Cuban
and Mexican Americans (Booth, Castro, & Anglin, 1990).

Regarding alcohol use, Latino youth as a group start drinking at a later age than Whites, and Puerto Rican adolescents begin later than other Hispanics (Alcocer, 1993). By age 18, only 46% of Puerto Rican adolescents have used alcohol compared with an estimated 50% of Mexican American and 53% of Cuban American adolescents. Even though Puerto Rican men begin to drink later than their White and Hispanic peers, heavy drinking is common among them. Alcocer (1993) also notes that Puerto Rican women have a lower rate of alcohol abstention and a higher rate of heavy drinking than Mexican or Cuban women. Caetano (1988) showed a relationship between acculturation and decrease in abstinence rates among Hispanic women. The Puerto Rican women on the mainland had the lowest rate of abstention (45%) in comparison with Cuban (48%), Mexican (71%), and South and Central American women (74%). Moreover, second-generation U.S.-born Hispanic women consistently reported even lower rates of abstention and higher rates of heavy drinking. These findings are not surprising given that the Puerto Rican island family and community are less accepting of heavy drinking by women and view such behavior as problematic, but at the same time accept that men can drink heavily and that such behavior is part of their *macho* role dynamic. On the mainland, however, Puerto Rican women who drink heavily experience less censure from their families and community because drinking is viewed as a by-product of their life stressors. Further research is needed in the areas of age, gender-specific issues, and degree of acculturation to better understand drug use among Puerto Ricans and within ethnocultural group differences.

CONCLUSION

This chapter addressed some of the social, political, and cultural forces that promote AOD abuse among Puerto Ricans: easy access to drugs, lack of economic opportunities, peer use, acculturation-related stress, changing gender roles, racism, and self-devaluation consistent with colonial status. This wide range of social, economic, psychological, and cultural dynamics produces serious substance abuse problems that affect individuals, families, and the Puerto Rican communities in the United States.

Within the Puerto Rican culture, treatment outcomes are closely related to the client's perception of the clinician's competence, the cultural relevancy of treatment to the client's situation, the availability of treatment resources (including insurance coverage), and family and community support in maintaining abstinence. The interplay among the various factors is key in developing appropriate treatment strategies. The clinician's understanding of an individual's culturally specific values as told in his or her narratives is especially important. The client and clinician should develop a mutual assessment of the multiple factors that affect AOD use and the impact of AOD use on the client's life. Puerto Rican clients intent on maintaining their culture, language, and other group-specific characteristics must be respected. The clinician must be instrumental in supporting the Puerto Rican family's and community's efforts to manage its tasks effectively and in harmony with its value system while acknowledging the realities of coping with the mainland urban environment and the ravages of the drug culture.

REFERENCES

Alcocer, A. M. (1993). Patterns of alcohol use among Hispanics. In R. S. Mayers, B. L. Kail, & T. D. Watts (Eds.), *Hispanic substance abuse* (pp. 37–49). Springfield, IL: Thomas.

Amahti-Mehler, J., Argentieri, S., & Canestri, J. (1993). *The babel of the unconscious.* Madison, CT: International Universities Press.

Amaro, H., Whitaker, R., Coffman, G., & Heeren, T. (1990). Acculturation and marijuana and cocaine use: Findings from HHANES 1982–84. *American Journal of Public Health, 80*(Suppl.), 54–60.

Anderson, E., & Rodriquez, O. (1984). *Conceptual issues in the study of Hispanic delinquency* (Research Bulletin No. 7). New York: Fordham University, Hispanic Research Center.

Berry, J. W. (1980). Acculturation as varieties of adaptation. In A. M. Padilla (Ed.), *Acculturation: Theory, models and some new findings* (pp. 9–26). Boulder, CO: Westview Press.

Bird, H. R. (1982). The cultural dichotomy of colonial people. *Journal of the American Academy of Psychoanalysis, 10*(2), 195–209.

Bonilla-Silva, E. (1997). Rethinking racism: Toward a structural interpretation. *American Sociological Review, 62*(3), 465–480.

Booth, M. W., Castro, F. G., & Anglin, M. D. (1990). What do we know about Hispanic substance abuse? A review of the literature. In R. Glick & J. Moore (Eds.), *Drugs in Hispanic communities* (pp. 21–43). New Brunswick, NJ: Rutgers University Press.

Buxbaum, E. (1949). The role of the second language in the formation of the ego and superego. *Psychoanalytic Quarterly, 18*, 279–289.

Caetano, R. (1988). Alcohol use among Hispanic groups in the United States. *American Journal of Drug and Alcohol Abuse, 14*, 293–308.

Centers for Disease Control and Prevention. (1995). *HIV/AIDS Surveillance Report, 7*(2). Atlanta: U.S. Public Health Service.

Cheung, Y. W. (1989). Making sense of ethnicity and drug use: A review and suggestions for future research. *Social Pharmacology, 3*, 55–82.

Comas-Díaz, L. (1982). Puerto Rican *espiritismo* and psychotherapy. *American Journal of Orthopsychiatry, 4,* 636–645.

De La Rosa, M. (1987, June). *Toward the development of better counseling approaches for Puerto Ricans.* Paper presented at the Annual Conference on Minority Issues of the National Association of Social Workers, Washington, DC.

De La Rosa, M. R., Khalsa, J. H., & Rouse, B. A. (1990). Hispanics and illicit drug use: A review of recent findings. *International Journal of the Addictions, 25*(6), 665–691.

Delgado, M. (1980). Consultation to a Puerto Rican drug abuse program. *American Journal of Drug and Alcohol Abuse, 7*(1), 63–72.

Diaz-Royo, A. (1976). *Dignidad y respeto: Dos temas centrales en la cultura puertorriqueña traditional.* Unpublished manuscript, University of Puerto Rico.

Fanon, F. (1965). *The wretched of the earth.* New York: Grove Press.

Fernandez-Mendez, E. (1970). *La identidad y cultura.* San Juan: Instituto de Cultura Puertorrequeña.

Garcia-Passalacqua, J. M. (1997, November 30). Dual citizenship is a step forward. *The San Juan Star,* p. 179.

Garcia-Preto, N. (1996). Puerto Rican families. In M. McGoldrick, J. Giordano, & J. K. Pearce (Eds.), *Ethnicity and family therapy* (pp. 183–199). New York: Guilford Press.

Garcia-Remis, M. (1993). Los celebros que se van y el corazón que se queda. In *La ciudad que me habita* (pp. 11–19). Rio Piedras, PR: Ediciones Huracan.

Gill, A. G., Vega, W. A., & Dimas, J. M. (1994). Acculturative stress and personal adjustment among Hispanic adolescent boys. *Journal of Community Psychology, 22,* 43–53.

Greenson, R. R. (1950). The mother tongue and the mother. *International Journal of Psycho-Analysis, 31,* 18–23.

Javier, R. A., & Munoz, M. A. (1993). Autobiographical memory in bilinguals. *Journal of Psycholinguistic Research, 22*(3), 319–338.

Loewald, H. W. (1980). *Papers on psychoanalysis.* New Haven, CT: Yale University Press.

Marin, G. (1993). Defining culturally appropriate community interventions: Hispanic as a case study. *Journal of Community Psychology, 21,* 149–158.

Marin, G., Posner, S. F., & Kinyon, J. B. (1991). *Alcohol expectancies among Hispanics and non-Hispanic Whites: Role of respondents' drinking status and acculturation* (Tech. Rep. No. 5). San Francisco: University of San Francisco, Social Psychology Laboratory.

Marsella, A. J. (1990). Ethnocultural identity: The new independent variable in cross-cultural research. *Focus, 4,* 14–15.

Mayers, R. S., & Kail, B. L. (1993). Hispanic substance abuse: An overview. In R. S. Mayers, B. L. Kail, & T. D. Watts (Eds.), *Hispanic substance abuse* (pp. 5–16). Springfield, IL: Thomas.

Melendez, E., & Melendez, E. (1993). *Colonial dilemma: Critical perspectives on contemporary Puerto Rico.* Boston: South End Press.

Memmi, A. (1968). *Dominated man.* Boston: Beacon.

162   CLIENTS OF NATIVE AMERICAN AND LATINO BACKGROUNDS

Mizio, E. (1983). The impact of macro systems on Puerto Rican families. In G. J. Powell, J. Yamamoto, A. Romero, & A. Morales (Eds.), *The psychosocial development of minority group children* (pp. 216–236). New York: Brunner/Mazel.

Montilla, A. (1997, November 28). Court ruling overlooks historical facts. *The San Juan Star*, p. 71.

Moore, J. W., & Mata, A. (1981). *Women and heroin in Chicano communities*. Los Angeles: Chicano Pinto Research Project.

Morgan, P. A. (1990). The making of a public problem: Mexican labor in California and the Marijuana Law of 1937. In R. Glick & J. Moore (Eds.), *Drugs in Hispanic communities* (pp. 233–252). New Brunswick, NJ: Rutgers University Press.

National Clearinghouse for Alcohol and Drug Information. (1993). *Prevention primer: An encyclopedia of alcohol, tobacco, and other drug prevention terms*. Rockville, MD: Author.

National Institute on Drug Abuse. (1989). *National household survey on drug abuse: 1988 population estimates*. Rockville, MD: U.S. Department of Health and Human Services.

National Institute on Drug Abuse. (1992). *National household survey of drug abuse population estimates, 1991* (DHHS Publication No. ADM 92-1887). Washington, DC: U.S. Government Printing Office.

Navarro, M. (1998, July 26). Marking a Puerto Rico anniversary. *The New York Times*, p. 24.

Novas, H. (1994). *Everything you need to know about Latino history*. New York: Plume.

Obeso, P., & Bordatto, O. (1979). Cultural implications in treating Puerto Rican females. *American Journal of Drug and Alcohol Abuse, 6*(3), 337–344.

Oetting, E., & Beauvais, F. (1991). Orthogonal cultural identification theory: The cultural identification of minority adolescents. *International Journal of the Addictions, 25*(5/6), 655–685.

Padilla, A. M. (1980). The role of cultural awareness and ethnic loyalty in acculturation. In A. M. Padilla (Ed.), *Acculturation: Theory, models and some new findings* (pp. 47–84). Boulder, CO: Westview Press.

Pariser, H. S. (1997). *Adventure guide to Puerto Rico* (3rd ed.). Edison, NJ: Hunter.

Phinney, J. S. (1990). Ethnic identity in adolescent and adults: Review of research. *Psychological Bulletin, 108*, 499–514.

Rodriquez, O. (1988, March). *A conceptual approach to Hispanic adolescent drug use*. Paper presented at the meeting of the Society for Research on Adolescence, Alexandria, VA.

Rodriquez, O., Recio, J. L., & De La Rosa, M. (1993). Intergrating mainstream and subcultural explanation of drug use among Puerto Rican youth. In M. De La Rosa & J. L. Recio (Eds.), *Drug use among minority youth: Advances in research and methodologies* (NIDA Research Monograph No. 130; pp. 8–31). Washington, DC: U.S. Department of Health and Human Services.

Rogler, L. H., Cortes, D. E., & Malgady, R. G. (1991). Acculturation and mental status among Hispanics. *American Psychologist, 46*(6), 585–597.

Ruiz-Guitierrez, P. (1996, September 28). Florida's McCollum asks Clinton to add funds for drug war. *The San Juan Star*, p. 2.

Russell, C. (1996). *The official guide to racial and ethnic diversity*. Ithaca, NY: New Strategist.

Stevens, E. (1972). Machismo and marianismo. *Transaction-Society, 10*(6), 57–63.

Substance Abuse and Mental Health Services Administration. (1995). *National Household Survey on Drug Abuse: Main findings 1993*. Rockville, MD: Department of Health and Human Services.

Sue, D. W., & Sue, D. (1990). *Counseling the culturally different: Theory and practice* (2nd ed.). New York: Wiley.

Szapocznik, J., Kurtines, W., & Fernandez, T. (1980). Biculturalism and adjustment in Hispanic youths. *International Journal of Intercultural Relations, 4*, 353–375.

Thomas, P. (1967). *Down these mean streets*. New York: Knopf.

Thomas, P. (1997). Brothers under the same skin. In J. De Jesús (Ed.), *Growing up Puerto Rican: An anthology* (pp. 63–68). New York: Morrow.

U.S. Bureau of the Census. (1991). The Hispanic population in the United States: March, 1990. *Current Population Reports* (Series P-20, No. 449). Washington, DC: U.S. Government Printing Office.

U.S. Bureau of the Census. (1995). The Hispanic population in the United States: March 1995. *Current Population Reports* (Series P-20, No. 501). Washington, DC: U.S. Government Printing Office.

U.S. Department of Justice. (1997). *1997 Statewide strategy: Puerto Rico drug and violent crime control*. Washington, DC: White House Office of National Drug Control Policy.

Vega, E. (1997). Foreword. In J. L. De Jesús (Ed.), *Growing up Puerto Rican: An anthology* (pp. xiii–ix). New York: Morrow.

Vega, W. A., & Amaro, H. (1994). Latino outlook: Good health, uncertain prognosis. *Annual Review of Public Health, 15*, 39–67.

Vega, W. A., & Gil, A. G. (1999). A model for explaining drug use behavior among Hispanic adolescents. In M. R. De La Rosa, B. Segal, & R. Lopez (Eds.), *Conducting drug abuse research with minority populations: Advances and issues* (pp. 57–72). New York: Haworth Press.

Vega, W. A., Hough, R., & Romero, A. (1983). Family life patterns of Mexican Americans. In G. W. Powell (Ed.), *The psychosocial development of minority group children* (pp. 194–215). New York: Brunner/Mazel.

Vega, W. A., & Miranda, M. R. (Eds.). (1985). *Stress and Hispanic mental health: Relating research to service delivery*. Rockville, MD: National Institute of Mental Health.

Velez, C. N., & Ungemack, J. A. (1989). Drug use among Puerto Rican youth: An exploration of generational status differences. *Social Science and Medicine, 29*(6), 779–789.

Wagenheim, K. (1975). *Puerto Rico: A profile* (2nd ed.). New York: Praeger.

Zayas, L. (1988). Puerto Rican familism: Considerations for family therapy. *Family Relations, 37*(4), 260–268.

IV

Working with Clients
of European Background

The paradox of writing about substance abusers of European background is that they are a group that is believed to be *the* group for whom the traditional alcohol and other drug treatment models have been developed, and yet they are a group whose unique treatment needs and treatment approaches have rarely been explored.

Despite the common observation that the French drink differently from the Irish, recent literature on such differences among their descendants in the United States is nonexistent. To what degree does understanding the original cultures of the European Americans help us make treatment more effective? What about the needs of the more recent European immigrants, who tend to be lumped as "Whites" together with the descendants of the early British colonists and who, by and large, tend to be subjected to the traditional 12-step-based substance abuse treatments? Is this homogeneous approach in the best interest of the clients? The six chapters in this section focus on the different "White" populations that are evident yet ignored when it comes to exploring their unique treatment needs.

8

Substance Abuse among Americans of British Descent

Katherine Stuart van Wormer

More than 70 million people in the United States, approximately one fourth of its population, are descended from the early English colonists who settled the so-called New World (McGill & Pearce, 1996). These descendants are variously called Anglo Americans, British Americans, White Anglo Saxon Protestants (or WASPs), or persons of Old American stock. And even though there is no clear name for them, the descendants of the English colonists and the more recent British emigrants do compose a cultural entity all their own.

Although culture is not static and the level of congruity between British and British Americans has faded over the centuries, certain British cultural characteristics, such as emotional restraint and individualism, can commonly be seen among their American cousins (Katz, 1985). These and other cultural values that are discussed in the following section bear on substance abuse in this population and on its treatment. Moreover, the ethos of the early Puritans who migrated from 16th-century Britain and their influence on values, if not on specific attitudes toward alcohol, are a major variable affecting substance abuse treatment in the United States today.

The purpose of this chapter is to show that even the category of Americans most taken for granted—the one that is included in the vague category of *White* on most application forms—is not without its cultural attributes and uniqueness. This chapter explores the cultural dynamics of British

Americans, the peculiar form that the Puritan heritage took on American shores, the role of alcohol and other drugs in contemporary Britain, and the implications for treatment for British Americans in the United States.

CULTURAL CHARACTERISTICS
OF BRITISH AMERICANS

Because culture and substance use interact and shape each other, as Amodeo and Jones (1997) remind us, they are inextricably connected. Therefore, it is important to understand the cultural characteristics of British Americans. In many ways, in fact, members of what we might think of as the dominant culture stand apart from other Americans: One thinks of the relentless status seeking, the isolated nuclear family, subdued emotions, the inhibitions about bodily functions, sexual prudery, and homophobia. On the positive side, one thinks of the hard work ethic, self-discipline and self-reliance, resourcefulness, integrity, and a perennial sense of optimism. As for any culture, this hodgepodge of traits woven together inextricably must be understood holistically as the key to the larger pattern.

The Values of Early British Americans

Fischer (1989) and McGill and Pearce (1996) delineate four distinct regional British-derived folk cultures in the United States: the Puritan New Englanders, the Anglicans of the Tidewater South, the Quakers of the mid-Atlantic states, and the Southern mountain people. Many of the Anglicans of the Tidewater South derive from the Puritan founding fathers (and mothers) who moved southward. Although the histories of the Quaker and Southern mountain people are culturally distinct, the uniting theme that transcends the differences among these disparate British American groups is individualism, or even what McGill and Pearce term "hyperindividualism." A second major theme is emotional restraint. Both of these dynamics derive from our Puritan heritage and both play a role in the use of mood-altering substances.

Like the very language that shapes our every thought and deed, the present-day American value system in general and of British Americans in particular is rooted in the foundation laid within the religious colony in Massachusetts Bay. The essence of this foundation was the holy experiment known to the world as Puritanism. In his classic *Wayward Puritans: A Study in the Sociology of Deviance* (1966), Kai Erikson provides a colorful portrait of this society and of the dissenters among them. Although, back in England, the English had found their narrow liberalism and lack of humor baffling, to the Puritans who reached Massachusetts the truth was perfectly clear: God had chosen an elite few to represent Him on earth. Influenced by the doctrines of Calvinist predestination, the Puritans believed that persons were either to be saved or condemned. Those who were destined to be condemned would inevitably sink to the lowest echelons of society. In accordance with the will of God, punishment for offenders was harsh (Erikson, 1966).

The peculiar ethos of Puritanism is highly visible in American society today. Despite modern secularism, the Puritan ethic manifests itself in the moralism pertaining to substance abusers, in the severity of punishment for users of illegal substances, and in many of the policies affecting alcohol and drug abusing clients today. Sexual prudery and enforced abstinence from drink, however, were not a part of the original Puritan system. These attributes were added later (Bryson, 1994).

Other current American values that originated with our British forebears are discussed in the following sections.

Individualism and Independence

Individualism and independence are major British American cultural attributes. The root of these cultural variables goes back to the Puritans, who tended to look within and to draw on their own resources, as informed by their individual and collective interpretation of the Bible. In the 1830s, the French social philosopher and most renowned commentator on the American psyche, Alexis de Tocqueville (1835/1966), characterized the people on this continent as individualists. The risk to the American character, said de Tocqueville, was that in the future isolation might prevail. This trait of individualism is still the primary value dimension that sums up the cultural climate in the United States today. British Americans have been taught that the meaningful issues and genuine struggles of life all lie within the self and that few external constraints cannot be overcome by individual effort (McGill & Pearce, 1996). "I can take care of myself," or "I can quit drinking/using drugs if I want to," are common responses to substance abuse problems. Although not always effective, such resourcefulness and optimism are important aspects in the treatment of British American substance abusers.

Emotional Restraint

The British are noted, sometimes even ridiculed, for the extent of their emotional restraint (Bryson, 1997). Although British Americans are apt to seem impatient and ill-tempered to the even more reserved Britons, they are among the most restrained and stoical of ethnic groups in the United States. Personal pain tends to be understated. For example, in his study of cultural patterns in response to pain in a hospital setting, Zborowski (1981) describes the behavior of the "Old Americans" as noncomplaining, seeking approval, and avoiding being a nuisance on the ward.

The Work Ethic

The work ethic, widely regarded as one of America's overriding characteristics, harks back to the Puritans and their association of prosperity with salvation. Long after the religious fervor faded, the capitalist, competitive thrust lingered on. Such views are internalized by many British Americans—to be on welfare or even unemployed is to feel a sense of failure and shame.

A value related to work is the perpetual desire to "get ahead," to move upward and onward and "to keep up with the Joneses." Workers are expected to climb the corporate ladder and to be willing to relocate if necessary for career advancement. The subsequent loss of community support and loneliness are also associated with excessive drinking (Goodwin, 1988).

Moreover, because one measure of parental success in an achievement-oriented society is the success of one's children, children reared in British American households may grow up with an inordinate sense of failure. Clients with addiction problems are especially susceptible to feelings of inadequacy. And certainly, the loss of control and other problems due to substance abuse exacerbate the sense of unworthiness.

Isolation of the Nuclear Family

Modern-day British American families tend to be small. Usually consisting of one-generation households, such families are frequently characterized by a limited sense of connection to elderly parents or other family members. An exception must be made for the American Deep South and Appalachian regions, where more of an extended-family pattern prevails. As pointed out by McGill and Pearce (1996), British American families cope well with success but not with troubles or failure. Brought up to be self-sufficient, British Americans usually hesitate to turn to their families of origin for economic or emotional support, even in times of severe stress.

Moralism

What is striking about the British American expression of moralism—undoubtedly a carryover from Puritan times—is the tendency to be judgmental about matters pertaining to pleasure, the so-called social vices, including drug and alcohol abuse. The tendency to equate the condition of intoxication with sin and the meting out of harsh punishments to drug users exemplify the moralistic ethos.

TREATMENT OF BRITISH AMERICANS

British pragmatism (in the case of reducing the spread of AIDS, for example) contrasts sharply with American punitiveness that reflects its Puritan heritage. So whereas the British harm-reduction model favors setting up needle exchanges to provide clean needles for drug users and even allows for the provision of a safe drug supply under medical supervision, the United States turns to its military might to eliminate the supply side of drugs. This approach is bolstered by harsh punishment not only of drug dealers but also of drug users.

As mentioned previously, the traditional British American cultural attributes include emotional restraint, individualism and independence, work and socioeconomic mobility, moralism, and primacy of the nuclear family. Each of these attributes has implications in terms of both risk substance abuse and treatment consideration.

Of all the common British American traits, the one with the most overriding consequences in the treatment of substance abuse is related to restraint of emotions and direct expression of feelings. Drugs, legal and illegal, are used to cope with emotional pain by boosting and numbing feelings. Ironically, substance abuse can be regarded as an attempt to seek control—the control of painful emotions in persons so emotionally repressed as to be unable to express them in healthy ways.

In counseling substance abusers of British heritage, the clinician is likely to find that clients from this background more commonly intellectualize their experiences than show their emotions. The area in which the most work is needed—intimacy—is the area that will inspire the most resistance and antagonism.

Addressing Communications Issues

Inasmuch as the typical substance abuse treatment program is geared to elicit interpersonal intimacy through intensive group work, British American clients may become psychologically alienated and experience extreme difficulty with group exercises. For example, in some therapy groups a female client may call out, "I need a hug," and almost ritualistically, the group leader will instruct all members to hug each other. The client who balks may then come under relentless group pressure to display affection. Inhibitions and shyness in one client may lead to hurt feelings in another, who feels rejected by the refusal to hug. With clients of British background, three major risks exist in this common practice of forced touching (even disregarding the sexual complications that may arise from these endeavors). The first is the risk of losing this client from the treatment setting altogether. The second risk is setting up an already sensitive person to be misunderstood by the group, who may interpret his or her reserve as coldness and/or an air of superiority. Finally, the client of British stock, already inclined to internalize his or her problems, may experience high performance anxiety and a sense of failure. Such feelings of negativism may induce a relapse and render the group encounter worse, in fact, than no treatment at all.

Instead, therapists would be well advised to show a cultural sensitivity toward the British American's communication style. Comments such as, "I sense your caring" or "I wonder if you don't have a lot more feeling than you're letting on," when said with kindness, will help endear the client to a group whose members may otherwise mistake reserve for indifference. When dealing with an inexpressive male client, a group discussion on mainstream upbringing in our society can open the door to self-understanding and sharing. Similarly, fill-in-the-blank group exercises of the nature of "My father always encouraged me to (or not to) _____" may be helpful in imparting self-awareness.

Communication skills work is especially effective in couples counseling and when working with family members. British Americans, who tend to be task oriented, usually react well to an organized format that describes appropriate means of confronting each other in a nonthreatening way. "When you do/say _____, I feel _____" practice schemes are an excellent means of enabling clients to express their feelings to each other in a productive fashion. "Rules for fighting fair" programs may be provided in the form of a homework assignment.

Clinicians from more demonstrative ethnocultural backgrounds frequently assume that love must be verbally or physically expressed. Often overlooked are the many subtle forms of expression that love can take among British Americans. A handshake in the Smith or Elliott household, for example, may be the equivalent of a bear hug in the Gomez family. In ethnically mixed marriages, the clinician may need to help each partner translate the culturally distinct body language of the other. For example, the clinician needs to help the couple, or even other patients, understand that the Anglo-American's standoffishness may be a sign of respect, not lack of caring.

In a similar vein, counselors who themselves are from highly expressive cultures may mistake the British American social distance or reserve for prejudice. Another common error is to presume that people who act emotionally cold are, in fact, devoid of caring feeling. Utilizing a strengths perspective, clinicians need to seek out the internal or external resources on which to base a treatment plan. The clinician who exudes warmth and genuineness and who manages to reinforce the positive in the British American client who tries to hide his or her pain may find that the warmth and genuineness may rub off on the client. Such dynamics can be seen in the following case.

> Denise, a 21-year-college student living at home with her parents, was brought into treatment by court order for a DWI (driving while intoxicated). In addition to excessive drinking, Denise had a history of bulimia. Her compulsive dieting and binge eating followed by forced vomiting was threatening her health. She was referred to a doctor who prescribed antidepressants to reduce her compulsive behavior and unmanageable cravings for food and alcohol. She was also put into a woman's therapy group that helped her develop a more realistic female body image and accept herself the way she was.
>
> Despite her progress, Denise had several relapses, both with bulimia and with drinking. Her therapist suggested family counseling, and after initial resistance, Denise returned with her parents. It soon materialized that there was a family secret, so forbidden as never to have been mentioned since Denise's childhood. The unmentionable secret was that Denise had been molested by her uncle, her father's brother. Throughout the years, Denise thought her parents blamed her and rejected her for being "tainted." The parents, in turn, thought that if they didn't talk about what happened, the issue would just go away. In explaining the matter directly, the therapist helped the parents communicate their love and acceptance for their child. Getting this family secret out in the open was the final step that needed to be taken to help Denise accept herself as a lovable and whole person. Talking about the buried past also helped to alleviate her parents' sense of guilt about what had happened to their daughter.

Individualism and Independence

Cox and Ephross (1998) discuss how what they call "ethnic" populations (as if descendants of English-speaking immigrants lack ethnicity) may have difficulty with the "nonethnic" emphasis on autonomy and individual resourcefulness. However, these interrelated traits, when not carried to the extreme, provide possibilities for a discovery of strengths.

The very focus on "turning one's life over" to a power greater than the self and the focus on group treatment can be viewed as an attempt to offset the hyperindividualism—the egotism, loneliness, and guilt feelings—often associated with abuse of chemicals. Guilt feelings are skillfully managed within the framework of Alcoholics Anonymous (AA) parlance that the bad behavior was all a part of the disease. "You had to hit your bottom," they say. What this model does *not* allow for is trust of the clients' own perceptions, either about the nature and extent of addiction or about its origins. Thus it is important that the client's status as an independent person is reinforced in a treatment relationship in which counselor and client are allies rather than antagonists in some sort of power struggle.

The Work Ethic

Given the previous discussion of the British American work ethic, it is easy to see how 12-step programs, with their emphasis on "working the program," on goal setting, and on regular and punctual attendance at meetings, are made to order for individuals reared to strive toward success in all avenues of life. Although the ready use of slogans such as "one day at a time" and "easy does it" tempers the addict's tendency to go to extremes, the achievement drive can still be satisfied in other ways. For example, sobriety anniversaries are given public recognition: The more years of sobriety the better. The hard work of recovery that begins at the treatment center extends to AA or Narcotics Anonymous (NA) activities, starting with the "90 meetings in 90 days" slogan. The 9th and 12th steps require further work in making direct amends to persons harmed and by helping other alcoholics and addicts. These issues can be seen in the following case.

> Don, a 36-year-old methamphetamine addict, had a history of extensive use of "uppers" to help him carry an intense work load and exceed his limits of endurance. Having lost his wife, who left him, taking their two children, and suffering from premature heart problems, Don had hit bottom and sought treatment at an outpatient clinic.
>
> Don liked the 12-step group his therapist recommended, and he worked hard on setting realistic goals for himself, taking "one day at a time" and securing the aid of a sponsor to help him deal with his workaholic tendencies. An underlying problem for Don was his sense of failure with regard to his hard-driving father. In his individual sessions, Don was able to come to see that his father loved him even if he did not verbalize this fact, that the only way his father knew to express his love was through taking care of his family financially and through fixing things in the house, such as the plumbing. Once he was able to accept his father and to feel better about himself, Don was able to

make amends to his former wife and children and to become a sponsor to other young men.

Isolation of the Nuclear Family

A serious challenge to the clinician working with substance abusers of Anglo descent is that they are not always able to renew their family ties; sometimes their family members have virtually disowned them due to their irresponsible behavior. Such a reaction may seem strange for clinicians from other ethnic groups: "I can't work with these clients; there's nothing to work with" was the reaction of one African American outreach center worker to the lack of extended family ties and the rejection by some White Anglo Saxon family members of relatives who had gotten into trouble with alcohol or other drugs. Although not easy, it is important to work on restoring these estranged family relationships. A persistent appeal by the therapist can often result in the cooperation of even the most recalcitrant family members in attending nonthreatening psychoeducational lecture sessions or in simply providing background data on the client. Often the parents and siblings of substance-abusing clients had themselves been reared in an alcoholic home and are eager to learn about the biological and social aspects of alcoholism. The value of the disease concept in alleviating family members' sense of guilt should not be underestimated.

> Kathy was a strong-willed and highly competitive 29-year-old northern White woman of Anglo heritage married to an African American from Mississippi; together, they had two small children. Both Kathy and her husband were alcoholics. Isolated from her family and lacking friends, Kathy was dependent on her husband; at the same time she was constantly belittling him in order to make herself appear in a more favorable light. Work with this couple entailed teaching them techniques of conflict resolution and improving their communications skills. In the end, the couple decided to separate.
>
> Kathy was able to maintain her sobriety only after she began to restore her ties with her family of origin. With the help of her mother, who agreed to come to a psychoeducational lecture at which she revealed that her own father was an alcoholic, Kathy and her children were gradually welcomed back by her family.

Moralism

Given the British American tendency to be moralistic and judgmental, the clinician can anticipate strong guilt feelings and defensiveness from clients who are loath to acknowledge their loss of control over substances and their failure to act as responsible members of society. A focus on the client's strengths and utilizing a modified disease model that incorporates a client-centered and low-keyed harm-minimization approach is perhaps the best strategy for helping clients who are wrestling with issues related to morality and for decreasing their feelings of self-blame and depression.

TREATMENT ISSUES FOR
OTHER BRITISH AMERICANS

As mentioned previously, British Americans include not only those descendants of the New England Puritans but also three other groups, each with its distinct culture and specific treatment needs.

Mid-Atlantic Quakers

Although few of the descendants of the early Quakers outside of Philadelphia are members of this religion today, Quakers were an important formative influence in the East and Midwest (McGill & Pearce, 1996). Quaker descendants tend to have the same attributes as other British Americans, stressing the work ethic, moralism, and emotional restraint. However, compared with other British Americans, the Quaker tradition is egalitarian as opposed to competitive and nonpunitive. Forgiveness and reconciliation are stressed over justice.

However, there is little tolerance of drunkenness or other addictions, such as gambling or smoking, among the Quakers. Historically, Quakers, along with Methodists, established themselves as one of the earliest religious groups to promote temperance. Today, consistent with Quaker individualism and belief in privacy, there is little direct guidance on alcoholism intervention offered in either the religious literature or by members of the meeting. For example, in researching an article for *Friends Journal* (van Wormer, 1986), I uncovered a handout about the experiences of Ann Bohan, a Quaker and a recovering alcoholic. In a disturbing and moving report, Bohan chided her Quaker group for failing to confront her or help her when she "turned to the bottle" following a personal crisis. After the crisis was over, individual members continued in their minimization of her earlier problem.

What may be especially helpful to substance-abusing members of this special population is a focus on the disease model. Once reframed as a disease, the alcohol or other drug abuse problem can be acknowledged, and the person's well-being can be placed above personal privacy to provide the help that is needed.

Southern Tidewater Region

In contrast to the egalitarianism of the Quakers, a rigid race and class hierarchy prevailed in what is referred to today as the Old South and among the British Americans living there. Such cultural characteristics provide the source for great literature such as the writings of William Faulkner, Tennessee Williams, and Pat Conroy. An additional theme running through such literature is the unwritten rule of avoiding certain topics, coupled with the understanding that family secrets must be kept at all costs.

Counselors working with Southern Whites of planter heritage will need to go to great lengths to help them communicate about the issues that matter. Again, the focus on the disease model can help clients feel less shame and guilt so that they can address the issues that need to be dealt with in treatment.

Appalachian or Southern Mountain People

The settlers of Appalachia are often referred to as the Scotch–Irish. Migrating from Northern Ireland in the 1700s, these zealous Protestants settled in the mountains of the southeast. This is the culture, as McGill and Pearce (1996) note, that we know from "country and Western music." At the opposite end of the social class spectrum from the Tidewater Southerners, Appalachian culture is associated with poverty, drinking, and fatalism and reflected in the stereotype: "steely eyes, glinting rifles, and clear white moonshine" (Edwards, 1985, p. 131). The manufacture of illegal alcohol or moonshine is an Appalachian tradition harking back to Scotch–Irish independence. However, those unable to control their use of alcohol are thought to be sinners and rarely get help from family members. Their presence is tolerated nevertheless. Edwards (1985) attributes this laissez-faire attitude to the fatalistic belief that this is "just the way things are."

Because a strong family orientation is a key trait of Southern mountain people, people may seem clannish and very reluctant to complain to outsiders about one another, particularly about such issues as domestic violence and child abuse. Clinicians may need to form an alliance with the extended family network in order to help a substance-abusing individual (R. Condon, personal communication, June 15, 1999). According to Edwards (1985), the Appalachian native is not inclined to put faith in abstractions or in people's credentials and titles. What counts is a person's moral character and friendliness. The clinician is thus well advised to engage in a certain amount of small talk and to establish a personal relationship first before getting to the business at hand.

CONCLUSION

For clients of Anglo-Saxon descent, the core British American values—emotional restraint, individualism and independence, hard work, nuclear family orientation, and moralism—can be problematic and yet can play an important role during recovery. The struggle to achieve success, for example, in the absence of group support can lead to depression and anxiety. The individual may abuse substances to lessen the pain. In turn, however, the success and the hard work of recovery can be self-reinforcing.

The stress management aspects of the 12-step approach, in conjunction with the emphasis on self-improvement, are clearly culturally relevant to this population. The disease concept has been very helpful in reducing self- and societal blame of alcoholics and addicts. However, many of the punitive aspects of programs designed for involuntary, court-ordered treatment, with their invasive urinalysis tests and harsh confrontation aspects, may be culturally alienating to persons brought up to value independence and personal pride.

The growing emphasis on harm reduction, well established in Great Britain, is a promising development for this population. Pragmatic and client centered, this model focuses on helping people minimize the harm they do to themselves with drugs and alcohol and to take responsibility for their own treatment progress—values that are clearly in line with the British American culture.

REFERENCES

Amodeo, M., & Jones, K. (1997, May/June). Viewing alcohol and other drug use cross culturally: A cultural framework for clinical practice. *Families in Society*, 78(3), 240–254.

Bryson, B. (1994). *Made in America*. London: Minerva.

Bryson, B. (1997). *Notes from a small island*. New York: Avon Books.

Cox, C., & Ephross, P. (1998). *Ethnicity and social work practice*. New York: Oxford University Press.

de Tocqueville, A. (1966). *Democracy in America*. New York: Harper & Row. (Original work published 1835)

Edwards, G. T. (1985). Appalachia: The effects of cultural values on the production and consumption of alcohol. In L. Bennett & G. Ames (Eds.), *The American experience with alcohol: Contrasting cultural perspectives* (pp. 131–146). New York: Plenum Press.

Erikson, K. (1966). *Wayward Puritans: A study in the sociology of deviance*. New York: Wiley.

Fischer, D. H. (1989). *Albion's seed: Four British folk ways in America*. New York: Oxford University Press.

Goodwin, D. (1988). *Alcohol and the writer*. New York: Penguin.

Katz, J. (1985). The sociopolitical nature of counseling. *Counseling Psychologist, 13*, 615–624.

McGill, D. W., & Pearce, J. K. (1996). American families with English ancestors from the colonial era: Anglo Americans. In M. McGoldrick, J. Giordano, & J. K. Pearce (Eds.), *Ethnicity and family therapy* (2nd ed., pp. 451–466). New York: Guilford Press.

van Wormer, K. (1986). Quakers and alcoholism. *Friends Journal, 32*(10), 10–11.

Zborowski, M. (1981). Cultural components in response to pain. In P. Conrad & R. Kern (Eds.), *The sociology of health and illness: Critical perspectives* (pp. 126–138). New York: St. Martin's Press.

9

Substance Abuse Treatment with Clients of French Background

Ann A. Abbott

For centuries, the French have been celebrated for superb wines and for their renowned ability to enjoy them, for their leadership role in diplomatic and economic communities, and for their strong nationalism and stoic self-control. What has not been celebrated is their pervasive alcohol abuse and the personality characteristics that may either impede or facilitate successful substance abuse treatment. This chapter is intended to enhance understanding and provide intervention skills to be used with substance-abusing clients of French background. It includes a brief historical overview of the immigration patterns of French and French Canadians to the United States and their assimilation into American culture. It also discusses French cultural characteristics, including communication and decision-making patterns, the development of relationships, family dynamics, gender roles, and sense of time.

This background material should facilitate understanding of the French view of substance use and abuse, particularly of alcohol, and the implications for ethnoculturally sensitive treatment of clients of French background. Similar to other ethnic groups, there is great diversity among clients of French origin. Particular attention will be directed to differences between two major immigration groups—French and French Canadians.

Collectively this information should serve as essential background for engaging in successful ethnoculturally sensitive clinical practice.

FRENCH IMMIGRATION TO THE UNITED STATES

French immigration to the United States has been small but continual. France, with its current population of approximately 60 million, ranks among the world's most economically advanced nations, playing a major role in the European community. Despite a recent high rate of unemployment, France continues to offer a protective social safety net for its citizens that includes health care and old-age pensions. Given these factors, and in the absence of other compelling forces such as religious persecution, current French interest in emigration to the United States is minimal.

Due to unique immigration patterns, it is difficult to determine accurate immigration rates. Higonnet (1980) notes that the French frequently enter the United States via another country, such as Germany, the French Caribbean, and, in particular, Canada; Hillstrom (1995), on the other hand, notes that people from other countries frequently migrate to the United States via France. Given these factors, it is difficult to determine accurate immigration figures for the French because, when asked their country of origin, immigrants frequently note their last country of residence.

Immigration via Canada

Prior to the latter half of the 18th century, the majority of Frenchmen emigrating to Canada were Catholics, whereas French Protestants tended to come directly to the United States. After the French Revolution, an increased number of Catholics sought shelter on U.S. shores, as was the case following the French and Indian War (1754–1763). The bulk of those coming via Canada settled in the New England states. During the last half of the 19th century and later, these French-Canadians tended to become more dispersed throughout the United States; however, their largest concentration continues to be in New England. Currently, those of French Canadian descent compose 34% of the population of Vermont, 30% of that of New Hampshire, 28% of that of Maine, and 17% of the population of Massachusetts (Parrillo, 1994). As of 1990, it was estimated that more than 2.17 million people of French Canadian descent were residing in the United States.

As a group, the French Canadians, most of whom migrated from the French-speaking province of Quebec, have reflected a strong commitment to preserve French as their primary language and to maintain Catholicism as their major religion (Barkan, 1980; Hillstrom, 1995; Langelier, 1996). On the whole, the French Canadian family is more nuclear and autonomous than its counterpart in France. Historically, French Canadian women appear to have higher status and authority than their French counterparts (Barkan, 1980; Hillstrom, 1995), although in both groups, traditional male-dominated sex roles have prevailed (Langelier, 1996).

French Canadian emigration to the United States ebbed and flowed over the years, with peaks occurring during the latter part of the 19th century and just prior to the Great Depression. The bulk of this later migration was directly related to economic opportunities and was part of an apparently contagious groundswell of immigration to the United States from Europe via Canadian ports of entry (Barkan, 1980; Fedunkiw, 1995; Hillstrom, 1995). Like their counterparts from France, French Canadian immigrants gradually began to marry outside their cultural group, with each subsequent generation moving toward greater erosion of their ethnocultural heritage.

The Role of Religion, Economics, and Politics

Migration to the United States, to a large extent, has been influenced by political, religious, and economic developments. For example, the French Revolution encouraged the flow of French Catholics to the United States in the latter part of the 18th century, whereas some French Jews immigrated to the United States after the fall of France to the Germans in 1940 (Higonnet, 1980).

To a larger extent than even religious or political freedom, economic possibility was the driving force behind much French immigration. Typically, many French immigrants have been skilled, middle-class workers, a profile that reflected the French nation as a whole. Primarily a rural nation, France entered the modern industrial era slowly but later progressed with vigor. The pull of economic possibility abroad enhanced the flow of French immigration to America.

Assimilation into American Culture

Initially, early French immigrants to the United States were determined to set up their own communities in which French was the spoken language and French customs prevailed; this ideal was short-lived. Although some French immigrants attempted to create Frenchtowns, the bulk of the immigrants were committed to assimilating into larger American society—

something that they appeared to do with ease and skill. Rather than congregating in a few major cities, immigrants from France have dispersed throughout the United States, although the French subculture of New Orleans is one example that suggests the contrary. The New Orleans culture is unique and does not appear to truly reflect the continuation of the culture of their French forefathers, because the bulk of those of French ancestry living in Louisiana were deported from Canada by the English beginning approximately in 1755 (Langelier, 1996).

In spite of the fact that even today French nationalism remains high within France (Kaplan, 1993), French immigrants in the United States have assimilated more quickly into the mainstream than many of their non-English-speaking counterparts (Higonnet, 1980). However, French Canadian immigrants have assimilated at a much slower rate and with an apparently stronger commitment to maintaining their ethnocultural heritage and native language (Langelier, 1996).

Assimilation and dispersal may have been easier for immigrants from France, given the fact that their economic philosophy and cultural orientation have been highly compatible with those of mainstream American society. Ease of assimilation may also be directly related to social class. For the most part, immigrants from France have reflected higher social status than that of their working-class French Canadian counterparts (Langelier, 1996). In spite of their general assimilation, remnants of French cultural heritage must be recognized as both contributing to behavior and influencing the course of clinical intervention with substance-abusing clients.

CULTURAL CHARACTERISTICS OF THE FRENCH

The French culture is not static—it evolves each day, but, like every other culture, it retains unique characteristics (Glazer & Moynihan, 1970; Steinberg, 1981). To better understand clients of French background, one must have an awareness of French cultural characteristics and the responses they evoke in oneself. Some of these characteristics are discussed in this section.

French Social Class and Decision Making

For generations, the French have had a rigid class system, ranging from aristocratic to working class (Hall & Hall, 1990). The concept of class is carried throughout French organizations. Within a broad range of organizational structures, authority is at the top, and decisions are made at that level. Those in the know understand the importance of getting to top-level individuals if a decision is required, and they are well aware of the avenues necessary for arriving there. In addition, the French carefully classify types of relationships; personal life and professional life are kept totally separate (Hall & Hall, 1990). On the whole, the French are viewed as low risk takers, tending to stick more to protocol than to reach out for unknown heights. They tend to defer to the status quo, to the proper and the predictable, and are known for their attention to detail (Gannon & Associates, 1994; Hofstede, 1980).

The Role of Catholicism

Over 85% of the French refer to themselves as Roman Catholic, although fewer than 15% report actively practicing their religion (Gannon & Associates, 1994). Although the majority do not actively practice their religion, to understand French culture, it is absolutely essential to recognize the influence of their religious roots. Catholicism, with its strong emphasis on duty and its authoritarian structure, has played a major role in shaping the French conservatism and rigidity. The French have been taught to defer to power—to God, the pope, the parish priest, the father, the boss. In addition to expectations for religious life, the parameters of sexual behavior were clearly dictated by the Church, with high priority placed on "early marriage and the begetting and raising of children" (Langelier, 1996, p. 478).

On the more positive side, Catholicism, with its sacrament of confession, presents the gift of forgiveness and the opportunity to start over anew. The dimensions of this important component of Catholicism have definite implications for mental health and substance abuse treatment and will be discussed later.

THE FRENCH FAMILY

To the French, family is very important. Although France has been classified as a "feminine society" with less emphasis on such masculine traits as aggression and material possessions (Gannon & Associates, 1994), the growth of the women's movement in France has been very slow. For example, French women were not granted the right to vote until 1945.

Clearly defined roles exist within families, and each role comes with specific rules and expectations. As with the Church, within the family the French also tend to defer to power, with the father or husband maintaining the position of greatest authority. In traditional sex-specific roles, the mother or wife is responsible for overseeing daily domestic affairs and taking care of the children. She serves as the family mediator and social director. The father's responsibility is not just one of authority but also of economic provider, moral leader, and purveyor of both affection and security (Langelier, 1996).

Parent–child relationships follow similar hierarchical patterns. Child management by punishment prevails over that of positive reinforcement. Of parent–child subsystems, those between cross-sex pairs (father–daughter, mother–son) seem to be stronger; in dysfunctional families, these pair relationships are overly intense. On the whole, relationships among siblings are strong, supportive, and highly valued (Langelier, 1996).

In general, anger is not an acceptable emotion. True feelings are frequently evidenced by passive–aggressive behavior, such as withdrawal or prolonged silence. Excessive drinking or other substance abuse also may be indicative of underlying emotional masking.

In his studies of the French, Carroll (1987) found most to be very private individuals, a characteristic reinforced by their closed shutters, drawn drapes, walled courtyards, and manner of inviting only close friends into their home space. Langelier (1996), in discussing French Canadians, noted similar value placed on privacy. In time of need, French families tend to rely on one another, on close friends, or on the local priest. They are reluctant to go outside those parameters for help. "Personal problems, especially family issues, are considered too intimate or private for a stranger (therapist)" (Langelier, 1996, p. 486). When they do seek help outside familiar avenues, only intense crises may open the door to outside help—and even then family secrets remain paramount. Given these characteristics, one can imagine the difficulty in establishing a professional therapeutic relationship, especially one designed to address substance abuse.

French Communication Patterns

The French are known for their great love of debate. In fact, at times they have been classified as "argumentative" (Morrison, Conaway, & Borden, 1994). In general, they tend to approach knowledge from an analytical or critical perspective; however, they follow specific rules of debate, based on authority and role, and tend to be intolerant of anything that runs counter to the cultural norm (Morrison et al., 1994).

Conversation is very important to the French (Carroll, 1987). Hall and Hall (1990), in describing communication patterns of French businessmen, note that the French are known for making small talk. They constitute a "high context" society, with much sharing of information among those in close relationships. Hall and Hall state that many French businessmen choose to be obscure so as not to appear naive. Many support specific rules for discussion and negotiation, which include being polite, formal, low key, scrupulously correct, carefully prepared, logical, and thorough. In addition, they are well prepared for and open to interruptions, debate, and long negotiations.

Development of Relationships

Gannon and Associates (1994) noted that for the French, relationships take a long time to develop, but once they have developed, they become very important and enduring. Like the French, the French Canadians place great value on family relationships and obligations. Outsiders are viewed with suspicion and distrust; however, once one enters the inner sanctum of close friendship, commitment and responsibility ensue (Langelier, 1996).

French Definition of Time

Hall and Hall (1990) see the French as being "polychronic," or having the capacity to do many things at once. Typically they can tolerate interruptions and loose schedules; however, the French pace is quick, with decisions frequently being made with gusto.

FRENCH VIEW OF SUBSTANCE USE AND ABUSE

The French have had a long-standing appreciation of alcohol, with wine being their beverage of cultural choice (Babor, 1992). Both French and French Canadians continue to view drinking favorably, and its place as a cultural artifact and its role within French history have been increasingly recognized and studied (Brennan, 1988, 1989). Its cultural importance is reflected in its association with the essential and major milestones of life—with birth, with fertility, with death (Bianquis-Gasser, 1992). All one has to do is spend a few days in Paris, the French countryside, or the province of Quebec to see these cultural influences at play.

In spite of the fact that France has an extremely high rate of cirrhosis of the liver, until recently excessive drinking has not been recognized as a problem. Rather, wine had been advanced as being essential for good health and a necessary ingredient of life. Daily drinking was espoused and abstinence ridiculed. It was not uncommon for many Frenchmen to consume wine on an ongoing basis throughout the course of a typical day. On such a schedule, with a daily consumption rate of two or more liters per day, they showed little overt evidence of drunkenness; however, they displayed symptoms of withdrawal if the schedule were altered significantly (Kinney & Leaton, 1995; Ray & Ksir, 1999). The dynamics evident here are those described by Jellinek (1960) in his classification of "delta" alcoholism: increased tissue tolerance develops and withdrawal symptoms occur when intake is discontinued. The drinker does not lose control over the amount consumed, but he or she does lose the ability to abstain for even one day. Jellinek (1962) referred to this type of drinking as "alcoholism without drunkenness" (p. 384). Typically no distressing social problems result; however, health problems may be evident (Babor et al., 1986; Jellinek, 1960; Rivers, 1994; van Wormer, 1995). The major contributors to the development of the delta alcoholic are thought to be sociocultural and economic factors, not psychological ones (Babor, Wolfson, Boivin, Radouco-Thomas, & Clark, 1992; Jellinek, 1960, 1962).

In contrast to the delta drinker, is the "gamma" alcoholic, who, in addition to developing increased tissue tolerance and withdrawal symptoms, also exhibits loss of control over his or her drinking (Jellinek, 1960, 1962). The gamma alcoholic is frequently intoxicated and uses alcohol to escape underlying psychological problems. This type of drinking more closely reflects the drinking patterns in the United States and other primarily Anglo-Saxon countries (Babor et al., 1992).

Canadian drinkers tend to fall in between these two categories and could be classified as "delta-gamma" alcoholics. It is important to note that the French Canadians tend to be more representative of the delta dimension and the Canadian Anglo-Protestants more reflective of the gamma dimension, supporting the underlying influence of ethnocultural heritage (Babor, 1992; Babor et al., 1986).

Kissin (1977) contends that the degree of psychopathology associated with the development of alcoholism is inversely related to the level of acceptance of drinking within the specific culture. As indicated previously, the French, as a society, are significantly more accepting of alcohol use than many other cultures. This may explain their greater preponderance of delta rather than gamma alcoholism, with its underlying psychopathological attributes.

Alcohol Consumption in France and Canada

Although production and consumption of alcohol in France remain among the highest in the world, the more recent trend has been toward maintaining levels of production and decreasing levels of consumption (d'Houtaud,

Adriaanse, & Field, 1989; Mosse, 1992; Sulkunen, 1989). This trend also is reflected to a much lesser degree in Canadian consumption statistics (Rush & Ogborne, 1992), which tend to parallel those of the English (Babor et al., 1992).

Although production of alcohol in France increased by almost 200% in less than a century, Brennan (1989) hypothesized that consumption did not increase proportionately; rather, the number of consumers increased as production increased. More recently, per capita alcohol consumption levels have shown a general reduction (Sulkunen, 1989). In examining drinking patterns based on occupational status and type of beverage consumed, Sulkunen (1989) found that there were definite shifts in beverage of choice. He explains the shifts on the basis of "cultural competition," stating that people in lower socioeconomic and ethnocultural positions tend to emulate the drinking patterns of the elite, frequently leading the elite to move to new patterns. The current fashionable pattern espoused by the French elite involves lowered consumption of alcohol and a shift toward nonalcoholic substitutes, such as flavored water, coffee, or juices, a shift supported by the research of d'Houtaud and colleagues (1989). A current concern might be the impact of the increased use of drugs such as cocaine, heroin, prescription drugs, and their various combinations by the so-called elite (Facy & Verron, 1989).

In a major policy shift developed in response to the fact that 40% of French highway fatalities are related to drunken driving, the French government lowered the blood alcohol limit to be used to determine drunk driving, effective September 15, 1995. The full impact of this policy has yet to be determined (Kole, 1995).

The Influence of Gender

In additional to overall cultural differences in the use and abuse of alcohol, it is essential to examine gender differences within cultures. In examining individuals' views of alcoholism, Babor and colleagues (1986) found that culture generally took priority, with females responding more like their male counterparts within each culture than like their female counterparts across cultures. However, in a later study analyzing the presence of primarily biologically based symptoms of psychopathology among French, French Canadians, and Americans, Babor and his colleagues (1992) found that gender took priority over culture, with females exhibiting similarities across cultures rather than sharing them with their male cultural counterparts. In their comparison of all three cultures, they found a shared disapproval of women drinking heavily. They also found that regardless of culture, the prevalence of psychopathology was higher among female alcoholics than among male alcoholics. Among males presenting symptoms of psychopathology, antisocial personality was the most frequent diagnosis; among females, it was depression. Babor and colleagues note that "although greater proportions of the males than the females were diagnosed as having 'alcoholism only' (i.e., no psychiatric comorbidity), there were no significant differences in the average number of psychiatric diagnoses between the sexes within each sample" (p. 189). They also suggest that the etiology and pattern of alcoholism among women is more complex than that among their male counterparts. Onset of alcoholism for males occurred typically 5 years earlier than for females, and both French males and females reported onset 6 years later than their French Canadian counterparts. In their Canadian study, which included a large number of French Canadians, Rush and Ogborne (1992) noted an increasing number of women seeking treatment. In 1970, the ratio of men to women seeking treatment was 5:1; by the early 1990s it was less than 3:1. They also noted a lowering of average age of those presenting for treatment during that time period. These figures parallel those found in the United States.

In a study comparing French female alcoholics with a comparable sample of nonalcoholics, Remy, Soukup-Stepan, and Tatossian (1988) found the female alcoholics exhibiting increased difficulty in communication and much-reduced utilization of their social support networks. The social networks of French alcoholic women were found to be comparable in size to but more limited to family members than those of the nonalcoholics. When they were able to connect with existing support systems, their prognoses for recovery were greatly enhanced.

Other Drug Usage

Although alcohol remains the major drug of choice among the French and their French Canadian counterparts, the use of other drugs, especially tobacco, is on the rise (Rush & Ogborne, 1992). Paralleling the U.S. experience, drug abuse, as we know it in today's treatment context, first appeared as being problematic in France during the 1960s. Initially the major drugs consumed were cannabis, LSD, and other hallucinogens. Heroin use, which as in other industrialized nations diminished after the 1930s, reappeared in the mid- to late 1970s. Heroin was reported as the primary drug of choice by 69% of identified drug users during that time period. As of the late 1980s, cocaine, alone or in combination with other drugs, became the more prevalent drug (Facy & Verron, 1989).

IMPLICATIONS FOR TREATMENT OF PEOPLE
OF FRENCH DESCENT IN THE UNITED STATES

The French, and to a lesser degree the French Canadians, tend to find it difficult to view alcoholism as a disease in need of treatment. Moreover, as a cultural group, they tend to resist going outside the immediate family for help, a perspective that certainly adds to the challenge of engaging someone in substance abuse treatment. Furthermore, the French are well known for the slow pace at which relationships mature, a factor that also influences the development of the professional relationships necessary for treatment. These factors have to be kept in mind when dealing with a substance-abusing individual of French descent.

In addition, given their strong acceptance of the hierarchical structure of the Catholic Church, the French place greater emphasis on external than internal control. Therefore, when working with French clients, a clinician should assess how they perceive their locus of control (Sue & Sue, 1990). Does the client believe that he or she can orchestrate change from within or that outside influences have primary control over outcomes? Sue and Sue (1990) note that locus of control frequently is determined by social class, ethnic group membership, and gender. Sue and Sue also emphasize the need to understand locus of responsibility (individual or sociocultural) as defined or identified by each individual. What standard of responsibility does the client hold for himself or herself? What view of the client does the clinician harbor? Culture plays a major role in determining the answers (Amodeo & Jones, 1997; Devore & Schlesinger, 1999). By deferring to a higher power, many French tend to relinquish or negate their sense of individual responsibility. They may avoid assuming responsibility for their drinking problems, attributing them to cultural expectations regarding alcohol consumption. On the other hand, they may more readily commit to a "power greater than oneself," thus supporting the philosophy and popularity of Alcoholics Anonymous (AA) as a viable treatment alternative. Given the hierarchical structure, successful treatment may hinge on having members of the family hierarchy or employment hierarchy demand and/or fully support any treatment initiatives.

Self-Help Groups

Given the typical way French people's relationships unfold, one might expect that self-help groups would not be well received; however, this has not been the case. The French have viewed self-help programs such as AA within their own country quite favorably. The fact that minimal pressure is put on AA members to share information may allow the reticent Frenchmen ample time to enter relationships slowly. Moreover, the anonymity of AA offers an inviting scenario for active and easy participation. Once a relationship with the group is established, it is likely to be enduring, and the likelihood of ongoing participation is strong. The following case illustrates this point.

> George, a middle-aged French Canadian who worked for a U.S. company, was mandated to treatment for alcohol abuse by his company's employee assistance program (EAP). He followed the directive of his EAP counselor by attending a designated treatment that consisted of a Monday-through-Thursday evening program that was run by a recovering alcoholic and a male nurse who had many years of military experience working in a dispensary. Both of these group leaders were assertive and demanding in their expectations of participants. Their demanding nature was quickly replicated by the majority of group members. George felt pressured by their abrasive style. Rather than engaging in treatment, he passively resisted addressing his own alcohol problem. During the 3rd week of his attendance, George started talking to another participant, Marc, who also appeared to be passively resisting the treatment program. Marc told George that this program was nothing like the AA meetings that he had attended in the past. Over the next few sessions, they continued to talk and finally decided to attend an AA meeting together. They both savored the anonymity of the AA group and the flexibility with respect to sharing. Over time, as George became more comfortable with the other members, he began to address the alcohol problem that had been interfering with many aspects of his daily life. The AA members encouraged George to confront his EAP counselor about his dissatisfaction with the mandated treatment program. With their support, George was able to renegotiate his contract and use the AA group as an alternative to the treatment program. He continued to attend meetings and to function better at work and at home.

As might be expected, George followed the directive of his EAP counselor, respecting his authority and opinion; however, he could not relate to the designated program because it failed to address his personal needs for establishing relationships. Once George connected with the appropriate vehicle, his motivation increased, as did his commitment to actively pursue recovery.

Had a culturally sensitive practitioner been involved in George's initial assessment, the length of time between initial contact and actual engagement in successful treatment might have been shortened considerably. Fortunately, George was eventually introduced to a helping approach that addressed his specific needs and dynamics.

Treatment Issues

One factor contributing to the reluctance to enter treatment may be the traditionally slow pace that the French employ in establishing relationships. This could affect both the relationships with others in a treatment program and the relationships with the various professional helpers.

Because of the traditional hierarchical decision-making structure typical of France, the French may be inclined to look to the professional or group leader for answers, many times hoping for authoritarian directives. Given this need, the French client may be somewhat frustrated by the egalitarian or nonhierarchical nature of many treatment programs, including self-help groups.

The respect for authority and the importance of nondirective, nonthreatening relationships may seem contradictory; however, they represent two strong characteristics of French culture—its hierarchical structure and its preference for slow, unfolding development of relationships. Structured, well-defined treatment—at times mandated by authority figures such as work-based programs, parents, or legal or medical authorities—should include a deliberate approach that allows relationships to unfold as a critical component of treatment.

Whereas the case of George illustrates the strong importance he placed on interpersonal relationships and the slow pace required for their development and maturation, the following case illustrates somewhat different treatment needs and dynamics.

> Marie, a 44-year-old French-born woman divorced from an American businessman, was eager to attend AA. It had been recommended by her family doctor, whom she saw after her children begged her to do something about her excessive drinking. Once there, however, she was quite disappointed. She longed for a definite leader who would move the group along and would tell her what she specifically needed to do to cut back on her drinking. She did not want to share her experiences with the other members; rather, she wished to keep her identity private and to be instructed by a person with credentials and authority. She also strongly resented the fact that most of the members in the group were male and that many of them lived in her immediate community. She stopped going to meetings and felt controlled by her drinking. Only later, when referred by her doctor to a culturally sensitive practitioner who was more responsive to her cultural background and per-

sonal needs, including those stemming from her gender, was she able to stop drinking.

Family Treatment

From one perspective, family treatment may be the treatment of choice, considering the importance the French assign to family and their tendency to seek help from within. However, the risk of family collusion is always present, and the strength of traditional French gender roles may interfere with essential communication. For example, alcoholism typically is shrouded by denial on the part of both sexes. French wives frequently tolerate heavy drinking on the part of their husbands, especially if they continue to assume financial responsibility for their families (Langelier, 1996).

Given the importance of family among the French, the therapist must attempt to utilize and build on family cohesiveness. Because the French typically operate with clear delineation of sex roles and accompanying rules of behavior, it may be useful for the therapist to define therapeutic tasks as essential ingredients for good sex-role or family-role performance, for example, helping the client to see the need to address the problem of alcohol or drug abuse as part of his or her responsibility of being the "good" parent or the "good" spouse. In addition, given the French preference for clear assignments and orders, therapeutic assignments should be straightforward, direct, and consistent. Therapeutic recommendations should be measurable and tied to positive reinforcement (Langelier, 1996). For example, telling clients that they must avoid people, places and things associated with drinking may not be enough. It is better to specify that this means not associating with particular individuals—coming directly home from work rather than stopping at the local pub or quitting a particular activity, such as bowling, because heavy drinking is involved. The specific positive reinforcement may include better relations with one's spouse and children or retaining a job that may have been in jeopardy due to alcohol abuse.

The Role of Religion

It is incumbent on the practitioner to assess the cultural influence of religion on a client's behavior. For clients of French background, one cannot address treatment without understanding the dynamics of Catholicism and the influence it might have. As noted earlier, the sacrament of penance, which includes the act of confession, fosters the luxury of forgiveness, as well as the ability to start over, both of which are important issues for substance-abusing clients. The process of confession encourages the act of telling all and of confronting one's most shameful actions, with the ultimate goal of being forgiven and moving on to a new, better level of functioning. Such confession is an important aspect of traditional substance abuse treatment programs, as well as of self-help groups. Considering that confession is an ongoing process, with a religious obligation of participating at least once per year, the edge is taken off any fear or embarrassment of relapse. It is important to note that although this dynamic sets the tone for ongoing encouragement and hope, it may also leave room for deviation from a proposed treatment plan and the acceptance of relapse.

In addition, French clients with a Catholic background have the potential of transferring onto the therapist the role typically filled by the parish priest: the role of confidant, omnipotent advisor, distributor of penance or other avenues of restitution, purveyor of the parameters of acceptable behavior, and patriarch with higher authority. Although some of these aspects may lead to positive therapeutic outcomes, the clinician must anticipate and address these dynamics and their implications.

Culturally Shaped Treatment Approaches

Not only must the clinician assess the influence of culture but he or she also has the responsibility of shaping treatment to accommodate identified cultural (and gender) diversity. The clinician must keep in mind that most treatment programs were developed by and for White males of European ancestry (Abbott, 1994, 1995; Hayton, 1994). Thus some programs may be appropriate for French males but totally lacking in appropriateness for their female counterparts. Treatment protocols may be employed with successful outcomes in many cultures but be totally ineffective in others. For example, in a culture that is accepting, almost demanding, of everyday use of alcohol, a culture with a higher incidence of delta than gamma alcoholism, how can treatment address the concept of abstinence?

To a person of French heritage whose family has always incorporated wine as a key component of any social and business gathering, the idea of abstinence may seem totally contradictory to the basic tenets of life. A gradual, eye-opening exploration and assessment of the negative impact of alcohol may be necessary to alter a lifelong belief that alcohol is an essential component of daily living. The involvement of peers who have tackled alcohol abuse may help to generate commitment and ease the path to recovery. It may also be more tenable to the client to start with an approach based on "controlled," gradually diminishing drinking.

The skill of the practitioner comes in his or her ability to understand the role that the French cultural heritage plays in contributing to, maintaining, and overcoming a substance abuse problem with each individual client.

In treating George or Marie it would be essential to understand the role assigned to alcohol in their respective cultural, familial, and personal contexts, the conflicts created by substance abuse in each context, and the impact a change would render in each context. It would be important to identify their views on locus of control and locus of responsibility. Marie, for example, viewed locus of control and locus of responsibility as being primarily housed in others. She believed she drank because others in specific situations expected it and that she could not change without rigid external help. George, on the other hand, believed he could change but felt that the external world held the key to unleashing his abilities. He initially responded to a hierarchical demand that he engage in treatment, but instead of rigid control he sought warm acceptance and reinforcement.

To expect both of these clients to fit the same treatment mold would result in less than desirable outcomes (Abbott, 1994, 1995). The fact that treatment options were available to address their unique needs was of critical importance; what was of greater importance was a clinician who could recognize their cultural and individual differences, develop responsive treatment strategies, or refer them to viable existing alternatives.

CONCLUSION

The French, and others from French-derived cultures such as the French Canadian, have a unique and varied history, one that differs greatly from other European countries. To be effective with clients of various cultural backgrounds "requires that workers develop the means to understand the salient aspects of culture for the individual in treatment. . . . In substance abuse treatment, multiculturalism is the perspective that the client can best be helped to overcome substance abuse problems by understanding the unique cultural heritage of each individual" (Dyer, 1994, p. 33). For example, different strategies may be warranted when working with clients from cultures that forbid or challenge the use of alcohol than those that endorse or encourage its use.

Some general parameters for understanding behavior were introduced in this chapter; however, it is up to the clinician to assess how each individual client manifests his or her cultural heritage. One can use generalization to guide overall program development and intervention design; however, to be effective, one must translate generalizations to necessary culturally sensitive, gender-specific, individually relevant interventions. The content presented in this chapter should help the clinician move toward achieving the goals of ethnoculturally sensitive practice with substance-abusing clients of French origin.

REFERENCES

Abbott, A. A. (1994). A feminist approach to substance abuse treatment and service delivery. *Social Work in Health Care, 19*(3/4), 67–83.

Abbott, A. A. (1995). Substance abuse and the feminist perspective. In N. Van Den Berth (Ed.), *Feminist practice in the 21st century* (pp. 258–277). Washington, DC: National Association of Social Workers Press.

Amodeo, M., & Jones, L. K. (1997). Viewing alcohol and other drug use cross culturally: A cultural framework for clinical practice. *Families in Society 78*(3), 240–254.

Babor, T. F. (1992). Cross-cultural research on alcohol: A quoi bon? In J. E. Helzer & G. J. Canino (Eds.), *Alcoholism in North America, Europe, and Asia* (pp. 33–52). New York: Oxford University Press.

Babor, T. F., Hasselbrock, M., Radouco-Thomas, S., Feguer, L., Ferrant, J.-P., & Choguette, K. (1986). Concepts of alcoholism among American, French-Canadian, and French alcoholics. In T. F. Babor (Ed.), *Alcohol and culture: Comparative perspectives from Europe and America* (pp. 98–109). New York: Academy of Sciences.

Babor, T. F., Wolfson, A., Boivin, D., Radouco-Thomas, S., & Clark, W. (1992). Alcoholism, culture, and psychopathology: A comparative study of French, French Canadian, and American alcoholics. In J. E. Helzer & G. J. Canino (Eds.), *Alcoholism in North America, Europe, and Asia* (pp. 182–195). New York: Oxford University Press.

Barkan, E. R. (1980). French Canadians. In S. Thernstrom (Ed.), *Harvard encyclopedia of American ethnic groups* (pp. 388–401). Cambridge MA: Harvard University Press.

Bianquis-Gasser, I. (1992). Wine and men in Alsace, France. In D. Gefon-Madianou (Ed.), *Alcohol, gender, and culture* (pp. 101–107). London: Routledge.

Brennan, T. E. (1988). *Public drinking and popular culture in eighteenth-century Paris.* Princeton, NJ: Princeton University Press.

Brennan, T. E. (1989). Toward the cultural history of alcohol in France. *Journal of Social History, 23,* 71–92.

Carroll, R. (1987). *Cultural misunderstandings: The French-American experience.* Chicago: University of Chicago Press.

Devore, W., & Schlesinger, E. G. (1999). *Ethnic-sensitive social work practice* (5th ed.). Needham Heights, MA: Allyn & Bacon.

d'Houtaud, A., Adriaanse, H., & Field, M. G. (1989). Alcohol consumption in France: Production, consumption, morbidity and mortality, prevention and education in the last three decades. *Advances in Alcohol and Substance Abuse, 8*(1), 19–44.

Dyer, L. (1994). Problems of definition. In J. U. Gordon (Ed.), *Managing multiculturalism in substance abuse services* (pp. 22–41). Thousand Oaks, CA: Sage.

Facy, F., & Verron, M. (1989). Drug abuse in France: A review of statistical data. *Drug and Alcohol Dependence, 24*(1), 1–9.

Fedunkiw, M. (1995). French-Canadian Americans. In J. Galens, A. Sheets, & R. V.

Young (Eds.) & R. J. Vecoli (Contributing Ed.), *Gale encyclopedia of multicultural America* (Vol. 1, pp. 546–564). Detroit, MI: Gale Research.

Gannon, M. J., & Associates. (1994). *Understanding global cultures: Metaphorical journeys through 17 countries.* Thousand Oaks, CA: Sage.

Glazer, N., & Moynihan, D. P. (1970). *Beyond the melting pot: The Negroes, Puerto Ricans, Jews, Italians, and Irish of New York City* (2nd ed.). Cambridge, MA: MIT Press.

Hall, E. T., & Hall, M. R. (1990). *Understanding cultural differences.* Yarmouth, ME: Intercultural Press.

Hayton, R. (1994). European American perspective: Some considerations. In J. U. Gordon (Ed.), *Managing multiculturalism in substance abuse services* (pp. 99–116). Thousand Oaks, CA: Sage.

Higonnet, P. L. R. (1980). French. In S. Thernstrom (Ed.), *Harvard encyclopedia of American ethnic groups* (pp. 379–388). Cambridge, MA: Harvard University Press.

Hillstrom, L. C. (1995). French Americans. In J. Galens, A. Sheets, & R. V. Young (Eds.) & R. J. Vecoli (Contributing Ed.), *Gale encyclopedia of multicultural America* (Vol. 1, pp. 533–545). Detroit, MI: Gale Research.

Hofstede, G. (1980). *Culture's consequences.* Beverly Hills, CA: Sage.

Jellinek, E. M. (1960). *The disease concept of alcoholism.* New Haven, CT: Hillhouse Press.

Jellinek, E. M. (1962). Cultural differences in the meaning of alcoholism. In D. J. Pittman & C. R. Snyder (Eds.), *Society, culture and drinking patterns* (pp. 382–394). New York: Wiley.

Kaplan, A. (1993). *French lessons.* Chicago: University of Chicago Press.

Kinney, J., & Leaton, G. (1995). *Loosening the grip: A handbook of alcohol information* (5th ed.). St. Louis: Mosby.

Kissin, B. (1977). Theory and practice in the treatment of alcoholism. In B. Kissin & H. Begleiter (Eds.), *Treatment and rehabilitation of the chronic alcoholic* (pp. 1–51). New York: Plenum Press.

Kole, W. J. (1995, September 16). A new limit on drinking and driving. *Philadelphia Inquirer,* p. A2.

Langelier, R. (1996). French Canadian families. In M. McGoldrick, J. K. Pearce, & J. Giordano (Eds.), *Ethnicity and family therapy* (2nd ed., pp. 477–495). New York: Guilford Press.

Morrison, T., Conaway, W. A., & Borden, G. A. (1994). *Kiss, bow, or shake hands.* Holbrook, MA: Bob Adams.

Mosse, P. (1992). The rise of alcohology in France: A monopolistic competition. In H. Klingemann, J. P. Takala, & G. Hunt (Eds.), *Cure, care, or control: Alcoholism treatment in sixteen countries* (pp. 205–221). Albany: State University of New York Press.

Parrillo, V. N. (1994). *Strangers to these shores: Race and ethnic relations in the United States* (4th ed.). New York: Macmillan.

Ray, O., & Ksir, C. (1999). *Drugs, society, and human behavior* (8th ed.) Boston: WCB/McGraw-Hill.

Remy, M., Soukup-Stepan, S., & Tatossian, A. (1988). Study of social support in a sample of French alcoholic women. In R. Nordmann, C. Ribiere, & H. Rouach (Eds.), *Alcohol toxicity and free radical mechanisms* (pp. 331–335). New York: Pergamon Press.

Rivers, P. C. (1994). *Alcohol and human behavior: Theory, research, and practice.* Englewood Cliffs, NJ: Prentice Hall.

Rush, B. R., & Ogborne, A. C. (1992). Alcoholism treatment in Canada: History, current status, and emerging issues. In H. Klingemann, J. P. Takala, & G. Hunt (Eds.), *Cure, care, or control: Alcoholism treatment in sixteen countries* (pp. 253–267). Albany: State University of New York Press.

Steinberg, S. (1981). *The ethnic myth: Race, ethnicity, and class in America.* New York: Atheneum.

Sue, D. W., & Sue, D. (1990). *Counseling the culturally different: Theory and practice* (2nd ed.). New York: Wiley.

Sulkunen, P. (1989). Drinking in France 1965–1979: An analysis of household consumption data. *British Journal of Addictions, 84,* 61.

van Wormer, K. S. (1995). *Alcoholism treatment: A social work perspective.* Chicago: Nelson-Hall.

10

The Irish and Substance Abuse

Philip O'Dwyer

The production and use of alcohol is embedded in the cultural fabric of the people of Ireland. The use of other drugs enjoys no such cultural accommodation and, as a result, is proportionally in minimal evidence. But culture, like patterns of substance use, is not a static entity (Cheung, 1993). In Ireland profound cultural changes are discernible, whereas among Irish Americans, the level of cultural affinity to Ireland varies as generations grow more distant from the Emerald Isle. It is difficult to predict the configuration of cultural traits or the level of ethnic affinity that may influence a client's behavior. Yet it seems essential for the clinician to have a sense of the dominant themes of the cultural heritage that may enter the therapeutic process. It is equally important to realize that Irish Americans, as an ethnocultural group, represent a variety of subgroups associated with "the Ireland" they left.

Although the heavy-drinking Irishman is a cultural stereotype, some researchers question the influence of ethnicity as determinative of drinking patterns. They claim that demographic variables such as education, income, age, and marital status may have a significant influence on ethnocultural drinking patterns (Wilson & Williams, 1989). Nonetheless, the values and perceptions that surround alcohol and drug use in any culture seem important, although demographic variables may facilitate or hinder their expression at various times.

This chapter introduces the clinician to the Irish people and to the key cultural features of their history and offers insight into the role of alcohol in Irish life and the current use of other substances in Ireland. Common treatment issues are reviewed and clinical guidelines are recommended. An understanding of why the Irish tend to abuse alcohol may provide clues to effective prevention strategies.

Although the entire history of Ireland cannot be reviewed, some historical events will be recounted because of their imprint on the Irish psyche. This chapter chiefly focuses on the Catholic Irish, for whom their ethnic identity is still a highly significant aspect of their lives.

HISTORY AND CULTURAL HERITAGE

Ireland is a small island, about the size of Indiana, yet its cultural influence in the world seems out of proportion to its total population of slightly over 5 million. McGoldrick (1982, 1996) describes the Irish people as being full of paradoxes: They are verbally skilled yet are tongue-tied on emotional issues; they assume responsibility yet are quick to blame; they are jovial and friendly yet avoid tenderness and affection. These paradoxes capture both the appeal and the anguish of the Irish, as this brief look at Irish historical and cultural characteristics shows.

British Occupation

The character of the Irish people was formed by centuries of political unrest and uncertainty. For more than eight centuries the British sought to dominate Ireland and its people. Once they captured regions of the country, they replaced many of the Irish farmers with loyal Protestants from London and other cities. This practice was called plantation. The plantation of Ulster in the 17th century had left the six counties of Northern Ireland predominantly Protestant and its people seeking to remain under the aegis of the British government. A 1921 treaty created a division of the island, with Northern Ireland remaining a province of the United Kingdom, whereas the remaining 26 counties formed the Republic of Ireland, whose population is 92% Catholic.

Although many prominent Protestant Irish contributed greatly to the Irish culture through the arts and politics, most do not see themselves as Irish. Protestant Irish immigrants to the United States tended to marry outside of their ethnic group (Fallows, 1979) and to avoid the designation of "Irish" by using the description of "Scots-Irish" (Griffin, 1992). Many have lost their sense of Irish identity, unlike most Catholic Irish.

Famine and Emigration

Disaster struck in 1845 when the potato crop failed due to a plant disease called "the Blight." Famine, exacerbated by the confiscation and exportation of available food by the British (Woodham-Smith, 1963), stalked the land. Consequently, more than 1 million people died of starvation and another million emigrated to North America and elsewhere. A new trend emerged in Irish history: Emigration became tradition. Since 1845, more than 7 million people have left the shores of Ireland for distant lands (Neill, 1979).

Family Dynamics

A common Irish cultural characteristic is the experience of guilt associated with success and material goods. Any display of opulence or pretense to success incurs withering disapproval. Those who prosper have been viewed as being deceptive in some way, such as receiving money as a reward for supplying information to the British. Many of the Irish saw consorting with the enemy as more reprehensible than being the enemy itself. Strong tendencies to preserve privacy, especially with regard to family issues, are common, and few people outside the priest can be trusted with such information. This trait creates difficulty for many clinicians.

Even within the family, it is common that family problems go undiscussed, especially if there is perceived shame associated with the problem (McGoldrick, 1982, 1996). Behavior that threatens the moral respectability of the family, such as a wife's drinking or a son's drug abuse, will likely be shame inducing and, when possible, will be withheld from others in the family. Unresolved problems create distance and resentment and, finally, the unspoken sentence of isolation. Pride and the need to keep up appearances forces many to choose to suffer alone rather than cause embarrassment to the family (McGoldrick, 1982, 1996).

Intergenerational and gender boundaries are strong, and, as a result, communication is more likely to occur within the same generation and gender (Hines, Garcia-Preto, McGoldrick, Almeida, & Weltmann, 1992). It is important that clinicians appreciate the impact of this dynamic on data gathering.

Use of Language

Like many oppressed people, the Irish tend to use metaphor, innuendo, and ambiguity to obscure and disguise their meaning (McGoldrick, 1982,

1996). Thus, although they have an engaging style, the Irish often speak a language that can easily confuse the outsider. As noted by Morton (1978), "Talk in Ireland is a game with no rules" (p. 20). Clinicians who are accustomed to directness may find that their Irish clients exhibit a mastery of indirect use of language. Objective truth is less significant than telling a story with flair. Clients may provide little information when questioned and try to distract the questioner from an unacceptable line of discussion. O'hEithir (1987) claims that for the Irish, words become a form of action that ultimately renders action unnecessary. Therapeutic issues that have been discussed may seem to many Irish clients to be resolved—without requiring any behavioral change.

Role of the Church

It is difficult to overstate the power of the Catholic bishops in Ireland. The bishops ensured that the laws of the land were consistent with Catholic teaching, especially on issues such as divorce and abortion. Dissident voices were quickly silenced.

The Church effectively controlled education for decades. Although these schools were outstanding, male and female roles were clearly defined and kept separate. The Church's teachings on sex and sexuality focused on "sins of the flesh." The consequent sexual repression resulted in the avoidance of overt tenderness and affection among many Irish couples. The emphasis on sexual acts rather than on relationships has been viewed as resulting in feelings of guilt regarding sexuality and the inability of many Irish Catholics to have fulfilling intimate relationships (Buckley, 1994). Drinking alcohol has been seen as providing a temporary remedy for this guilt (Teehan, 1988).

Traditional Catholic theology's view of the world as a "valley of tears" offered comfort to a population who suffered under brutal penal laws and frequent famines. Suffering was to be accepted as a natural consequence of one's sinful nature. This may explain the general fatalistic tendency of the Irish (McGoldrick, 1982). This metaphysical approach to life may provide a coherent way of understanding suffering but does little to reduce its sting. Alcohol appears to be the elixir of choice to dispel the gloom and make painful situations tolerable (Teehan, 1988).

Irish Culture in Transition

Since the 1960s, major changes in Irish society have occurred that have led many to describe the Ireland of the late 1990s as a "new Ireland."

The reforms of the Catholic Church in the early 1960s converged with improved access to advanced education, increased economic opportunities, and an expanding media—the result being the development of the "new Ireland."

THE IRISH IN THE UNITED STATES

The Irish frequently claim that St. Brendan, an Irish abbot, was the first European to arrive in America, almost 1,000 years before Columbus. Although this claim remains in dispute, Irish immigration to the United States since the Great Famine is well documented. More than 43 million Americans now consider themselves to be of Irish descent (Griffin, 1992).

Almost 2 million Irish Catholics settled along the East Coast of the United States between 1830 and 1860. By 1870, one in five voters in New York City had been born in Ireland. Their living conditions were unpleasant; the Irish were subjected to massive social discrimination and were generally viewed with derision (Lender & Martin, 1982). Familiar with institutional violence and injustice at the hands of the British, the Irish knew how to resist it. They deepened their allegiance to the Catholic Church, shaped its growth in America, built their own parochial schools, and established their own civic organizations (Lender & Martin, 1982). These actions served to keep the Irish cohesive as a group and made them a force to be reckoned with once they entered the political process.

During the 1980s, Irish immigration to the United States began to increase following a decline during the previous 20 years (Griffin, 1992), although numerous undocumented immigrants make it difficult to get precise numbers. These immigrants from the "new Ireland" are more educated, articulate, self-confident, and self-directed than their predecessors. They are not given to the guilt of their ancestors. Gone, too, is the limiting concern about what the neighbors will think. Many see themselves as citizens of the world who have warm feelings for the land of their birth. They still have the lilting brogue and are only slightly more direct in expression. Many still like to drink; however, they are more open to therapy.

ROLE OF DRINKING IN IRISH CULTURE

That the Irish who drink drink heavily seems beyond dispute, yet the cause of this phenomenon, as well as the full scope of the problem, has received little scholarly attention (Greeley, 1981; Stivers, 1976). *Uisce beatha* is the

Gaelic term for whiskey, generally translated as "blessed water." Alcohol in all its forms has played a significant role in Irish life.

In the early 18th century, the invention of gin led to a period of heavy drinking throughout Britain and Ireland (Stivers, 1976). For the next 100 years, abstinence movements made significant progress in containing this gin epidemic, and it is estimated that more than half the people of Ireland were total abstainers prior to the Great Famine of the late 1840s (Greeley, 1981). However, heavy drinking became a widespread method of coping with the devastation of the famine. Moreover, young males displayed their masculinity by "drinking like men," implying a demonstration of tolerance for alcohol. Such excessive male drinking has been seen as a form of compensation for the scarcity of opportunity to attain adulthood through land ownership or marriage (Stivers, 1976).

Concern about giving legitimacy to the stereotype of the Irish as heavy drinkers has caused the extent of drinking problems among the Irish to be discounted or minimized. For example, the low reported death rates from liver disease and cirrhosis (Stivers, 1976) may be explained by the reluctance of many physicians to identify these conditions as the cause of death on death certificates in order to spare families perceived embarrassment associated with the stigma of alcoholism. Yet, when consumption rates are analyzed, taking into consideration that 11% of Irish men and 23% of Irish women are lifetime abstainers and that a high percentage of the population of Ireland is under the age of 15, we can conclude that a large percentage of Irish men drink heavily (Harrison, Carrhill, & Sutton, 1993).

The Role of the Pub

The pub in Ireland serves as a social center. There neighbors meet, exchange stories, and celebrate whatever is topical. As a symbol of manliness, acceptance, and affirmation, there is an obligatory practice of "treating" or "standing your round" in Irish pubs (Stivers, 1976). In practical terms, this custom means that if five people enter a pub together, each one in turn is expected to purchase a round of drinks and therefore to consume five drinks. This practice often results in individuals consuming more alcohol in order to avoid being labeled as "not standing."

The Pledge

During the early part of the 19th century, some Church leaders grew concerned about the excessive use of alcohol (Malcolm, 1986), and through the tenacity of Father Theobald Matthew, the Pioneer Total Abstinence Association was founded in 1835. The movement gave spiritual meaning to abstaining from alcohol and required its members to recite certain prayers for the sins of intemperance. It became common for adolescents to take a pledge to abstain from alcohol until at least age 21; most children still make that promise today.

An unintended consequence of the Pioneer movement to this day is the Irish tendency to view alcohol in extreme terms—that is, good versus evil; abstinent versus drunk. For this reason, the Irish are likely to deal with an alcohol problem by embracing abstinence more easily than other ethnic groups do (Valliant, 1983). Ireland has a higher proportion of lifetime abstainers than almost any country outside the Islamic world (Malcolm, 1986).

Use of Other Drugs

Ireland is similar to most countries in that a wide variety of drugs have become available in the past 20 years. Unlike alcoholism, drug addiction is largely unacceptable in the Irish culture. It exists in the major cities chiefly among unemployed youth and is frequently associated with youth violence. It is now estimated that there are 5,000 heroin abusers in Dublin (Cusack, 1996), and marijuana use is common in urban areas, but the preference for alcohol is so dominant that all other addictions pale by comparison. Vigilante groups have been known to violently put drug pushers out of business. Some authors have claimed that the drug problem in the major cities of Ireland is more extensive than is generally acknowledged (Henderson, 1994) and is enhanced by the Irish tendency to avoid talking about it.

Irish Women and Their Use of Alcohol and Other Drugs

In the Irish family women play a dominant role, which they execute skillfully. They tend to make all significant decisions while giving the appearance that the father is the authority and head of the house. The mother in the home, like the priest in the community, enforces the moral code (Stivers, 1976).

Traditionally, Irish women received equal educational opportunity, which may account for their high representation among the professions (Greeley, 1981). Their role is generally more empowered than in other cultures, and they seem to be aware of that power. It is common for young Irish women to be convinced that they can change the drinking behavior of a fiancé once they are married. When this plan becomes unattainable, they are generally praised for "putting up with himself" and fall into the role of martyr. For these Catholic women, leaving an alcoholic husband is not seen as an option —these wives have "made their bed" and now they "must sleep in it."

Drinking patterns among Irish women have dramatically changed since 1960, resulting in substantial increases in consumption (Corrigan & Butler, 1991). Traditional Irish women seldom drink, but when they do it is usually done at home, alone. Contemporary Irish women drink with men in social situations, although problem drinking for women is severely sanctioned by the culture. Social disapproval of alcoholism among women is very strong, leading to very high levels of denial. In one study (Corrigan & Butler, 1991), 53% of the female patients attempted to deny their drinking, even though they were in treatment for the problem, and fully 61% had prior inpatient treatment. Fifty-eight percent of these women also used tranquilizers, 55% used sleeping pills, and 13% used marijuana (Corrigan & Butler, 1991).

Irish Adolescent Drinking

Although the Irish accept heavy drinking in men as being normal, in general, parents tend to insist on abstinence from their adolescent children, who often drink secretively. Adolescent access to alcohol in Irish pubs is restricted by government legislation, although it is not uniformly enforced. There are scant data on high school drinking patterns in Ireland. In one study by Grube, Morgan, and Kearney (1989), 47% of high school students reported using alcohol at least once in the previous 30 days, which is slightly below comparable studies of adolescent behavior in the United States. This study identified significant gender differences with regard to alcohol use: Males were six times more likely than females to have used alcohol.

Intravenous Drug Use and AIDS

During the early 1990s, there were close to 1,500 documented cases of HIV seropositivity in Ireland (Bradley, Bury, O'Kelly, & Shannon, 1993; Henderson, 1994). These numbers may have been understated because AIDS is still considered a "gay disease," and many infected people attempt to keep their condition secret (Henderson, 1994). Ireland has a much higher proportion of HIV transmission through intravenous drug use than do many other European countries (Johnson et al., 1994). Between 1990 and 1992, intravenous (IV) drug use accounted for 89% of all HIV patients who presented for treatment (Desmond, Murphy, Plunkett, & Mulcahy, 1993), and a needle exchange program in Dublin found that one in six participants were HIV seropositive (Johnson et al., 1994).

The rate of AIDS infection among women and children has been rising dramatically (Henderson, 1994). The stigma associated with IV drug use by women socially inhibits them from purchasing sterile syringes and needles; thus needle sharing is more common among women, placing them at increased risk of developing HIV and hepatitis C (Barnard, 1993; Smyth, Keenan, Dorman, & O'Connor, 1994).

ALCOHOL AND DRUG USE
AMONG IRISH-AMERICANS

Evidence of alcohol problems among the Irish in America in the second half of the 19th century and the early and mid-1900s can be seen in the numbers of arrests for drunkenness and disorderly conduct and of alcohol-related deaths. In these categories, the Irish ethnocultural group outranked all other nationalities. A study of admissions to all hospitals in New York between 1929 and 1931 concluded that alcohol-related admissions of Irish people were substantially higher than those for all other ethnocultural groups (Stivers, 1976). Moreover, a 1950 study of arrests for "drunkenness" in the state of Connecticut showed that Irish Americans had the highest percentage of arrests among the 10 ethnocultural groups studied, and studies of alcohol consumption rates during 1960 placed those of Irish background above all others with regard to heavy drinking (Stivers, 1976). Yet another study found that 51% of the Irish-born males admitted to New York psychiatric hospitals had alcohol-related diagnoses, whereas only 4% of Italian-born men had similar diagnoses (Muhlin, 1985).

Despite these findings, some people believe that the Irish have been unfairly stereotyped as heavy drinkers and that this stereotype emerged from Irish immigrants in England and the United States in the early part of this century. These immigrants were frequently overrepresented by young, single males who were hard workers, drank excessively, and were not strangers to the police (Walsh, 1987). Some later studies even showed that the Irish American drinking patterns were within the norm for all Americans (Stivers, 1976).

Current data on drinking problems among Irish Americans are scarce because more recent studies tend to investigate drinking and drug use patterns among African Americans, Hispanic Americans, Native Americans, and Caucasians in general and do not focus on distinctions among ethnic Caucasians. However, a recent study by the National Opinion Research

Center found that 40% of Irish Americans indicated that a drinking problem existed in their homes during their childhoods (National Opinion Research Center, 1997), reflecting a very high rate of alcohol-related problems.

Studies also indicate that the Irish consume alcohol to relieve stress and that they frequently deliberately seek intoxication (National Opinion Research Center, 1997). These findings confirm those of an earlier comparison study of alcoholics in treatment in Ireland and Canada by Teehan (1988). Teehan found that the Irish drank for relief from painful feelings or for mood alteration, whereas the Canadian alcoholics drank for social facilitation and sexual enhancement (Teehan, 1988). The "painful feelings" that were identified by the Irish included guilt, low self-esteem, and anxiety.

Nonetheless, the impact of negative stereotyping on drinking among Irish Americans cannot be overlooked, because it is both imposed and accepted. Irish Americans may drink more than the native Irish in large part because they are expected to do so to fulfill the prevailing cultural stereotype. They seem to accept these expectations—making it a self-fulfilling prophecy (Greeley, 1981; Stivers, 1976). The Irish in Ireland have no such stereotype to fulfill and so are spared this method of demonstrating their "Irishness." It is theoretically possible that the Irish American stereotype may extend back to Ireland in the future—the result of tourism, telecommunication, and the appeal of the stereotype itself.

For the Irish Americans, the pub continues its role as a social center in the United States. Irish immigrants and their offspring find hospitality, exchange leads on employment opportunities, meet fellow Irish people, and are regaled with Irish music and song in these pubs. Because the pub has such a significant social dimension, it is difficult for those in recovery programs to avoid the feeling of isolation associated with not going to the pub. This is an important issue that has to be addressed during treatment.

CLINICAL INTERVENTIONS

The development of a therapeutic relationship is central to all effective therapy. In dealing with the Irish, it is essential to keep a friendly distance. The first step should be to determine the level of cultural identification. Individual clients of Irish background may range from those who hold to traditional Irish values to those who may have minimal knowledge of either

Ireland or its culture. Those who were raised in Irish enclaves in the United States are more likely to have significant exposure to their Irish heritage and to have a close psychological attachment to their Irish ethnicity.

Clients influenced by the more traditional culture are usually older and more restricted in sharing their feelings. When working with such clients, the clinician should avoid exploring feelings and adopt a more didactic approach. For example, appealing to the client's sense of responsibility is usually a more effective, culturally syntonic strategy. Every opportunity should be taken throughout treatment to affirm the client and bolster self-esteem. The use of instructional videotapes that highlight priests in recovery may help to reduce the sense of guilt and shame likely to be felt by many such clients. Many find Alcoholics Anonymous (AA) appealing and helpful. Shy, cynical, and even supercilious people seem miraculously unembarrassed at AA meetings (O'Faolain, 1996).

The clinician should be particularly attentive to understatements by clients of Irish background. Any reference to physical pain or emotional discomfort should be closely evaluated, because it is likely to be much more severe than the client is willing to admit. In general, male clients may resist family involvement, wanting to handle things on their own. This preference enables the client to deemphasize the effect of the problem on others. When families do participate, their learning about addiction and recovery should be the first objective. Some family members may resist going to Al-Anon due to a strong reluctance to talk about family issues with strangers.

Direct confrontation may alienate the client of Irish background. In many cases it will be unnecessary, because Irish clients tend to invest the clinician with great expertise and are likely to comply, although at their own pace. However, the compliance may be a gesture of politeness rather than a sign of genuine change. The so-called intervention (Casolaro & Smith, 1993; Johnson, 1986) whereby a group of family members and friends, under the guidance of the therapist, confront the client is usually seen as an ambush. It often increases the sense of shame and may be greeted with intransigence. Support, not confrontation, will yield superior results. It may be productive to apply the adage: "You are not responsible for your addiction, but you are responsible for your recovery."

Tests for alcohol dependence should be carefully chosen. The CAGE assessment test (Ewing, 1984; Straussner, 1993) is useful and nonthreatening, and its use in Ireland has shown it to be a more effective screen for alcohol problems than the Michigan Alcoholism Screening Test (Schofield, 1991).

As indicated earlier, patterns of indirect communication are frequently more natural to the Irish; therefore, the clinician who is specific and direct is likely to be seen as impolite or rude. The challenge then becomes one of adaptation to a more subtle verbal communication with constant need to "read between the lines."

Time and space are also important considerations in the therapeutic process. Clinicians follow a schedule of appointments and must usually end at specific times. However, Irish clients who sense that they are being rushed may interpret this as a reflection of their unimportance. Managing each therapeutic session so that the client feels that he or she is welcome and is a priority becomes important. A warm handshake at the beginning and conclusion of each session and the use of the client's preferred version of his or her first name could convey that sentiment. In addition, respect for personal boundaries is highly valued among the Irish. Such respect may be reflected through the level of eye contact. Culturally, the Irish are likely to see constant eye contact as overly intrusive, penetrating, and ultimately disrespectful. A more casual and distant approach is generally less threatening.

Although confidentiality is always important, it is especially critical when working with Irish clients. The undocumented immigration status of some only adds to their sensitivity to this issue. Usually the concern about confidentiality declines when clients become more accepting of their alcohol or drug problems.

The notion of "paying to talk" is troublesome to many traditional Irish. In a curious paradox, those of Irish background revere the art of language usage yet may see little value in talking about problems. The expectation that they should pay for such talk challenges their sense of propriety. This issue is further complicated by a cultural theme that prohibits talking about problems lest they "become worse in the talking." This superstitious belief causes many to avoid using words such as "cancer" when referring to someone's diagnosis. Instead, euphemisms such as "the lad" or "the lodger" are used in order to avoid the perceived negative implications of the word itself. In the same vein, it is best to avoid words such as "alcoholic" or "addict," and references to alcohol or drug problems should be used sparingly.

It is suggested that clinicians distance themselves from collecting professional fees and, when possible, allow office staff to handle this aspect of treatment provision. Although the private practitioner can bill the client, it is important not to imply any concern that the bill will go unpaid. A hint of doubt about the client's integrity will usually damage the therapeutic relationship and may end it without explanation. If an explanation is offered, it will be a positive face-saving reason unrelated to the truth, which the clinician may never discover.

Clinicians dealing with clients from the modern Irish culture or those acculturated to American values will find them more willing participants in therapy. Direct focus on substance abuse as the key problem and involvement of family members will be accepted much more readily. Feelings, relationships, and communication patterns can be explored gently but more directly.

Because AA is a useful adjunct to treatment, it can provide an important alternative to the pub. In addition, any concern regarding social isolation can be countered by encouraging participation in Irish social events such as those designed to provide financial assistance to Irish missionaries in Third World countries. These events are common in most major cities in the United States. There are also branches of the Irish Pioneer Total Abstinence Association throughout the country. Interventions that enable clients to deal with emotions or the daily stresses of life are likely to be important in preventing relapse.

A CLINICAL VIGNETTE

Pat is a 57-year-old Irish-born electrician who presented for treatment for alcohol problems following his third arrest for drunk driving. He was ordered by the court to participate in treatment, and failure to do so would result in a jail sentence.

Pat had immigrated to the United States 37 years before and still retained a distinctive Tipperary accent. He was driven to therapy by his wife of 25 years. When the clinician asked Pat to describe his reason for coming to therapy he replied:

> "A brat of a cop tried to tell me that I was drunk and shouldn't be driving. You know these people [Americans] don't know who we [the Irish] are at all. They don't know when to mind their own business. By the way, the young lady you have in the office is doing you no good, you wouldn't believe all the signing of papers I had to do. . . . You see, the judge sent me over to have a word with you for a few minutes and then everything would be the finest."

It was clear to the clinician that Pat was putting him on notice that:

1. He had no problem with alcohol and it would be disrespectful to accuse him of having such a problem.
2. The clinician was likely not to understand the Irish drinking pat-

terns and may therefore conclude that a problem existed when it was just "normal" drinking.

3. He had reinterpreted the judge's decision in a benign fashion.
4. He was offering advice to the clinician regarding his office staff to deflect discussion from himself.

The culturally aware clinician then casually asked, "Pat, tell me about your family," as though ignoring the alcohol problem. Midway through the session the clinician circled back to the drinking issue in a nonthreatening manner. Now that some level of comfort had developed in the relationship, the therapist asserted, "Well, I know, Pat, that if a problem existed with alcohol you would be the first to want to take care of it." This was followed by a short lecture from Pat on his belief about "doing what's right." This opened the door to explore the quantity and frequency of Pat's consumption of alcohol. This was a slow process due to Pat's stories. When the therapist indicated that he would like to speak with Pat's wife, he was quickly told "don't let on to herself about how much I have been drinking . . . this was just between me and you."

As the interview verified, Pat's wife had no knowledge of how much he drank but could identify the many hours he spent in the pub. Her primary concern was helping Pat "get out of the trouble with the judge—I would die if he had to go to jail. No one knows about this problem . . . we have one kid in college and two kids graduated from college and they don't know a word about daddy's drinking problem." "It must be hard to deal with all that," said the clinician, showing great understanding. Mrs. B straightened up in her chair and said, "Well, that is a cross God sent us and we must accept it. Pat is a good man." She did not want to discuss her feelings about Pat's drinking.

At the conclusion of the first session the clinician saw both Mr. and Mrs. B together for a brief summary, taking time to assure both of confidentiality and of the main focus of doing what the judge wanted, and finally suggesting a willingness to join forces with Pat to see if in fact there may be a little problem with alcohol. A final handshake and a scheduled second appointment concluded the session. Meanwhile, Pat agreed to "stop drinking for the moment until we see what's what."

By the third session, Pat was willing to go to an AA meeting—"for educational purposes." Within a short time, Pat embraced recovery, not because he was "an alcoholic" but because he was "too old to be drinking like that." The therapeutic approach consisted of a brief, solution-focused therapy with strong didactic elements that did not focus on exploring Pat's feelings.

CONCLUSION

Addiction to alcohol or drugs is a complex issue to treat in itself. It can be further complicated by cultural factors that may serve as a barrier between client and clinician. The Irish have more than their share of alcohol problems, but when handled with sensitivity they will embrace abstinence more easily than other ethnic groups. The key is to appreciate indirect language so that a therapeutic relationship can be established. A willingness to "talk around" an issue will usually be beneficial. Over time, the therapeutic process can become more direct, although increasing emotional awareness may be a slow process.

REFERENCES

Barnard, M. (1993). Needle sharing in context: Patterns of sharing among men and women injectors and HIV risks. *Addiction, 88*, 805–812.

Bradley, F., Bury, G., O'Kelly, F., & Shannon, W. (1993). Irish general practice and the human immunodeficiency virus. *Irish Medical Journal, 86*(5), 152–153.

Buckley, P. (1994). *A thorn in the side*. Dublin: O'Brien Press.

Casolaro, V., & Smith, R. J. (1993). The process of intervention: Getting alcoholics and drug abusers to treatment. In S. L. A. Straussner (Ed.), *Clinical work with substance-abusing clients* (pp. 105–118). New York: Guilford Press.

Cheung, Y. W. (1993). Approaches to ethnicity: Cleaning roadblocks in the study of ethnicity and substance abuse. *International Journal of the Addictions, 28*(12), 1209–1226.

Corrigan, E. M., & Butler, S. (1991). Irish alcoholic women in treatment: Early findings. *International Journal of the Addictions, 26*(3), 281–292.

Cusack, J. (1996, May 22). Heroin worth 1 million pounds seized as big drug link cut. *The Irish Times*, p. 1.

Desmond, N., Murphy, M., Plunkett, P., & Mulcahy, F. (1993). Use of a Dublin inner city hospital A & E department by patients with known HIV-1 infection. *International Journal of Studies on AIDS, 4*(4), 222–225.

Ewing, J. A. (1984). Detecting alcoholism: The CAGE questionnaire. *Journal of the American Medical Association, 252*, 1905–1907.

Fallows, M. (1979). *Irish Americans: Identity and assimilation*. Englewood Cliffs, NJ: Prentice-Hall.

Greeley, A. (1981). *The Irish Americans*. New York: Harper & Row.

Griffin, W. (1992). This distant land: The Irish in America. *Ireland of the Welcomes, 41*(4), 26–31.

Grube, J., Morgan, M., & Kearney, K. (1989). Using self-generated identification codes to match questionnaires in panel studies of adolescent substance use. *Addictive Behaviors, 14*(2) 159–171.

Harrison, L., Carrhill, R., & Sutton, M. (1993). Consumption and harm: Drinking patterns of the Irish, the English and the Irish in England. *Alcohol and Alcoholism, 28*(6), 715–723.

Henderson, C. (1994, April 11). Dublin AIDS groups call for government funding. *Ireland: AIDS Weekly*, p. 23.

Hines, P., Garcia-Preto, N., McGoldrick, M., Almeida, R., & Weltmann, S. (1992) Intergenerational relationships across cultures. *Families in Society, 76*(6), 323–339.

Johnson, V. (1986). *Intervention.* Minneapolis, MN: Johnson Institute Books.

Johnson, Z., O'Connor, M., Pomeroy, L., Barry, J., Scully, M., & Fitzpatrick, E. (1994). Prevalence of HIV and associated risk behaviour in attendees at a Dublin needle exchange. *Addiction, 89*(5), 603–607.

Lender, M., & Martin, J. (1982). *Drinking in America.* London: Macmillan.

Malcolm, E. (1986). *Ireland sober, Ireland free.* Dublin: Gill & Macmillan.

McGoldrick, M. (1982). *Irish families.* In M. McGoldrick, J. K. Pearce, & J. Giordano (Eds.), *Ethnicity and family therapy* (pp. 310–339). New York: Guilford Press.

McGoldrick, M. (1996). *Irish families.* In M. McGoldrick, J. Giordano, & J. K. Pearce (Eds.), *Ethnicity and family therapy* (2nd ed., pp. 544–566). New York: Guilford Press.

Morton, H. V. (1978). *The magic of Ireland.* London: Arrow Books.

Muhlin, G. (1985). Ethnic differences in alcohol misuse: A striking reaffirmation. *Journal of Alcohol Studies, 46,* 172–173.

National Opinion Research Center. (1997). *Understanding alcohol and other drugs: A multimedia resource.* New York: Facts on File.

Neill, K. (1979). *An illustrated history of the Irish people.* Dublin: Gill and Macmillan.

O'Faolain, N. (1996, January 15). Opinion. *The Irish Times*, p. 6.

O'hEithir, B. (1987). *This is Ireland.* Dublin: O'Brien Press.

Schofield, A. (1991). The prevalence of alcoholism in an Irish general hospital. *Irish Journal of Psychological Medicine, 8*(1), 33–36.

Smyth, B., Keenan, E., Dorman, A., & O'Connor, J. (1994). Gender differences in needle sharing behaviour patterns. *Addiction, 89*(1), 96–97.

Stivers, R. (1976). *A hair of the dog: Irish drinking and American stereotype.* University Park: Pennsylvania State University Press.

Straussner, S. L. A. (1993). Assessment and treatment of clients with alcohol and other drug abuse problems: An overview. In S. L. A. Straussner (Ed.), *Clinical work with substance-abusing clients* (pp. 3–30). New York: Guilford Press.

Teehan, J. (1988). Alcohol expectancies of Irish and Canadian alcoholics. *International Journal of the Addictions, 23*(10), 1057–1070.

Valliant, G. E. (1983). *The natural history of alcoholism.* Cambridge, MA: Harvard University Press.

Walsh, D. (1987). Alcohol and alcohol problems: Research 15. Ireland. *British Journal of Addiction, 82,* 747–751.

Wilson, R. W., & Williams, G. D. (1989). Alcohol use and abuse among U.S. minority groups: Results from the 1983 National Health Interview Study. In D. L. Spiegler, D. A. Tate, S. A. Aitken, & C. M. Christian (Eds.), *Alcohol use among U.S. ethnic minorities* (pp. 399–410). Rockville, MD: U.S. Department of Health and Human Services.

Woodham-Smith, C. (1963). *The great hunger.* New York: Harper & Row.

11

Italian Culture and Its Impact on Addiction

Pia Marinangeli

More than 14 million Americans of Italian ancestry are currently living in the United States (U.S. Bureau of Census, 1990), making them one of the more numerous of the many racial and ethnocultural groups that make up the American people. In fact, in New York City alone, 12% of the population is Italian American (Milione, 1996-1997). Consequently, many clinicians are presently working with Italian American clients, including those who are affected by substance abuse.

Among Italian Americans, there is a broad spectrum of differences in ideas, in lifestyles, in the way they perceive themselves, in the extent to which they feel group membership, and in how they are perceived by others. It is therefore essential that clinicians have an understanding of individual clients, the cultural heritage of these clients, and the implications of these dynamics on the therapeutic process. This chapter focuses on the character, traditions, and beliefs of Italians and Italian Americans, discusses the use and abuse of alcohol and other drugs among this population, and provides a framework for treatment of Italian American substance abusers.

HISTORICAL BACKGROUND
AND NATIONAL CHARACTER

For centuries, due to its strategic location on the Mediterranean Sea, Italy has served as a crossroads from western to eastern Europe. It was continually invaded, leaving Italians often in the presence of hostile foreigners. In addition, as the center of the Catholic Church, Rome was the destination of numerous pilgrims, adding to the influx of strangers. Much of the extraordinary suspiciousness of anyone outside of blood relations that is so common to many Italians can be traced to this constant influx of foreigners (Rotunno & McGoldrick, 1982).

With little protection or support from the state or the Church, Italians turned to their families, close neighbors, and their own internal resources: It was dangerous to be too trusting of anyone with whom they did not have personal connections. The need to rely on the family was compounded by the many natural disasters, such as floods, earthquakes, and droughts, endured by Italians throughout the centuries. For most Italians, the importance of the family supersedes that of country, state, region, town, or even the Church. More so than in some other cultures, the extended family is placed first and is seen as a primary source of protection and safety—an important dynamic to consider in treatment.

Italians have lived together as one nation for only little more than the past 100 years. Consequently, although the Italians absorbed and adapted a diverse range of cultural influences, they tended to maintain their regional dialects, traditions, customs, and practices. It was not until after World War II, with the introduction of the radio and then television, that all Italians began to speak standardized Italian. Even today, regionalism remains a strong force in Italy, and many people identify more strongly with their region, even their town, than with the concept of nationality.

Because of their geography and economy, southern Italians, who constitute the vast majority of Italian immigrants to the United States, developed different customs, lifestyles, nuances in language, and food preferences from their northern Italian neighbors. In contrast to the relatively prosperous existence of the northerners, the southerners, who lacked sources of energy and raw materials, relied on farming for their livelihood and tended to be poorer, less educated, and somewhat more fatalistic in their outlook on life (Giordano & McGoldrick, 1996).

Centuries of living within political and religious authoritarian structures that oppressed the values and needs of individuals have forced Italians to become shrewd and self-reliant in order to survive. Having to deal with and adjust to quick political changes and foreign conquerors required a flexible mentality and encouraged a certain detached attitude toward political institutions and regimes. In general, Italians tend to be very tolerant people, mainly concerned with the lives of their family members and reluctant to become involved in other people's business. Personality traits such as resilience and adaptability are highly valued. Italians tend to be optimistic, hard working, and resourceful and to have a good sense of humor. They tend to take great pleasure in the present and to experience intense enjoyment, whether in eating, celebrating, fighting, loving, or drinking (Giordano & McGoldrick, 1996).

Eating together has always been at the center of Italian life, and even today, food is considered a primary source of emotional and physical solace (Giordano & McGoldrick, 1996). Although famous for their wines, Italians have historically viewed drinking as only an accompaniment to the eating ritual. It is commonly believed that the historically low rate of alcoholism among Italians was due to the fact that drinking was usually done in context—at the family table. This issue is addressed later in the chapter.

THE ITALIAN IMMIGRANTS

The majority of Italian immigrants to the United States came from southern Italy between 1900 and 1910 in order to escape hunger and poverty. Most were peasants who were often illiterate and suspicious of foreigners or "strangers." It is important to note, however, that not all Italian immigrants were southern or poor. There were also the young, the adventurous, the middle class, and the educated and professionally trained. Most of these came from central or northern Italy, as is true for many of the more recent Italian immigrants (Giamatti, 1987).

The major barrier for the early Italian immigrant was language. English was difficult to learn; thus most immigrants retained their native language. They also retained their native dialects as a security blanket and as proof of their identity. These immigrants quickly discovered that in America, individualism, independence, and personal achievement were emphasized over family and group affiliation—values that contrasted greatly with their Italian experience. Consequently, the Italian migration had one of the highest proportions of returning immigrants (Rotunno & McGoldrick, 1982).

Psychologically, the early Italian immigrants seem to have been less afflicted with feelings of inferiority than their offspring were. Ethnotherapists have found that as second- and third-generation Italian Americans became assimilated into American society, the White Anglo-Saxon Protestant ethic became their cultural ideal, whereas their own ethnocultural background was devalued, lowering their self-esteem (Mangione & Morreale, 1992). A study by Sirey, Patti, and Mann (1985) found that even though the participants were an upwardly mobile, high-achieving group of Italian Americans, they still struggled with the feeling that they were "outsiders," "different," and "less than" other Americans and had to work hard to prove themselves worthy. Exploring the roots of such feelings, participants recalled that their parents communicated feelings of lower self-esteem when they felt conscious of the differences between themselves and the *Americane* who emphasized class status and educational achievement (Sirey et al., 1985). Lower self-worth and feelings of shame also could be due to unconscious identification with negative Italian American stereotypes frequently portrayed in the mass media. A study of television programs during the early 1980s revealed that "denigrating presentations of Italian Americans outnumbered positive ones by a margin of nearly two to one" (Mangione & Morreale, 1992, p. 219).

Overall, the third-generation grandchildren of Italian immigrants have had a far easier time in the New World than their second-generation parents, despite the effects of the persistent negative stereotypes about Italian Americans. In increasing numbers they have acquired college degrees and professional status. However, as Italian Americans become acculturated, they also became susceptible to many of the problems found among the rest of the U. S. population, including the abuse of alcohol and other drugs.

COMMON CULTURAL CHARACTERISTICS
OF ITALIAN AMERICANS

As indicated previously, Italian values emphasize the importance of the family. Among Italian Americans, divorce, separation, and desertion are less common than among other ethnic groups (U.S. Bureau of the Census, 1990). Moreover, compared with the general population, few Italian Americans remain unmarried. According to the 1990 census, 57.2% of Americans of Italian ancestry over the age of 15 were married, and only 27.2% have never married. Young adults tend to remain in the family home until they marry, and extended family members tend to live near each other.

Although the traditional Italian American family structure has been changing (Milione, 1996-1997), many of the traditional values have remained. For example, although most Italian American nuclear families tend to be financially independent, on an emotional level they remain inextricably intertwined with their extended families. In general, the needs and desires of the traditional Italian American family supersede those of the individual. Occupational, financial, and educational achievement is often measured by the extent to which it benefits the extended family. A combination of love, a sense of duty, obligation, and guilt tends to push many Italian Americans to sublimate their personal needs and wants for the sake of the family (Tardi, 1996-1997).

The Italian family is often characterized by its closeness and strength, its heightened and uninhibited emotionality, and strong ties between mothers and sons and among siblings. A study by Tardi (1996-1997) in which 60 Italian Americans living in New Jersey were interviewed found that both close parent–child and sibling bonds continue to be emphasized in these families. The traditional Italian American family is in many ways a matriarchal culture in which feminine strength is accepted. Though the father may be the head of the family, the Italian mother is its heart. The mother plays a significant role in the important decisions of the family. She is largely responsible for raising the children, seeing to their religious education, preparing them for marriage, and establishing social relationships with friends, relatives, and neighbors. The mother also plays a very powerful role in her son's affections. According to Rosatti (1990), the close childhood bond between mothers and sons rarely changes in adulthood and continues to be reinforced by the all-giving mother. This all-pervasive nurturance is experienced as both supportive and controlling by the sons. In his adult relationships, the Italian male has been described as searching for this ideal mother who is willing to give up anything for him and put his wishes first (Rosatti, 1990).

The Italian American woman, on the other hand, faces different issues than the Italian American man does. Within the complex relationship between mother and daughter, the "daughter often feels the crush of impossible standards, criticism and competition rather than the oppressive overprotection experienced by her brothers" (Sirey et al., 1985, p. 20). Italian and Italian American mothers appear to have a less nurturing attitude toward their daughters, whom they frequently choose to be confidantes, to share complaints about their husbands. As the historian Andrew Rolle states, "daughters became substitute husbands, acting out the unexpressed anger of the passive–aggressive mother," and enabling the mother to remain "the idealized Madonna in the eyes of the sons" (as cited in Mangione & Morreale, 1992, p. 237). These daughters often feel burdened by the traditional caretaker role as they become the guardians of their aging parents and in-laws.

Although not as strong as that between mothers and sons, the tie between fathers and daughters is also important. Italian men seem to feel comfortable expressing their warm and nurturing feelings toward their young daughters and often coddle and protect them. However, as the daughters reach puberty, this overt affectionate behavior is dramatically stopped and is replaced by rigid rules. Due to the many restrictions imposed on daughters during adolescence, mostly having to do with sexual matters and courtship issues, many Italian American women rebel and strive to separate from their parents to start a family of their own (Sirey et. al., 1985). At times, drugs and alcohol may become a component of this rebellion.

The Role of Education

Despite their growing numbers in the professions, Italian Americans continue to be underrepresented in prestigious occupations (Elmi, 1996). In the past, formal schooling beyond the fundamentals was not seen as a priority in accomplishing the goal of maintaining the welfare and tradition of *la famiglia*. The high priority placed on working to assist their families who were still mired in poverty can offer some explanation as to why many Italian immigrants were reluctant to invest time and resources in education. Italian male children were often trained in carpentry, barbering, tailoring, and other skills that would provide sustenance for themselves and for the family. Girls were trained, mostly by the mother, in the skills necessary to assume the roles of wife and mother. More recently, Italian American children under the age of 16 have been found to have a very high rate of school attendance, 93.3% (Worrall, 1993, as cited in Elmi, 1996); however, older Italian American children in large cities have been found to "have the highest school drop out rates among White ethnic groups" (Calandra Institute, 1990, as cited in Giordano & McGoldrick, 1996, p. 570), putting them at high risk for substance abuse.

The Role of the Church

Most Italians are Roman Catholics who appreciate Church rituals for their pageantry, spectacle, and value in fostering family celebrations and rites of passage (Giordano & McGoldrick, 1996). Traditional Italian Catholicism was artistic, theatrical, and sensual; it also contained strong moral precepts, such as charity, forgiveness, and reverence for life, that exerted a tremendous force on Italian life (Gesualdi, 1997).

Italian Americans always have had a very personalized relationship with religion and many, especially women, were deeply religious. Prayer could take place anywhere and with anyone. Some traditional Italian Americans continue to have strong belief in and fear and awe of the supernatural, such as the power of the evil eye and a belief in magic spells (Mangione & Morreale, 1992). Their deep spiritual belief makes it easier for many Italian Americans to grasp the 12-step programs and their reference to a higher power.

Current Alcohol and Other Substance Consumption in Italy by Native Italians

It is often believed that Italians have a very low rate of alcoholism due to the fact that they begin to drink wine early in life and in the context of a family setting. Researchers in the 1950s had remarked that "Italians rarely become intoxicated and that Italy was virtually free of the psychological, social, economic and legal difficulties that are associated with drinking in the United States and other countries" (Lolli, Serianni, Golder, & Luzzatto-Fegiz, 1958, p. 33). Even during the 1990s, Cooper (1993) described drinking in Italy as a "normal, wholesome enjoyable aspect of everyday life." Drinking was seen in very much the same way as eating and was not used for relaxation, for relief from psychic stress, for escape, or for delusions of power. Theorists such as Lolli and colleagues (1958) suggested that Italian cultural values and attitudes toward drinking serve as inoculation against alcohol dependence and drinking problems. Nonetheless, during the past 30 years, extensive changes have taken place in the drinking patterns among the Italians as wine has become more and more a drink used for celebrating and socializing and less as a component of daily meals (Pisani, 1991).

Recent data on alcohol consumption patterns among the Italians are lacking. There are several reasons for this absence, including the lack of social recognition of the existence of alcohol problems, the economic cost of research studies, and the general distrust of Italian culture toward social surveys. Available studies tend to focus on the drinking of adolescents rather than of the general population (Poldrugo & Stratta, 1993). Nonetheless, the health consequences of constant heavy alcohol consumption among Italians are serious. According to LaVecchia, Decarli, Mexxanotte, and Cislaghi (1986), alcohol-related diseases represented a much larger proportion of all causes of deaths in Italy than in many other developed countries. Alcohol consumption in Italy is believed to be responsible for over 30,000 deaths per year. Half of these deaths are related to cirrhosis of the liver, followed by alcohol-related accidents and cancer (Patussi et al., 1993).

The long-standing Italian tradition of social tolerance toward drinking not only promotes the daily use of alcohol but also discourages people, especially the young, from perceiving alcohol intake as a potentially serious social or psychomedical problem. Such acceptance of drinking may reinforce the denial system among Italians and Italian Americans struggling with alcohol-related disorders.

The long Italian tradition that views wine as a prized alimentary element with unique social, medicinal, and nutritional values explains why wine and other alcoholic beverages are perceived as socially acceptable even when used by children and adolescents. Not infrequently, wine is offered to young Italian children as a normal part of the family life. According to Poldrugo and Stratta (1993), "the administering of alcoholic drinks often takes place in the first few months of a child's life when wine is added to the baby's bottle to make him sleep" (p. 74). A 1985 survey conducted in schools by Federazione Italiana Silvestrelli per l'Alcoholismo showed that many children drink wine "when they feel lonely, when they are afraid, or surreptitiously to overcome family arguments" (as cited in Poldrugo & Stratta, 1993, p. 74). Moreover, studies of patients at the Psychiatric Hospital of Verona showed that "in 56 percent of cases the beginning of the alcoholisation process could be traced back to childhood" (p. 74).

In contrast to earlier studies that found that young Italians, though starting to drink earlier, got drunk less often than young people from Anglo-Saxon countries and had fewer personal problems, recent studies found that young Italians, particularly in the south, were consuming more alcohol than previously and experiencing more social problems (Poldrugo & Stratta, 1993). In addition, there has been a general transition from a "pub" to a "bar" culture. Whereas the pub (*osteria*) has been a traditional meeting place for young and old, young people today are more likely to frequent the bar, where alcohol is used to ease social relationships (Poldrugo & Stratta, 1993).

In addition to alcohol, other substances are also abused in Italy. Research "on the use of cannabis derivatives in the last three years of Italian high school students indicates that between 25–30 percent of these students have sporadically or occasionally taken the drug" (Bruno, 1994, p. 702). However, cocaine and heroin use are also problems in Italy. According to Bruno (1994), "the most reliable statistics indicate there are approximately 250,000 opiate addicts, and an equal, if not even larger, number of cocaine consumers. In addition, the number of people who misuse legalized psychotropic substances (tranquilizers, hypnotics, and antidepressants) to better their personal performance and control anxiety is increasing" (p. 702). Mortality data from 1990 reveal that AIDS is the fourth leading cause of death in Italy among men between the ages of 25 and 44 years (Conti, Farchi, & Prati, 1994). The average prevalence of HIV infection in the population of drug users is 30–40% (Bruno, 1994).

ALCOHOL AND OTHER DRUG
USE BY ITALIAN AMERICANS

Culturally, Italians would be expected to consume rather large per capita quantities of beverage alcohol but without attendant alcohol problems.

Traditionally, this pattern resulted from the integration of alcohol use into the everyday life of most Italians and Italian Americans—an integration that can be traced back to the values of responsibility, duty, and moderation espoused by Italian families. This integration, however, does not protect those of Italian descent from alcohol dependence.

The current generation of Italian Americans are experiencing a distinct shift away from the culturally functional patterns of alcohol use toward more negative ones. A study done by Klein (1990) concluded that Italian American college students no longer enjoy the "protection" afforded them by their ethnocultural background when it comes to their drinking patterns. These students were more likely than their non-Italian peers to be drinkers and drank significantly more wine and beer than any other ethnic group. "Although the Italian students surveyed still drink frequently and fairly heavily, as has been true for Italians in general over the years, they no longer seem to be able to do so without experiencing the adverse consequences of drinking" (Klein, 1990, p. 185). As Italian Americans become increasingly Americanized in their drinking practices, we can expect that their alcohol problem rates will increase in the years to come.

Although alcohol abuse is believed to be the major substance abuse problem for Italian Americans, illicit drug abuse is also prevalent. One of the few studies that focused on drug-abusing Italian Americans was conducted by Kaufman and Kaufmann (1979). They looked at the dynamics of 78 heroin-abusing and heroin-dependent youths from mostly Italian and Jewish families in New York City and Los Angeles. The families were treated for 6 months. The authors found that 88% of the mothers were "emotionally enmeshed" with their drug-abusing children (mainly sons) to the extent that their emotional states were totally dependent on the behavior of and their closeness with these children. They also found a relatively high percentage (41%) of fathers who were overinvolved with their drug-abusing daughters.

Dynamics of Substance-Abusing Italian Americans

The dynamics of Italian American families appear to play an important role in substance abuse, particularly in the use of drugs among adolescents and young adults. The strong emotional ties in Italian American families often result in nearly symbiotic relationships between parents and children. Italian families tend to be "enmeshed" (Minuchin, 1974), with unclear, diffuse boundaries among family members. Drug and alcohol use are thus seen as a way for Italian Americans to differentiate and separate from the family of origin (Kaufman & Kaufmann, 1979).

The low level of tolerance for uncomfortable feelings may be another factor in substance abuse among Italian Americans. A study done in a health care setting by Zborowski (1969, as cited in Glasscote, Sussex, & Jaffe, 1972) indicated that Italian patients were much more preoccupied than members of other ethnocultural groups with obtaining immediate pain relief. Unlike Jewish patients, who were worried about the long-range effects of drugs given to relieve pain, Italians had little such concern. They wanted medication immediately. "Low threshold for frustration, disappointment and pain, and seeking immediate gratification have been identified in a great many if not most drug abusers" (Glasscote et al., 1972, p. 22). This could be an important dynamic to consider when working with Italian American substance abusers.

It is also important to note that Italians typically do not discuss problems publicly. According to Giordano and McGoldrick (1996), "Hot issues are not openly discussed and Italians do more sidestepping than most in the initial stage of therapy" (p. 576). This "dancing" around issues fits into the Italian cultural context of feeling ashamed for having to go outside the family for help and may exacerbate the natural stages of denial in both the substance abuser and the family. Thus it is very important to attend to what is *not* being said.

TREATMENT OF SUBSTANCE-ABUSING ITALIAN AMERICANS

Italian American clients with alcohol and drug problems are seen in many different treatment settings. In order to treat them effectively, each client needs to be carefully assessed, taking into account his or her culture, as well as individual, familial, and substance use background.

Assessment

A comprehensive assessment is an important first step in substance abuse treatment. The clinician must determine the nature and extent of the substance abuse and carefully assess its specific consequences. Because Italian Americans tend to sidestep hot issues, it is helpful to pinpoint what brought them to treatment at this particular time. Is a spouse finally fed up and threatening to leave? Is the client being mandated to treatment through the job or courts? In addition, reviewing past treatment attempts and exploring what was or was not helpful to maintaining sobriety can help determine what level of treatment the client needs. The assessment must also include medical and psychiatric status, legal issues, educational level, social support network, family history of substance abuse, and current family functioning. It is also very important to assess the history of childhood physical, sexual, and emotional abuse, as well as any other past and current family violence.

When working with Italian Americans, a clinician must explore clients' support systems and interactions with important people in their lives. The clinician needs to assess the level of contact with and whereabouts of relatives, as well as the level of emotional separation of the substance abuser from family members. It is crucial to differentiate between intense, culturally sanctioned closeness and pathological enmeshment: Does family involvement interfere with the individual's ability to function and develop independent life skills? Can the family dynamics be utilized to break through denial and help sustain recovery?

It is also important to explore the client's self-esteem, as low self-esteem makes one more susceptible to continuing alcohol and drug abuse, which further decreases one's sense of self. As pointed out previously, Italian Americans are vulnerable to lower self-esteem in comparison with other European Americans (Sirey et al., 1985).

Intervention

Substance abuse is a severe disorder that pervades an individual's mental, physical, and spiritual existence. It is rare that so intensive an illness can be helped by individual therapy alone. Thus a combination of individual therapy, 12-step work, group therapy, and family treatment tailored to each client is recommended.

When working with clients in groups, as well as individually, the clinician must maintain a level of frustration that is tolerable for the client. Given the cultural suspicion of strangers, it may take extra effort on the part of the clinician to form an initial trust and break through the denial. It is important to set limits and maintain boundaries, particularly in light of the tendency toward enmeshment found among families of Italian origin.

A common belief among some Italians is that illness can be caused by the suppression of emotions, as well as by stress caused by fear, grief, and anxiety, and that one may "burst" if unable to find an emotional outlet (Spector, 1996). This belief can be used positively during treatment to explore the role of the substance in clients' lives and to prevent future relapses. One of the goals of treatment is to help the Italian American client put his or her feelings into words without acting destructively.

Individual and Group Treatment

Group therapy has often been the treatment of choice for substance abusers. Groups reduce the sense of isolation by helping the individual to recognize that he or she is not alone. This is particularly helpful for Italian Americans, who often struggle with the feeling that they are "different." Sirey and colleagues (1985) conducted a research project using a short-term group experience in which Italian American participants explored issues of ethnic identity and self-esteem. They found that the group experience, which provided a sense of belonging and sharing with others, was very important for Italian Americans. In addition to structured group therapy in a treatment setting, 12-step programs such as Alcoholics Anonymous (AA) and Narcotics Anonymous (NA) are also recommended for substance-abusing Italian Americans. In these programs clients have access to individuals in long-term recovery who can serve as positive role models and can instill hope to the newcomer. The following case exemplifies some of the above dynamics.

Anthony is a 40-year-old overweight, divorced Italian American professional who came for individual therapy to a social worker in private practice at the recommendation of a friend in AA. He presented with an 8-year history of alcohol dependence and 1 year of sobriety through AA.

Anthony was born and raised in Italy by an Italian-born father and an Italian American mother. His parents separated when he was 6 years old, and he was brought to live in the United States with his mother and her family. He did not have any contact with his father, who had since died, and suspected that the father also had an alcohol problem. He described a difficult adjustment period following his migration, with difficulties with the language, making friends, and in school. He recalled always feeling "different" and not "fitting in." Because his mother never remarried, he became the "parentified" child and her surrogate husband and companion. Aside from experimenting with marijuana while in college, he did not use any drugs and did not drink heavily until after he got married at the age of 30.

Anthony's mother, with whom he was still very close, was described as a controlling, anxious woman who is guilt provoking, manipulative, and overprotective, yet at the same time nurturing, loving, and supportive. He met his ex-wife, who was not of Italian background, at work and married her despite the fact that his mother did not like her. Anthony viewed his drinking as an attempt to deal with his conflict between trying to please both his mother and his wife. It was only after his wife left him 2 years before he came to treatment that he "hit bottom" and started going to AA. It was the first time in his life that he found people with whom he could identify. He sought individual therapy in order to deal with his feelings of guilt, as well as anger at his mother, and with his general sense of loneliness, depression, and fear of resuming drinking.

Treatment of Italian-American Women

Poldrugo, Fiore, and Manzan (1988) found that one out of every four alcoholics admitted to the Psychiatric Clinic of the University of Trieste in Italy was a woman. In this study, the authors found that women had higher educational levels and higher occupational stability than men (Poldrugo et al., 1988). They also found higher frequencies of psychopathology and secondary alcoholism among the women. These Italian women have shown better treatment outcomes than men. Such findings were explained by "more stable living conditions, as demonstrated by high rates of married subjects, by occupational stability, and a better family income. Women requested help more often, reached a hospital at a younger age, and enjoyed higher involvement of significant others" (Poldrugo et al., 1988, p. 688).

There are no comparable data on substance-abusing Italian American women. As discussed previously, Italian American women struggle between feeling trapped in a maternal, caretaking, or dependent role or selecting a more independent path that may lead to feelings of conflict, betrayal, and disloyalty to the family. In light of the importance of the woman in the Italian American family and her responsibility for the welfare of its members, a chemically dependent woman is likely to be burdened by guilt and shame as a result of having failed to achieve the idealized gender image. Because there is much more stigma attached to Italian women who abuse substances than to men, women may try harder to hide their addiction. Moreover, as a cultural norm it is expected that women should rely economically on men and that they be protected from the consequences of their addiction by their husbands and parents. Therefore, by the time women present for treatment, their addictions have already done much damage. Thus it is important for the clinician to be sensitive to gender (Straussner & Zelvin, 1997), as well as to cultural dynamics.

> Maria, a 28-year-old Italian American married secretary, was referred to a private outpatient drug rehabilitation program by her company's Employee Assistance Program (EAP). She presented with a 12-year history of substance abuse that began at age 16 with alcohol and escalated to intranasal cocaine use by age 25. Her use progressed to the point at which she was spending up to $500 weekly on cocaine, resulting in a debt of over $20,000. She supported her drug habit by stealing

money from her husband and parents while pretending to pay household bills. She was referred to the EAP by her boss, who found her taking the petty cash money at work. Despite this theft, he continued to employ her and supported her treatment efforts.

Maria, who had two brothers, was an only daughter raised by second-generation Italian American parents. She was living with her Italian American husband of 5 years in an isolated Italian community in a large town. The couple resided in a two-family house owned by her parents, who lived upstairs. Maria was very close to her father and described herself as "daddy's girl." She did not feel as emotionally connected to her mother, whom she viewed as "not an affectionate person" who always preferred her brothers.

Maria was attractive and well kept. She spoke in a babyish voice and in general presented very child-like. The main men in her life—her husband, father, and boss—all treated her like a child, and she actually seemed to radiate a kind of helplessness that encouraged people to take care of her.

Maria was seen in individual and group treatment, and her husband and parents were referred to a psychoeducational group for family members, as well as to Al-Anon and Co-Anon. Although her mother continued to attend Al-Anon, the men refused to attend after one visit to each group.

In her groups, which she attended three times a week, Maria learned about the nature of addiction. She was able to talk about her shame over stealing from her elderly parents and worked on making amends to them. In a weekly women's group, she was also learning to say no and to realize that a woman can say no and still be a "nice" person or "good girl."

Maria was also seen together with her husband in order to explore the dynamics between them, to obtain his support for her ongoing treatment, and to develop a financial plan to repay her debts. The couple's counseling helped Maria to take responsibility for her actions and to accept the consequences of her drug use. It also helped her become aware of her husband's investment in keeping her a little girl and her need to act out with drugs instead of openly addressing her feelings of resentment.

Intervention with Family Members

The need for detachment and letting go of the need to control the addict are necessary for the recovery of both the substance abusers and their Italian American families. As indicated previously, it is difficult for Italian American families to emotionally disconnect because of the deep meaning of family to them. There is a strong belief that the family has control of its members, especially the substance abuser, whom they believe they can change.

Therefore, it is important for the clinician to help the family realize that they are not to blame, to educate them on the disease of addiction, and to give them a sense of hope.

The clinician should not label the Italian American's intense involvement with family members as pathological and inappropriate but should communicate that the closeness is a positive expression of the family's caring. The goal in treatment is to encourage the client to take responsibility for his or her behavior and to find ways to stay connected to the family without being enabled to continue drug use. It is important for the clinician to reinforce the family's problem-solving abilities and to affirm the value of protection and loyalty (Giordano & McGoldrick, 1996).

According to Kaufman and Kaufmann (1979), multiple-family groups can be very helpful in providing Italian families with the support they need to let their substance-abusing family member individuate. They found that "(g)iven the insularity of the Italian extended family, their willingness to open up and change in a group of other families is surprising. The use of an Italian co-therapist, their view of the doctor as respected expert, and other Italian families in the group who supported the letting go process were also helpful" (p. 163). Some of these dynamics can be seen in the following case.

Joey is a 17-year-old male brought to a substance abuse outpatient treatment center by both of his second-generation Italian American parents, who were concerned about his use of marijuana and pills. Initially, it was Mrs. G, Joey's mother, who called for an appointment. The therapist, sensing the enmeshment between the two, had asked the mother to have Joey call to make arrangements himself for his first session. Joey arrived accompanied by both of his parents. He was dressed in a typical teenage outfit—baggy jeans, T-shirt, and baseball cap. His well-dressed parents appeared anxious and very concerned about their inability to control the behavior of their only child. The parents complained about his staying out very late, hanging around a "bad" crowd of friends, dressing sloppily, and cutting classes. Joey had recently been arrested with a group of friends who stole a car to go joyriding. Joey's father, who owns his own business, was able to arrange for a lawyer to get the charges dismissed. Joey's mother was a housewife whose main activities consisted of caring for her house and her family and spending time with her sisters, who lived nearby. Both parents denied any substance abuse of their own aside from some experimentation during their teens.

During an individual assessment session, Joey admitted to a 4-year history of experimenting with various drugs and to current daily use of marijuana. He also drank beer and liquor on weekends and used various pills such as Ecstasy while going to clubs. He expressed minimal concern about his involvement with substances and the trouble it was getting him into. He shared how he had a secret hiding place in his room to put his "stuff," because on numerous occasions his mother would search his room and drawers looking for drugs. He would then get punished physically by his father and not be allowed to go out for a few days. He usually disobeyed these orders, leading to further physical punishment. Lately, he had started fighting back when his father threatened to hit him with a belt.

Joey expressed a desire to move out and get his own apartment to get his parents off his back. However, each time he would regain the trust of his parents, he would sabotage it by getting into further trouble, causing him to be punished by not being allowed to leave home. This interesting dynamic was explored with Joey. The close bond between mother and son was evident. When in trouble, he would call home to his mother to bail him out and would ask her not to tell his father.

His fear of separation from his home and family was clearly a major conflict for him. His substance abuse seemed to play a large part in the struggle between maintaining closeness and distancing himself from his family. On the one hand, by doing drugs he was rebelling and doing something neither his mother nor father could control. On the other hand, he would leave clues and get in trouble, thereby bringing him even closer to the family.

In addition to continued individual treatment for Joey, the family agreed to attend a 6-week multifamily group that included three other families. The group, led by two therapists, provided education regarding substance abuse and enabling behaviors, as well as mutual aid for the participants. Listening to the other parents and their teenage children helped Joey's parents, particularly his mother. She was able to identify her anxiety at letting her son grow up and gain his independence. She agreed not to look through his room and drawers, and both parents agreed to stop bailing him out of trouble, to let him take responsibility for his actions and to stop the "punishing game." Joey stopped smoking marijuana at home, and although he continued to go out to night clubs, he started hanging out with a "nicer" group of friends.

CONCLUSION

Understanding the unique characteristics and core values of Italian Americans and their families can enhance the clinician's sensitivity, aid in client retention, and improve substance abuse treatment effectiveness. The positive personal attributes common to many individuals of Italian background, such as their warmth, spontaneity, resilience, and hard work, enhances the clinician's positive countertransference despite any initial distrust on the part of the client.

Substance abuse clinicians need to be aware of the value placed by clients of Italian background on their family and close relationships with friends and of their focus on home life, as well as of their general respect for parental authority. They also need to be sensitive to the Italian cultural tendency to be mistrustful of strangers, to have a low tolerance for pain and frustration, and to stay safely within the family rather than to venture out and become their own separate person or to seek professional help.

Whether Italian American family dynamics are a cause of, a symptom of, or a contributing factor to substance abuse must be further researched. It will take time to develop effective ethnoculturally specific models of treatment. Such efforts will require the involvement not only of substance abuse experts who are sensitive to Italian American values but also of Italian American organizations and community leaders. The process promises to be both challenging and exciting.

REFERENCES

Bruno, F. (1994). Drug and alcohol problems in the workplace in Italy. *Journal of Drug Issues, 24,* 697–713.

Conti, S., Farchi, G., & Prati, S. (1994, December). AIDS is the leading cause of death among young adults in Italy. *European Journal of Epidemiology, 10*(6), 669–673.

Cooper, A. M. (1993). Italian drinking patterns: Model for theories and policies. *Modern Reading, 7*(2), 33–35.

Gesualdi, L. (1997). The religious acculturation of the Italian American Catholics: Cultural and socioeconomic factors. In *Topical Issues Series* [Booklet] (pp. 1–88). New York: John D. Calandra Italian American Institute.

Giamatti, B. (1987). Commentary. In A. Schoener *The Italian Americans* (pp. 9–24). New York: Macmillan.

Giordano, J., & McGoldrick, M. (1996). Italian families. In M. McGoldrick, J. Giordano, & J. K. Pearce (Eds.), *Ethnicity and family therapy* (2nd ed., pp. 567–582). New York: Guilford Press.

Glasscote, R. M., Sussex, J. N., & Jaffe, J. H. (1972). *The treatment of drug abuse: Programs, problems, prospects.* Washington, DC: American Psychological Association.

Kaufman, E., & Kaufmann, P. (1979). From a psychodynamic to a structural understanding of drug dependency. In E. Kaufman & P. Kaufmann (Eds.), *The family therapy of drug and alcohol abuse* (pp. 255–272). New York: Gardner Press.

Klein, H. (1990). Contemporary Italian American college student drinking patterns.

In J. Scelsa, S. LaGumina, & L. Tomasi (Eds.), *Italian Americans in transition* (pp. 177–187). New York: American Italian Historical Association.

LaVecchia, C., Decarli, A., Mexxanotte, G., & Cislaghi, C. (1986). Mortality from alcohol related disease in Italy. *Journal of Epidemiology and Community Health*, 40, 257–261.

Lolli, G., Serianni, E., Golder, G. M., & Luzzatto-Fegiz, P. (1958). *Alcohol in Italian culture*. Glencoe, IL: Free Press.

Mangione, J., & Morreale, B. (1992). *La storia: Five centuries of the Italian American experience*. New York: HarperPerrenial.

Milione, V. (1996-1997). The changing demographic of Italian Americans in New York State, New York City and Long Island: 1980 and 1990. *Italian American Review*, 5(2), 133–154.

Minuchin, S. (1974). *Families and family therapy*. Cambridge, MA: Harvard University Press.

Patussi, V., Quartini, A., Napolitano, G., Tedesco, A., Surrenti, C., Cecchi, M., & Berni, M. (1993). Alcohol: Knowledge and attitudes among adolescents and teachers at two junior high schools in Florence, Italy. *Alcoholism* (Zagreb), 29, 63–71.

Pisani, P. L. (1991). Historical aspects of the vine and wine in Italy. *Alcologia*, 3, 21–29.

Poldrugo, F., Fiore, A., & Manzan, L. (1988). *Alcoholic women: Background characteristics and treatment outcome*. Trieste, Italy: University of Trieste, Alcohol Research Center.

Poldrugo, F., & Stratta, P. (1993). Alcoholism among young people in Italy: An attempt to analyse the phenomenon. *Alcoholism* (Zagreb), 29, 73–79.

Rosatti, A. (1990). The Italians. In *Insight Guides* (pp. 64–71). Singapore: Hofer Press.

Rotunno, M., & McGoldrick, M. (1982). Italian families. In M. McGoldrick, J. K. Pearce, & J. Giordano (Eds.), *Ethnicity and family therapy* (pp. 340–363). New York: Guilford Press.

Sirey, A. R., Patti, A., & Mann, L. (1985). *Ethnotherapy: An exploration of Italian-American identity*. New York: National Institute for the Psychotherapies.

Spector, R. (1996). *Cultural diversity in health and illness*. Stamford, CT: Appleton & Lange.

Straussner, S. L. A., & Zelvin, E. (Eds.). (1997). *Gender and addiction: Men and women in treatment*. Northvale, NJ: Jason Aronson.

Tardi, S. (1996-1997). The traditional Italian family is alive and well and living in New Jersey. *Italian American Review*, 5(2), 2–14.

U.S. Bureau of the Census. (1990). *Census of population and housing*. Washington, DC: U.S. Department of Commerce.

12

Polish Identity and Substance Abuse

Jim Gilbert
Jan Langrod

$\mathbf{P}$olish Americans make up one of the largest White ethno-cultural groups in the United States, numbering approximately 6 million (U.S. Bureau of the Census, 1998). Substance abuse, particularly alcoholism, has historically been a challenge to this community. This chapter explores cultural and historical factors related to substance abuse in the Polish American community and discusses treatment approaches and implications for this population.

POLAND'S HISTORY

Polish jokes denigrate a culture rich in tradition and accomplishment. For the first 600 years of its existence, Poland was a major European power and exerted a profound influence on European history (Barnett, 1958; Curtis, 1994). For example, during the 16th and 17th centuries substantial segments of the Polish intelligentsia stressed freedom of religious thought, tolerance, education, and social equality for all people (Krzyżanowski, 1983). During the 18th century, even under the domination of foreign powers, free universal education for all social classes was maintained in certain areas of Poland (Thackeray, 1983).

Beginning in the 17th century Poland went into decline, culminating in a partition takeover in the 18th century by Prussia, Russia, and Austria. This virtually erased Poland from the map of Europe (Davis, 1992; Thernstrom, 1990). The Republic of Poland reemerged following World War I but was invaded by Germany in 1939 and occupied until the end of World War II. A period of socialism with strong Soviet Communist influence followed, ending in 1989 with the election of Lech Walesa and the Solidarity Movement.

Currently, Poland is struggling with the transition from socialism to capitalism. This transition has resulted in a dramatic increase in social problems, including increased unemployment, homelessness, and crime, as well as addiction and HIV (Sekiewicz, 1994).

POLISH CULTURAL DYNAMICS

Family and church are principal factors in Polish culture, the family being the center of Polish life. Polish women play an important role in the family, often at odds with traditional female roles. Although much has been said about Roman Catholicism as a repressive institution, the Catholic Church, for Poles, has had an overall positive effect in maintaining the culture. These factors have to be taken into consideration in treating substance abuse disorders among Poles.

The Role of the Family

In Polish culture it is the family, and not the individual's reputation, that is all-important—a value that has historically reinforced the unity of the family. According to Folwarski and Marganoff (1996), "strong measures of family social control were used to prevent deviation that might lower the family's reputation in the community" (p. 662). As a result, shame became a principal aspect of the Polish experience: One must not deviate from the expected in the areas of religion, family, and community. To do so brings shame to the family.

Mostwin (1980) suggests that cultural values among Polish families include "mutual respect, support, cooperation, financial and spiritual help, staying together and sacrificing . . . " (p. 110). Respect, rather than unconditional love, is the principal binding factor, and love within a family is expressed through cooperation and action (Mondykowski, 1982; Mostwin, 1980). For example, a Polish American client talked about how during his childhood in Detroit he was given the "job" of shining everyone's shoes for church on Sunday. He experienced this as a sign of status and respect within the family, even though some of his non-Polish friends used to make fun of this "job." He readily internalized his Polish family values, by which "doing" was more important than "being," work was highly valued, and cooperation was imperative.

The Role of Women

Male dominance has traditionally been a presence in Polish history (Folwarski & Marganoff, 1996; Tryzno, Pedagogic, Grudziak-Sobczyk, Prawn, & Morowski, 1989). However, the role of Polish women is not entirely subservient. By tradition, Polish wives brought a dowry to the marriage, and after marriage it was the wife who monitored those assets (Mondykowski, 1982). Moreover, despite Poland's close association with the Catholic Church, sex is not considered sinful in and of itself, and it is appropriate for women to enjoy it (Novak, 1975). Nonetheless, as in many other societies, there are double standards regarding extramarital and premarital sex. If men are unfaithful in marriage and are discreet about it, such behavior is tolerated without being condoned. However, the same behavior is not tolerated in women (Mondykowski, 1982).

In keeping with Polish cultural values, respect rather than the open display of affection is the noticeable trait in wife–husband relationships (Barnett, 1958). Such mutual respect is reflected in the division of labor and decision making in Polish families, in which historically, women worked alongside their husbands in harvesting and planting: "Doing heavy field work gave these women a higher status than their Western European counterparts, who contributed most of their labor in the home" (Mondykowski, 1982, p. 398). More recently, Poland, like most Communist countries, had offered women greater opportunities for work and education than have been provided by their Western European neighbors. By the 1970s, almost half of the Polish workforce was made up of women. In addition, between 1975 and 1983, the total number of Polish women with graduate degrees almost doubled to 681,000. Professions such as architecture, engineering, and university teaching have a substantially higher representation of women in Poland than in the West (Curtis, 1994). Yet women were virtually excluded from the highest positions in government in the Communist system and also in Solidarity, which took power from the Communists. In 1992, Hanna Suchocka was elected as the first woman prime minister of Poland; however, her coalition government contained no other women.

Women are completely excluded from another source of power in Poland—the Catholic Church. However, in the early 1990s Polish women set a precedent by organizing and demonstrating against the Catholic Church's position on abortion. This movement was sparked not only by the abortion question but also by the fact that unemployment increased dramatically following the transition from socialism to a market economy, and women were disproportionately represented among the unemployed (Curtis, 1994).

The Role of Religion

Although historically Poland has been the home of a sizeable Jewish population, being Polish has been described as synonymous with being Catholic (Folwarski & Marganoff, 1996).

The Importance of Catholicism

Polish ties to the Catholic Church go back to the 10th century. When Poland was fragmented by outside forces during the 18th century, the Church not only remained stable and intact but also expanded its role to combat social repression. During this time, the public use of the Polish language was forbidden by the Russian forces that had taken over a large section of the country. Consequently, religious practice was often the only means of national and social communication among Poles (Curtis, 1994). During the Nazi occupation, between 1938 and 1945, the Church suffered tremendous losses as its leadership was severely persecuted or killed, its schools closed, and its property seized or destroyed. In the years following World War II, the Church underwent a further revision, which was described as a "conversion from an aloof hierarchy with feudal overtones to a flexible, socially active institution capable of dealing with the adversity of the post-war years" (Curtis, 1994, p. 93). Roman Catholicism thus continued to provide a link between national and religious identity and, as a result, Poland was the only country in which the advent of Communist leadership had almost no effect on religious practice.

Although the Roman Catholic Church enhanced its power in post-Communist Poland, it also has begun to alienate significant sectors of the population due to its conservative stance on abortion and compulsory religious instruction in the schools. In addition, its support of programs of aid to the poor has been viewed by some anti-Communist Poles as a remnant of the Communist system (Curtis, 1994).

The Relationship between Christian and Jewish Poles

For approximately 800 years, until the first partition in 1772, Poland provided a safe haven for European Jews. Casimir the Great (1332–1370) and successive rulers encouraged Jewish settlement in Polish territories, thus invigorating Polish urban life and commerce (Lopata, 1975). For several centuries following Casimir's rule, Jews were given a home in Poland with semiautonomous rights that included freedom to practice their religion and to provide for their own education and local self-government. Ultimately, Jews suffered fewer restrictions in Poland than elsewhere in Europe, while establishing themselves as leaders in commerce and managers of noble estates (Curtis, 1994; Mondykowski, 1982). By the 17th century, Poland became home to 75% of the world's Jews. However, during the long period of the decline of Poland, anti-Semitism emerged and flourished. Despite the positive influence that the Catholic Church had on the Polish community, many Jews believe that the Church ignored anti-Semitism and overlooked its practice by individual clergymen.

During World War II, many non-Jewish Poles risked their lives in giving aid to Polish Jews, and numerous Polish families were murdered by the Nazis for protecting Jews. Nonetheless, some Poles collaborated with the Nazis against Jews, and after the war Jewish survivors faced anti-Semitic attacks in Poland (Werner, 1992). Following the war, the Communists who took power in Poland enacted laws against anti-Semitism but unfortunately did not eradicate it.

Since the 1990s, a minirevival of Jewish culture and religion has been taking place in Poland, much of it supported by American Jews. There has been an increasing dialogue between representatives of the Jewish community and the Polish government to return Jewish commercial property to the Jewish community (Greenberg, 1998). Nonetheless, the relationship between Poles and the Jewish community remains problematic. As stated by Folwarski and Marganoff (1996), "few subjects are more sensitive in Polish circles today than Poland's relations with her Jewish minority" (p. 665). Moreover, some Jews in the United States, whose families lived in Poland during the war, tend to hold negative views regarding Poles and Polish Americans. This attitude may be an unverbalized factor in the treatment of Polish American substance abusers by Jewish clinicians and vice versa.

POLISH IMMIGRATION TO THE UNITED STATES

Although there are anecdotal reports of Poles coming to the New World prior to 1600 on Viking ships and also traveling with Columbus, the actual documentation of Polish immigration starts with the Jamestown colony in the early part of the 17th century (Greene, 1961). These early immigrants were mainly artisans and craftsmen. For the next 100 years, small groups of relatively wealthy Poles settled in the various colonies (Folwarski & Marganoff, 1996). Two major uprisings against foreign dominance, one in 1830 and one in 1863, failed to win freedom for Poland and led to the first major exodus of Polish intellectuals, many of whom settled in the United States. The United States had a particular appeal to these Polish immigrants, who admired the constitutional foundation of its government and its revolutionary fervor (Thernstrom, 1990).

Beginning in 1870, a new type of Polish immigrant began arriving in the United States in large numbers. In Poland, these emigrants were called *za chlebem* (for bread). They were mostly very poor and illiterate peasants seeking economic opportunities unavailable at home. The estimated numbers of Polish immigrants who came to the United States between 1870 and 1913 vary from 2 to 3 million (Folwarski & Marganoff, 1996; Greene, 1961). Upon reaching the United States, they took the most menial jobs and lived and worked under deplorable conditions. Moreover, having lived under severe political oppression, they were not prone to trust or assimilate with outsiders. Consequently, they were treated with disdain by Americans and other immigrant groups. Davis (1992) describes Polish Americans during the latter part of the 19th and the early part of the 20th centuries as discriminated against socially and in housing and employment in most communities in the United States. He compared immigrant Poles to African Americans living in the Jim Crow South. Their high rate of illiteracy further contributed to severe discrimination and led to the stereotypical phrase of "dumb Polack."

Due to the ever-present discrimination, the survival of Polish American immigrants depended upon the strength and integrity of their families, their close association with the Catholic Church, and assistance based on mutuality and self-help. They bonded together in tightly built communities known as "Polonias" and were able to join together to work for their common interests with apparent ease. Under the circumstances, assimilation was slow, and family life among Polish Americans reflected little change over the years. Polzin (1973) described their way of life as "relatively distinct from that of the surrounding society" (p. 130). More recently, upward mobility among younger Polish Americans has apparently eroded some of the separateness of these communities and, like many other Americans, the more acculturated younger Poles have left the Polonias and moved to the suburbs (Folwarski & Marganoff, 1996). Initially, however, when Polonias were quite distinct from the surrounding society, Polish Americans formed mutual aid and self-help organizations ranging from insurance and banking to help widows and orphans (Greene, 1975).

From World War II until about 1960, Polish migration to the United

States consisted mostly of educated professionals. These immigrants apparently had an easier time assimilating than their earlier counterparts (Folwarski & Marganoff, 1996). More recently, due to the economic problems in Poland, there has been an influx of single, educated Polish women, as well as of working-class Polish men, who settled mainly in Chicago, New York City, and other cities with existing Polish communities. Many of them are here illegally.

Unable to get employment in their fields, many of the recent immigrant Polish women work off the books as baby-sitters, domestic workers, and nurse's aides earning a minimal wage. Their loss of status and homesickness makes them vulnerable to depression and substance abuse. Unlike these unmarried women, most of the recently migrating Polish men left their wives and children in Poland, hoping to save enough money to send for them or to return to Poland with their savings. With minimal education and language skills, these men tend to live in conditions of severe poverty with few social supports. They are even more susceptible to substance abuse, particularly alcoholism.

SUBSTANCE ABUSE

Alcohol abuse is the most serious substance abuse problem among Poles, both in Poland and in the United States (Folwarski & Marganoff, 1996; Knab, 1993; Morowski, 1992; Tryzno et al., 1989). However, since World War II, there has been a substantial increase in the use and abuse of other substances, as well as a growing awareness of treatment effectiveness.

Alcohol Abuse in Poland

Heavy drinking is common among Poles, and drinking is frequently seen as "a natural and positive part of life" (Folwarski & Marganoff, 1996, p. 663). In Polish culture, alcohol is considered a necessary part of life: It is used for sealing contracts, marking life events, and as a function of hospitality. Drinking among Poles has been characterized as an expression of personal freedom (Freund, 1985).

Despite the frequency of heavy drinking and a growing recognition of alcoholism as a serious problem, there is a strong cultural resistance to acknowledging alcoholism as a disease. Feelings of shame at not being able to handle the drinking, combined with the idea that drinking, even heavy drinking, is acceptable, leads to denial and enabling activities among many Polish families. Tryzno and colleagues (1989) report that alcoholism in Poland is a major cause of divorce and that 21% of Polish children are raised in alcoholic homes. These factors should be taken into consideration when treating Polish families, both in Poland and in the United States.

The Abuse of Other Drugs in Poland

The use and addiction to drugs began to emerge during the late 1960s, in parallel with the experiences of the "hippie" generation in the United States. Trichlorethylene, a hallucinogen commonly called "tri," became the most popular drug among young people. This and a variety of other hallucinogens, solvents, and glues are commonly consumed together with alcohol (Sekiewicz, 1994).

During the mid-1970s, following a brief period during which sedative hypnotics and stimulants were popular, a massive increase in the use of narcotics took place after a pharmacy student developed what became known as Polish heroin, or *kompot*. *Kompot* constitutes from 70% to 80% of all illicit drugs used by Polish addicts (Curtis, 1994).

Moreover, since 1991, Poland has become one of the largest world producers of illicit amphetamines. Amphetamines are generally used with *kompot* in intravenous injections (Sieroslawski, 1995). Between May 1991 and December 1992, law enforcement authorities confiscated more than 92 kilos of illicit amphetamine that was being exported from Poland (Holyst, 1994).

Substance Abuse and Polish Americans

According to Folwarski and Marganoff (1996), "when it comes to conflict and conflict resolution, Poles are stubborn and have a national and individual reluctance to yield or compromise" (p. 669). The authors see this dynamic as playing an important role in the use of alcohol by Polish Americans: "This inability to negotiate to achieve mutually satisfying goals probably is both a contributing cause and an effect of the pervasive use and abuse of alcohol in Polish American culture. The heavy drinking functions to allow the expression of weakness through crying or other forms of abreaction. If individuals are drunk they can disclaim responsibility for their words and actions" (pp. 669–670).

No available data exists regarding substance abuse among Polish Americans. However, anecdotal reports from two substance abuse programs that service Polish Americans suggest that crack and heroin abuse is growing among younger Polish Americans (R. Pabis & K. Troczynska, personal communication, September 15, 1998). Nevertheless, alcohol appears to be the principal substance of choice among Polish Americans. As in Poland, drinking, even heavy drinking, is accepted as the norm among Polish Americans. As pointed out by Folwarski and Marganoff (1996), two of the most common establishments in Polish American communities are bars and churches—with bars outnumbering the churches.

TREATMENT ISSUES FOR POLISH AMERICANS

Although there are no specific substance abuse treatment approaches for Polish Americans, there are certain specific considerations that should be taken into account when dealing with this population in any kind of treatment setting. Because Poles tend to be mainly action oriented in personal relationships, tangible and practical treatment goals should be applied in preference to insight-oriented approaches. Self-help approaches are highly valued.

Shame

Substance abuse as an illness has been described as "shame based" (Johnson, 1986), and, as mentioned previously, shame is a principal component of the Polish experience. Consequently, if not dealt with, the issue of shame, particularly as it is related to one's sense of identity, can be a detriment to successful treatment and may contribute to future relapse.

Lopata (1975) reports that Poles changed their names more often than members of any other ethnocultural group in the United States. Although most Poles who change their surname claim that the new names are easier to spell and pronounce, Folwarski and Marganoff (1996) believe that name changes are also related to feelings of shame resulting from a culture that has been "brutalized by historical events, distorted by the media and literature and ridiculed by countless Polish jokes" (p. 662). Such name changes often make it difficult for treatment practitioners to identify many of their clients as being of Polish background. Subsequently, this lack of identification may contribute to difficulties in addressing cultural identity conflict that may play a role in substance abuse.

An example of how the issue of identity and shame can be associated with substance abuse is demonstrated in the following case example:

> John O is a 61-year-old elementary school teacher who had a long history of heavy drinking until he joined Alcoholics Anonymous (AA) 6 years ago at the suggestion of his cousin. His mother was a first-

generation Polish American, and his father's family migrated from Poland during the 19th century, at which time they changed their name to a more American-sounding one. Both of his parents were alcoholics and were unable to raise him. Mr. O was raised by Polish immigrant relatives of his mother who lived in an Irish American neighborhood. During his childhood, he remembers feeling ashamed of being Polish and wanted to be Irish like his friends. When he discovered alcohol in his teens, he found a way to be more desirable, interesting, and at ease with himself and his peers. As an adult, Mr. O was glad that he did not have a Polish surname and that few people knew of his Polish background. It was not until after participating in ongoing therapy with a private practitioner that Mr. O made a connection between his intense feelings of shame and his Polish background. Mr. O now believes that the anti-Polish climate during his childhood contributed to his feelings of inadequacy and self-consciousness, which had such a tremendously negative impact on his life for many years.

Substance abuse in general, and alcoholism in particular, are generally seen as the result of a multifactorial process involving genetic, psychological, family, and cultural factors (Straussner, 1993). Frequently, however, there is a tendency to diminish, if not ignore, social or cultural factors related to substance abuse (Gilbert, 1998). In the case of Mr. O, it was not until the latter part of a relatively long treatment experience that he became aware of his shame related to being Polish. He did not have a Polish last name and could deny his Polish ethnicity with relatively little deception. However, it was only when Mr. O began to address his strongly negative feelings related to his Polish identity that the last hurdle in his treatment was addressed and overcome.

The use of a family genogram is particularly valuable in helping clients whose names have been changed to identify their Polish roots and to get in touch with any of their unconscious negative feelings about their background. Folwarski and Marganoff (1996) emphasize the value of a three- or four-generational genogram in order to open up such a discussion.

Oliver (1989) suggests that the use of historical information in interventions with young African American men has been an effective tool in addressing shame and self-hatred in this population. He argues that the knowledge of historical accomplishments in a population that has been stigmatized by much of society reduces self-hatred. This dynamic also has significant implications for clinical interventions with Polish Americans. For example, it is valuable for an individual who feels ashamed about being Polish to learn that for more than 600 years Poland was a leader among European countries in the fields of art, science, and commerce. Becoming aware of Poland's early historical emphasis on universal education can be used to provide a strong repudiation to the negative stereotypical image of the "dumb Polack."

Glen Curtis (1994) has completed a remarkable research document on Poland called *Poland: A Country Study* that covers the entire history of its existence. This book, and others like it, can be utilized to educate Polish Americans about their long history of trauma and survival and the numerous positive contributions of the Polish people.

Immigration and Legal Issues

An important issue affecting more recent Polish immigrants is their legal status in the United States, which may limit their treatment options. For example:

> Wojtek K is a 37-year-old chemical engineer. He was laid off from his job in Poland during the wave of privatization in the early 1990s. He and his wife, an elementary school teacher, and their two young children lived in a small one-bedroom apartment in Warsaw. Unable to find a job, Mr. K decided to come to the United States. He initially arrived on a 6-month tourist visa but then decided to stay longer. Because he was an undocumented immigrant with limited English skills, he took the first job that was offered, working for less than minimum wage in asbestos removal. Working overtime, he earned approximately $350 weekly and sent $300 of it each week to his family in Poland. In order to save money, he lived with two other Polish men in an abandoned apartment building in a city with a large Polish community.
>
> In Poland, although Mr. K drank regularly on weekends, he was able to control his drinking and to function well. However, once in the United States, his drinking escalated. He and his roommates would drink daily, sharing their liquor supplies. After a few months, Mr. K grew increasingly more depressed and had difficulty at work. He started complaining of pains in the abdomen and finally was taken to a local emergency room by a coworker. He was initially treated for a bleeding ulcer and was then diagnosed as alcohol dependent and transferred to an inpatient alcohol detoxification unit. Upon discharge, he was encouraged to attend a Polish-speaking AA group, where he found an important source of support and was able to maintain his abstinence. The absence of a prior history of depression suggests that his depression was secondary to his drinking and reflected adjustment difficulties.
>
> Unfortunately, with the change in immigration laws and policies, Mr. K was no longer able to obtain low-cost medications and treatment for his ulcer. Shortly afterward he returned to Poland. However,

the introduction to AA provided him with the tools of recovery. When he returned to Poland, Mr. K was able to utilize this experience by becoming an active member of AA in his hometown and continuing his recovery.

As indicated previously, mutual aid and self-help are important aspects of Polish culture. In keeping with these priorities, Poland was the first Eastern European country to establish AA groups in the early 1970s (Alcoholics Anonymous World Services, 1998). In addition to AA, Al-Anon, Alateen, and Adult Children of Alcoholics (ACOA) groups have also been established (Makela, Arminen, & Bloomfield, 1996).

Situations like Mr. K's are becoming increasingly more common in the Polish immigrant community in the United States. For example, four homeless Polish immigrants were found dead over the past 2 years in one New Jersey community alone (May, 1999). A newspaper report focused on the most recent death of a man who had a similar profile to that of Mr. K. A skilled carpenter who left his wife and children in Poland, this man came to the United States to find work but succumbed to alcohol abuse and homelessness. The report goes on to state that he lived in a community of homeless Polish men who declined outside assistance (May, 1999). Reflecting awareness of the cultural resistance to outside help and of the traditional self-help approach of the Polish American, segments of the larger Polish American community, including the Church, are attempting to address this problem.

It is evident that when culture and language are taken into consideration, the traditional substance abuse treatment approaches utilized in the United States can be readily applied with clients of Polish background. Although current policies may discourage illegal immigrants from seeking help, the availability of free and anonymous 12-step programs such as AA is an important and culturally appropriate source of help for Polish individuals in the United States.

Interventions with Family Members

Resistance to treatment may be encountered among Polish American clients because of difficulty in accepting the idea of substance abuse as a treatable problem. This leads to enabling behavior on the part of many Polish American families. However, the therapeutic utilization of Polish culture can be helpful in dealing with treatment resistance and enabling behavior. For example, children in Polish families tend to be raised in a rather strict disciplinary tradition. However, as noted by Mondykowski (1982), it is the "bad behavior" that is punished, without an implication of "personal bad-ness." It would be culturally uncharacteristic for Polish parents to punish a child simply to abate their own anger. The principle is that negative behavior results in negative consequences. This view is in keeping with a major principle of substance abuse treatment—that substance abuse results in negative consequences (Johnson, 1986). This approach can be readily understood by Polish families.

Once engaged in treatment, family members can be a significant resource in the treatment of Polish American substance abusers. In fact, segments of Polish communities, including the Church and extended families, can be utilized as part of a support network that would enhance treatment effectiveness.

> Mary L is a 58-year-old first-generation Polish American homemaker. She had been married to Richard L for 38 years. The couple had four grown children. Mr. L. had a progressive alcohol problem for 30 of those years, during which time he became increasingly more verbally abusive and at times even physically abusive to Mrs. L. In the past, when it was suggested by a neighbor or more recently by her married daughter that she seek outside help, Mrs. L would reply that she wasn't the one with the problem. She always maintained a good home for Mr. L and did her job bringing up their children. However, Mr. L was diagnosed with a severe alcohol-related liver disorder for which the prognosis was very poor unless he stopped drinking. Mrs. L, feeling depressed and scared, sought help from her parish priest. The priest suggested that she attend Al-Anon meetings held in their church basement. This time Mrs. L complied. Subsequently, with the support of her daughter and her priest, she began to encourage Mr. L to go to AA meetings held in the same church.

Tryzno and colleagues (1989) maintain that Polish families tend to resist outside help to a greater degree than many other groups. Mrs. L endured years of her husband's active alcoholism and also harbored feelings of hurt and resentment. She desperately attempted to keep up appearances, and in line with her cultural background, believed that as long as she did her job and held her family together, everything was fine. For years she was able to tolerate her own discomfort and pain, as long as her family's unity continued. Only when family unity was threatened by Mr. L's illness did she seek help from a source she could trust—her priest. Given the strong connection that many Poles feel toward the Roman Catholic Church, it is clear that the involvement and support of their priests is important in providing help to Polish American substance abusers and their family members.

CONCLUSION

People of Polish background generally reflect the cultural values of hard work, loyalty, and resilience, which are important dynamics given their history of heavy drinking and, more recently, other substance abuse problems. Getting a "little drunk" is not a shameful thing in itself, but if alcohol or other drugs interfere with work or home life, it can lead to intense feelings of shame that need to be addressed during treatment. Treatment providers may experience initial resistance among Polish clients, but once engaged, they are likely to work hard toward achieving treatment goals. AA-oriented treatment has been effective for this population and should be used when appropriate. Many Poles are deeply religious and have a strong collective identity with the Catholic Church. This characteristic reinforces their ethnocultural identity and should be encouraged by clinicians. Finally, Poles who are at odds with their ethnocultural identity should be encouraged to revisit their Polish roots. Folwarski and Marganoff (1996) speak of this process as "a way of going home, not again, but for the first time" (p. 672).

REFERENCES

Alcoholics Anonymous World Services. (1998). AA's growth in Eastern Europe. In *About AA* (pp. 1–4). New York: Author.

Barnett, C. (1958). *Poland.* New Haven, CT: Human Relations Area File Press.

Curtis, G. E. (Ed.). (1994). *Poland: A country study* (3rd ed.). Washington, DC: Federal Research Division, Library of Congress.

Davis, N. (1992). *Heart of Europe: A short history of Europe.* New York: Oxford University Press.

Folwarski, J., &. Marganoff, P. P. (1996). Polish families. In M. McGoldrick, J. Giordano, & J. K. Pearce (Eds.) *Ethnicity and family therapy* (2nd ed., pp. 658–672). New York: Guilford Press.

Freund, P. (1985). Polish-American drinking: Continuity and change. In L. Bennett & G. Ames (Eds.), *The American experience with alcohol: Contrasting cultural perspectives* (pp. 77–92). New York: Plenum Press.

Gilbert, J. (1998). *A comparison of African American and White addicts in methadone treatment program: The role of social causality in the development of addiction.* Unpublished doctoral dissertation, New York University, Ehrenkranz School of Social Work.

Greenberg, E. (1998, June 19). At last, Kaddish in Auschwitz. *The Jewish Week,* pp. 1, 15.

Greene, V. (1961). Pre World War I emigration to America: Motives and statistics. *Polish Review, 3,* 45–68.

Greene, V. (1975). *For God and country: The rise of Polish and Lithuanian ethnic consciousness in America 1860–1910.* Madison, WI: State Historical Society of Wisconsin.

Holyst, B. (1994). Drugs and crime in Poland. *Euro Criminology, 7,* 141–167.

Johnson, V. (1986). *Intervention.* Minneapolis, MN: Johnson Institute Books.

Knab, S. (1993). *Polish customs, traditions and folklore.* New York: Hippocrene Books.

Krzyżanowski, L. (1983). Exploring the roots of Unitarianism. *The Polish Review, 28*(1), 66–73.

Lopata, H. (1975). The Polish-American family. In C. Mindel & R. Habenstein (Eds.), *Ethnic families in America: Patterns and variations* (pp. 15–40). New York: Elsevier.

Makela, K., Arminen, I., & Bloomfield, K. (1996). *Alcoholics Anonymous as a mutual-help movement: A study in eight societies.* Madison, WI: University of Wisconsin Press.

May, T. (1999, July 17). Homeless man found dead is identified as Polish immigrant. *Hackensack Record,* p. A-13.

Mondykowski, S. (1982). Polish families. In M. McGoldrick, J. K. Pearce, & J. Giordano (Eds.), *Ethnicity and family therapy* (pp. 393–411). New York: Guilford Press.

Morowski, J. (1992). The odyssey of the Polish alcohol system. In H. Klingemann, J. Takala, & G. Hunt (Eds.), *Cure, care or control: Alcoholism treatment in sixteen countries* (pp. 238–248). Albany: State University of New York Press.

Mostwin, D. (1980). *Social dimension of family treatment.* Washington, DC: National Association of Social Workers.

Novak, M. (1975). *The rise of the unmeltable ethnics.* New York: Macmillan.

Oliver, M. (1989). Black males and social problems: Prevention through Afrocentric socialization. *Journal of Black Studies, 20*(1), 15–39.

Polzin, T. (1973). *The Polish Americans: Whence and whither.* Pulaski, WI: Franciscan.

Sekiewicz, J. (1994). *Janit Pompdiou Group/United Nations Community Development Project: Extension of the Multi-City Networks to Central and Eastern Europe.* Gdansk, Poland: City Report.

Sieroslawski, J. (1995, June). *Between aid and repression: The dilemmas of policy toward drug addiction in Poland.* Paper presented at the Annual Alcohol Epidemiology Symposium, Porto, Portugal.

Straussner, S. L. A. (1993). Assessment and treatment of clients with alcohol and other drug abuse problems: An overview. In S. L. A. Straussner (Ed.), *Clinical work with substance-abusing clients* (pp. 3–30). New York: Guilford Press.

Thackeray, F. (1983). N. N. Novosil'tsov: The Polish years. *Polish Review, 28*(1), 32–46.

Thernstrom, P. (Ed.). (1990). *Harvard encyclopedia of American ethnic groups.* Cambridge, MA: Harvard University Press.

Tryzno, W., Pedagogic, M., Grudziak-Sobczyk, E., Prawn, N., & Marowski, J.

(1989). The role of the family in alcohol education and alcohol abuse in Poland. *Medical Law*, *8*, 267–273.

U.S. Bureau of the Census. (1998). *Historical statistics of the United States*. New York: U.S. Department of Commerce.

Werner, H. (1992). *Fighting back: A memoir of Jewish resistance in World War II*. New York: Columbia University Press.

13

Russian-Speaking Substance Abusers in Transition

New Country, Old Problems

Helen Kagan
Kathryn C. Shafer

"Dad, now that vodka is so expensive, will you drink less?"
"No, my son, you will eat less."
—RUSSIAN JOKE

The Commonwealth of Independent States (CIS), formerly called the Union of Soviet Socialist Republics (USSR), has one of the highest incidences of alcoholism in the world (Segal, 1990). Concerns about alcohol consumption have been evident as early as 1917, when the Russian Czar Nicholas II implemented prohibition (Segal, 1987). The recent political changes in the CIS and the collapse of the Soviet ideology have radically changed the lives of its people and have led to an increase in social problems, including substance abuse, HIV, and AIDS (Specter, 1997a, 1997b). As the doors to the West opened, Soviet immigrants entered a world that had been previously forbidden, bringing their problems with them (Castex, 1992). Clinicians may thus find themselves dealing with recent arrivals from Russia and other republics while having limited experience, information, or guidance regarding such clients.

The purpose of this chapter is to explore the historical and cultural heritage of excessive drinking and drug use in the former Soviet Union and the impact of the Communist government and its downfall on the abuse of substances, particularly alcohol. We describe the common cultural, social, economic, and ideological aspects of the former Soviet citizen and the implications for therapeutic interventions with substance-abusing immigrants from the countries within the former Soviet Union.

BRIEF HISTORY OF THE FORMER SOVIET UNION

The former Soviet Union, now the CIS, is the largest country in the world. The vast area that makes up this country covers 8.6 million miles, which is larger than the United States and Canada combined. There are dozens of nationalities and hundreds of different ethnocultural groups. The most numerous are the Russians, although they make up only one half of this entire nation of people. In addition, there are the Ukrainians, the Byelorussians, and many other smaller ethnocultural groups, such as the Tartars, the Mongols, and the Chinese. The census bureaus officially recognize 112 different languages and numerous dialects (Moore, 1989).

In addition to political changes, the CIS is undergoing tremendous social upheaval. Until recently, central Moscow was filled with shoppers crowded into empty stores, waiting in lines for hours for a piece of meat for the family dinner. Today, there are still crowds but the shops are filled with bright colors and flashy fashions. Russians now have some money and are no longer at risk of being arrested by the secret service when they try to spend it. Russians, who were once worried about American nuclear bombs, are now more concerned about the possibility of their own nuclear weapons falling into the hands of former Communist leaders or about further power plant explosions such as Chernobyl. Lenin still lies in his Red Square mausoleum, but the line is now longer at the Moscow branch of McDonald's. Hundreds of monuments to the Soviet founder have been torn down, and the city of Leningrad has returned to its original name of St. Petersburg, after its founder, Peter the Great (Benn, 1997). Meanwhile, the former Communists are now free to practice their religions and are returning to the few remaining churches and other religious institutions.

For the ordinary person, the biggest change in this country has been the freedom to speak—and to starve. When Russian President Boris Yeltsin lifted controls on prices, which had been frozen for 30 years, inflation went wild. Suddenly, milk that had been sold for 30 kopecks was now selling for 2 rubles (200 kopecks)—if it could be found at all. A 5-kopeck bus ride rose to 50 kopecks. Elderly widows who had stashed 1,000 rubles under their mattresses for their funerals suddenly found that their life savings would not even buy a meal for the wake. For the first time, there are beggars in the streets, new wealthy Russians driving by in their Mercedes, and drug addicts seen daily in local neighborhoods.

Between the October 1917 revolution and March 1985, when Mikhail Gorbachev came to power and cracked open the wall of the Iron Curtain, the political life of the Soviet Union had been ruled by the Communist Party. Following the overthrow of the czarist rule of Nicholas II in 1922, Lenin, Trotsky, and the Communist Party established the Soviet Union as a federation under a complex division of republics and national areas. Although each subdivision was able to establish its own constitution and although the head of that republic would be a native, the deputy of the region would be a Russian with close links to Moscow and under the disciplined rule of the Communist Party (Moore, 1989).

It took Gorbachev 3 years to replace the old, hard-line Communists when he began his restructuring program, *perestroika*. In the spring of 1989, the Soviet people were allowed to vote in a multicandidate election. The Communist Party was still the only political party, but for the first time since 1917, the people could, and would, vote against it.

Recent Soviet History

Recent Soviet history can be divided into three major periods: (1) the period of general stagnation (or the period of slow erosion), associated primarily with the Brezhnev era; (2) the period of *perestroika* and *glasnost,* or reconstruction and openness (often referred to as the period of dismantling and dismay) under Gorbachev; and (3) the collapse of Communism and the Soviet Union (which can be viewed as a period of total disillusionment and disorientation) under the leadership of Boris Yeltsin. Each of these periods had an impact on the social attitudes, norms, behaviors, and values of the former Soviet citizens, as well as on their mental health and use of substances (Kissin, 1991).

The Stagnation Period

The "stagnation period" was a politically authoritarian period that lasted from 1960 until the mid-1980s. It was characterized by the cold war, social stagnation, and slow erosion of the economy. These dynamics led to mental conflicts and social isolation among the Soviet people. People felt mistrustful toward authority figures and society in general, while trying to maintain traditional family values and beliefs and hope for a better Communist way of life. On the emotional level, hostility was suppressed because it was unsafe to express it openly. Behaviorally, there was a tendency toward general passivity, along with attempts to utilize and manipulate the system to obtain basic human needs and services such as food, housing, and medical care. Intoxicating substances were used to cope with the pervasive feelings of powerlessness and insecurity.

The Dismantling Period

The period known as the era of *perestroika* and *glasnost* began with Gorbachev's rise to power in the mid-1980s and opened previously censored doors to the West. This opening led to the exposure and international awareness of the crimes and abuses of previous political leaders and of the problems perpetuated by the current one. Psychological reactions during this period included disillusionment with the Communist ideology and hope for the emergence of some democratic values. Emotionally, people had much fear and anxiety about the future of Russia, as well as feelings of being fooled, manipulated, and victimized by their leaders (Kissin, 1991). For the first time, many began to question traditional family values and ties and to openly express hostility toward authority. Physical confrontation and violence, both in the family and in the streets, became more prevalent. An increase in extramarital affairs, in substance abuse, and in drug addiction among teenagers also became evident. Greater freedom of sexual expression, sexual promiscuity, and prostitution increased the prevalence and contributed to the spread of HIV and AIDS (Specter, 1997b).

The Disorientation Period

The years between 1992 and 1997 were characterized by the total collapse of the Soviet system. The cognitive response to this development can be described as one of confusion and disorientation, with a corresponding emotional reaction of panic and fear. Behaviorally, this stage of disorientation has resulted in a hoarding of material possessions and an unprecedented desire (and opportunity) to flee the country. The decline of traditional beliefs and values, spiritual emptiness, and interrupted societal development have forced former Soviets to abandon their roots, ideologies, and ethics. These factors resulted in further increase in alcohol and drug abuse among the Russian population (Kagan, 1995-1996).

The Role of Religion

The atheist state propaganda attempted to keep the Soviet people from openly practicing their different religions. Consequently, many Russian Orthodox grandmothers kept their religious icons, Bibles, and candles hidden. They often took their children and grandchildren to be baptized in secret. Likewise, many Jewish families secretly tried to practice their religious traditions and observe their holidays at great risks to themselves and their families. The majority of the former Soviets, however, grew up without any religious or spiritual beliefs. Even Alcoholics Anonymous (AA) meetings, which emerged after *perestroika,* were held in secret because the "higher power" concept was viewed as quasi-religious by the Communist regime.

The Role of Russian Women

Although the Soviet regime empowered women to leave the home, obtain a college education, and enter the workforce, these "opportunities" also tripled women's responsibilities. With the downfall of the Soviet economy, despite 70 years of state propaganda during the Soviet era about the equality of the sexes, it became common to find the Russian husband at home, without work, socializing with other men over vodka, while the women worked like oxen, looking to their mothers and female friends for help with child care, friendship, and support. Women became family breadwinners, caretakers of the children and household—without any of the labor-saving household appliances available to their Western sisters—and responsible for managing the bureaucratic struggles of everyday survival.

At the same time, given the Communist ideology, which idealized feminine traits, they maintained an extravagant perception of femininity. The absence of feminist and women's liberation movements as seen in other developing countries has made it especially challenging for former Soviet women to assert themselves in relation to their men or the state. Since the doors to the West have opened, many Russian women are now seen wearing lots of makeup, smoking and drinking in bars, and spending their limited income on cosmetics, shampoos, clothing, and self-improvement items.

THE ROLE OF DRINKING IN RUSSIAN HISTORY

It has been said both that vodka is the lifeblood of the Russian culture and, conversely, that drinking is the Russian curse. For hundreds of years bingeing was characterized as a "Russian style" of drinking. Russia has been called the "land of the endless toasts" and "a nation of male bonding through the bottle." Although professional literature on Russian and Soviet *pianstvo* (drunkenness) is limited, drinking to get drunk is an important Russian custom that has been documented since ancient times (Kagan, 1992).

Drinking In Prerevolutionary Russia

In prerevolutionary Russia it was considered safer to drink alcohol than water. It was believed that rum, gin, and brandy were nutritious and healthy. "Spirits" such as vodka were viewed as being able to cure colds, fevers, and snakebite. Drinking alcohol enabled hard-working laborers to enjoy a moment of happy camaraderie, and public intoxication was customary. As pointed out by Segal (1990), "Communal intoxication was an important social custom among ancient Slavic tribes. All events of public significance—from wedding celebrations to religious holidays—were ritualized with alcohol. When a Slavic child was born, or when he grew up, when seeds were planted, or when the harvest was in, when the enemies were dispersed, or when the beloved died—at every point in the social cycle of a tribe, general drunkenness prevailed" (p. 1).

Whereas drinking in Muscovite Russia was fairly moderate and took place mainly at home, the Slavs who settled in Kievan Russia in the 9th century and became its rulers contributed a style of drinking in which people customarily drank until they became quite intoxicated. Segal (1990) states that according to legend, the Varangian Prince Vladimir, who reigned in 10th century Kiev and accepted Christianity in 988, had rejected Islam because the latter prohibited alcohol. " 'Drinking is the joy of the Rusi,' declared Vladimir; 'we cannot do without it.' His statement survives as a virtual slogan for Russian behavior through the ages" (Segal, 1990, p. 2).

Peter the Great, who ruled Russia between 1682 and 1725, was himself known to enjoy heavy drinking and insisted that his servants match him drink for drink (Segal, 1990). It is common knowledge that when a Russian wants a drink, he gestures by tapping his throat with his finger, signaling that the server should "set him up." This custom is believed to have originated during the time of Peter, who rewarded his loyalists with free drinking privileges by branding them under the chin. These men could then walk into any *kabak* (bar) and flick their throat, demonstrating their privilege to be "set up" for a free drink (Gibbons, 1992).

Throughout Russian history, its princes tried to maintain a firm control on alcohol production, and there were various czarist efforts to control drinking as a way of decreasing crime, violence, and poverty. Temperance

societies began as early as 1856 under the direction of the Russian Orthodox Church. However, according to Segal (1990), attempts at prohibition
turned out to be detrimental for the czarist, and later provisional, governments because they eliminated the traditional outlet for feelings of dissatis-
faction, envy, and rage.

Drinking in the Postrevolutionary Period

Following the October Revolution in 1917, the Communist Party and the
Soviet regime initiated and maintained a rigid revolutionary and atheistic
doctrine. Among the various proclamations was the theme that drunkenness could turn the country back to capitalism and that drinking was considered an "immoral behavior." However, neither the revolutionary consciousness nor the severe punishments given to public drunks had much
impact on the level of drinking among the Soviets (Segal, 1987).

   During World War II, Stalin, himself the child of an alcoholic father,
rationed the soldiers' daily intake of vodka. It became common practice for
Soviet servicemen to exchange their last piece of bread in order to get
vodka, and millions of soldiers got drunk to fight for their *matushka Rus*
(beloved mother-Russia). About 60 million Soviet citizens died during the
war. Following the war, Stalin and his *apparat* (cabinet) organized mass arrests for those who "betrayed" Rodina (the motherland) during the war.
These "betrayers," as well as innocent victims of his anti-Semitic campaign,
were persecuted and executed. Thousands of people were sent to labor
camps in Siberia, where they died due to malnutrition and forced labor.
The consequences of these events on the Soviet population were devastating: families were destroyed, the country was traumatized, and the quality
of life in the postwar Soviet Union remained extremely poor. Segal (1990)
claims that these factors made the country ripe for epidemic drinking of alcohol.

The Role of Drinking in Recent Soviet History

Throughout Russia's history, alcohol, primarily vodka, was used as an effective coping mechanism. The Soviet totalitarian regime emphasized the
loss of individuality and total immersion in the omnipotent societal group.
Opposition or deviation from this societal norm was punishable by execu-
tion, imprisonment, ostracism, or loss of employment and political restraint. This reality reinforced, and often dictated, a social style that is often
associated with prealcoholic personality traits (Segal, 1986). These traits
are characterized by passive–aggressive behaviors toward authority figures,

difficulties in interpersonal relationships, low self-esteem, and feelings of boredom, loneliness, and hopelessness.

In their efforts to control the feelings of isolation and alienation, Soviet citizens used alcohol and the social activities associated with its use as a means of creating an illusion of friendship when real companionship was politically dangerous. Because they were deprived of the freedom of expression and could not reveal their thoughts and opinions publicly, a drinking subculture emerged. A "kitchen culture" developed in which a night in the kitchen, accompanied by a bottle of vodka, was the only safe place to discuss political issues and to share one's personal problems (Kagan, 1997a).

Because the Soviets could not even imagine expressing their feelings openly, they did not learn the skills necessary to do so. One had to appear cheerful and enthusiastic and had to always demonstrate support and agreement with political and social issues, even if one genuinely disagreed with them. The Soviet system was always correct, and the capitalistic system, the enemy, was viewed as destructive, inhumane, and evil. This paranoid split view of the world was promoted in education and in the media. According to Olga Marlin, a Czechoslovakian psychologist who now works in New York City, growing up in this kind of atmosphere can make people feel dissociated, guilty, and ashamed (Marlin, 1990). The totalitarian society projected aggression onto other individuals, groups, or systems. There was a constant search for the external forces or outside enemies that were responsible for all the social and economic disadvantages of the nation and for the personal problems of individual citizens. The changing political and economic climate in the CIS has made life even more difficult and, as a result, further encouraged alcohol and drug use as an escape (Kagan, 1996).

In 1985, administrative measures were established to control individual alcohol purchases, as well as hours of operation for liquor vendors. History was repeated when criminal penalties were imposed on those identified as alcoholics. Purchasing a bottle of vodka in a liquor store required incredible endurance. People would stand from 3 to 5 hours in line, in rain, snow, and subzero temperatures, hoping that supplies of vodka would be available when their turn came. To meet the high demand, illegal "black markets" developed—one could simply go up an alley, walk into a park, or enter a taxicab and have well-stocked dealers in blue coats satisfy the demand. During this time of "controlled prohibition," many alcoholics drank perfumes, antifreeze, and household cleaning fluids. Illegal alcohol production increased sharply, with 40% of the *samogon* (moonshine) being manufactured in the cities (Segal, 1990). The ineffectiveness of the prohibition efforts and the lack of social, psychological, and medical services needed to address the high rate of alcohol problems forced the regime to stop enforcing these measures.

CURRENT ALCOHOL AND DRUG USE

Data on current per capita consumption of alcohol among the former Soviet republics are limited, and official statistics regarding social problems tend to be unreliable. From the 1950s to the 1970s, a group of Soviet researchers attempted to study the problem of alcoholism by conducting national surveys. However, this research was viewed as anti-Soviet propaganda, and the publication of its findings was censored (Segal, 1986).

It was estimated that the per capita consumption of alcoholic beverages in the USSR in 1985 was eight times higher than the per capita consumption had been prior to the 1917 Revolution and three times higher than the consumption in the United States. The rate of violent alcohol-related crimes was 10.5 times as high as that in the United States. The reduction of work productivity in the Russian economy due to alcoholic drinking is six times that of the United States (Segal, 1990).

More recent estimates indicate that 60% of the Russian workforce abuses alcohol (Anderson, 1992). Out of 148 million people, there are approximately 15 million "chronic alcoholics," and the number of "heavy drinkers" is three to four times that (Davis, 1994). In 1990, in St. Petersburg alone, a city of 4,672,000 people, there were approximately 80,000 substance abusers, predominantly alcoholics, and 60,000 suicides, many of which were alcohol related. Moreover, there were 19,000 deaths from acute alcohol poisoning, and of the 22,000 murders, 80% were alcohol related (Yandow, 1992). In Moscow, a city of 10,446,000 people, about 145,000 patients were registered in the city's largest narcological (alcohol and drug abuse) hospital during 1992. Of these, 95% were in the most severe stage of the disease and about 10% were women. One in every 10 was a teenager (E. Drozdov, personal communication, March 1992).

Since the collapse of the Soviet Union in 1991, the abuse of other drugs has reached epidemic proportions. Currently, use of marijuana, cocaine, heroin, and prescription drugs is increasing. In addition, significant increases have occurred among adolescents in sniffing inhalants such as glue, paint, and homemade synthetic drugs (Davis, 1994; Specter, 1997b). The recent changes in Russian economy and the globalization of trade have increased illegal drug traffic in the former Soviet Union. Officials document a general increase in cross-addiction due, in part, to the rapid rise of the Russian Mafia, who have acquired the technology and chemicals for producing heroin and other illicit drugs (Davis, 1994). According to Specter (1997a), with more than 2 million drug addicts, "Russia has become one of the world's great drug bazaars. Cheap liquid heroin often costs little more than an ice cream sandwich. Children as young as 12 regularly experiment with a special cut-rate and low-quality brand of heroin called Chornye, which means black, and originates mostly from the poorly guarded borders of Pakistan, Afghanistan and other countries in Central Asia." (p.5).

TREATMENT APPROACHES IN THE FORMER SOVIET UNION

Following the 1917 Revolution, alcoholics who were drinking on the job or displaying public drunkenness were picked up by the militia (police) and registered with the government, and the word "alcoholic" was stamped on their domestic passports (Segal, 1990). During the Soviet era alcoholics were involuntarily sent to "sobering-up stations." Such "stations" were unique Soviet creations for overnight detoxification, stabilization, and public humiliation. The family of the "captured" individual was made responsible for paying for the involuntary detoxification at the sobering-up station, and the person's photograph was posted at his or her place of employment as a warning to others (Kagan, 1994).

If a person displayed psychotic symptoms while intoxicated or in the state of withdrawal, he or she was transported to the local psychiatric institution. For medical complications due to alcohol poisoning, treatment options included admission to the narcological unit at the psychiatric facility or to a specialized narcological facility that was usually affiliated with a factory or plant. This type of inpatient treatment facility was known as a "Labor-Prevention-Rehabilitation" camp. It often included the use of "labor therapy," an important aspect of the Communist ideology (Kagan, 1992). Treatment also included the surgical implantation of "torpedoes" into the patients' backs. These torpedoes contained Antabuse-like drugs that created severe nausea and pain if the alcoholic drank again. At times, due to lack of proper medical supplies, surrogate drugs were utilized as placebos and dispensed to patients when supplies of the proper medications were not made available. Like the torpedoes, these medications also caused toxic consequences in the body. Alcoholics who refused treatment were labeled as "antisocial elements" and were required to do hard physical labor. Once discharged from the hospital, they were usually unable to find work, and, if caught drinking again, they were literally thrown back into the hospital, where they were injected with painful drugs to "discipline" them (Gibbons, 1992).

CURRENT TREATMENT APPROACHES

Current substance abuse treatment includes the use of alternative and herbal medicine. These techniques are based on the use of biological methods similar to the practices utilized in homeopathy, often associated with folk remedies. In addition, detoxification, psychotherapy, and pharmacotherapy such as Antabuse are commonly used. According to E. Drosdov, director of Narcology Hospital #17, treatment methods used at his facility include those that arouse the patient's disgust for alcohol through Pavlovian behavioral conditioning methods and recoding (hypnosis). These approaches are claimed to have effective treatment outcomes and no side effects (E. Drosdov, personal communication, March 1992).

Alcoholics Anonymous (AA) in Russia only emerged after *perestroika*, and meetings were usually held in secret. Many people resisted attending AA meetings because of the general mistrust toward organized activities that resembled the common practices of the "collective" ideology. Moreover, many people had a difficult time embracing the "higher power" concept, which was considered too religious, as well as associated with the negative power of the totalitarian regime. In addition, the expense of printing information about when and where meetings were held was prohibitive, and the necessity of relying on word of mouth to obtain meeting information compromised the anonymity of its members (Shafer, 1994).

Although some Russian clinicians have embraced the disease concept and the medical model of addiction treatment, they retain a general lack of knowledge and understanding of the social and psychological aspects of addiction, particularly as applied to family dynamics. For example, they lack knowledge of such concepts as enabling and codependency, terms associated with the family's response to substance-abusing members. Therefore, professionals tend to view the family members of the substance abuser as helpless victims. In general, no help or support is offered to the families of substance abusers. Moreover, confidentiality is a concept unfamiliar not only to persons receiving substance abuse treatment but also to clinicians. In the former Soviet Union as in other developing nations, alcohol and drug prevention efforts have not been viewed as an important priority of the central government (Kagan, 1998).

SUBSTANCE ABUSE AMONG FORMER SOVIETS IN THE UNITED STATES

According to the U.S. Immigration and Naturalization Service, almost one quarter of a million (247,764) former Soviets arrived in the United States between 1990 and 1994. The largest contingent of the immigrants were born in the Ukraine, followed by Russia, Uzbek, and Belarus (U.S. Immigration and Naturalization Service, 1997). During fiscal year 1996, 19,668 immigrants came to the United States from Russia, and another 21,079 came from the Ukraine (United States Department of Justice, 1997). There is no documentation available on the prevalence of alcohol and drug problems among CIS immigrants in the United States. However, because approximately 20–25% of the population in the former Soviet Union have alcohol and drug problems (Davis, 1994), it can be assumed that thousands of former Soviet citizens have problems related to alcohol and other drug use.

It is not unusual for immigrants to cope with the stresses caused by the discrepancies between their expectations and the realities of life in their new home by turning to alcohol and drugs. The greater availability, lower cost, higher level of alcohol concentration, and higher quality of alcoholic beverages in the United States results in increased drinking among those immigrants from CIS who were already reliant on the use of alcohol to cope with life. Additionally, due to years of poor diet and medical care, Russian immigrants often arrive in the United States with serious medical problems. Such problems may require prolonged use of prescribed medications and often result in abuse and dependency on the prescribed drugs. Some immigrants have become involved in illegal drug distribution in the United States.

Cocaine and heroin use appear to be increasing among younger immigrants from the CIS. Due to the lack of education and prevention efforts in Russia and the other former Soviet republics, young people are not familiar with the dangerous consequences of illegal drugs and often find their new American identity in the easily accessible drug culture, as exemplified in the following case:

Dennis is a 20-year-old Jewish male from Russia who was brought to a drug-free substance abuse clinic for help with his heroin addiction by a new friend who was a patient at the clinic. Dennis, who had been in the United States for only a few months, had emigrated in order to fulfill his dream of a better life than the miserable, hopeless existence he had had, living with his mother in a small Russian village. Dennis's parents divorced when he was a child, and he had had limited contact with his father since then. When Dennis was 17, he received a letter from his father, who had emigrated to the United States, inviting him to come to America. Dennis had to wait for 3 years before he was able to obtain his visa to enter the United States. Upon arrival in the United States, Dennis finally saw his father, whom he hardly recognized. He soon realized that his father was unable to provide any financial support or emotional care for him. In addition, Dennis reported that his father's new wife considered him a burden and a threat to the family's financial stability. Three months after his arrival, he left his father's apartment after a violent argument with his stepmother. Dennis was suddenly homeless, with no money, no food, and no ability to speak English. He lived on the streets of New York for 2 months, learning "street" language to survive. He made friends with drug dealers, who introduced him to heroin and the drug lifestyle. Initially, he felt welcomed and accepted. Soon Dennis started shoplifting to support his habit. Shortly after, unable to get enough money, he became suicidal. Dennis showed up at the treatment center half dressed and begging for help. He was taken to a psychiatric emergency room but was denied admission to an inpatient unit because he was not deemed to be in medical or psychiatric emergency. Moreover, he lacked insurance coverage and did not have the proper legal documents in his possession. Several days later, the friend who had initially brought Dennis to the center reported that he had been thrown from a second-floor window by a drug dealer. He suffered broken legs and an injured back, for which he required hospitalization. Two months later, Dennis was discharged and referred to a treatment program for Russian-speaking substance abusers.

TREATMENT ISSUES FOR FORMER SOVIETS

The pressures of immigration, cultural dissonance, mistrust of authority figures, and family problems all compound the treatment of the immigrant substance abuser. In general, immigrants from the former Soviet Union are not interested or willing to participate in therapy, especially substance abuse counseling ("Weaning Newcomers," 1993). Based on their experiences in "the mother country," they fear being stigmatized and punished for their problems. Most of all, they fear that exposing their substance abuse problems can affect their political and social status in the United States (Kagan, 1997a). The difficulties in working with Russian immigrants are exacerbated by the lack of awareness of the disease concept by family members, Russian professionals, and community leaders. Few of their employers, generally immigrants themselves, are knowledgeable about Employee Assistance Programs (EAPs) and effective ways to deal with problem employees. In addition, language barriers and lack of insurance benefits contribute to the difficulty of obtaining substance abuse services.

In treating substance-abusing clients from the former Soviet Union, the clinician needs to take into account such issues as impact of immigration, the existence of "double denial," issues of trust, importance of psychoeducation, understanding of spirituality and resistance to group treatment and

12-step programs, and gender role and family dynamics, particularly domestic violence (Kagan, 1994).

Impact of Immigration

The correlation between substance abuse problems and immigration, as related to adjustment, resettlement, and acculturation, must be taken into consideration when working with substance-abusing clients from the former Soviet Union. Immigration is experienced as a series of losses, including loss of homeland, loss of family and friends, loss of professional and social status, and loss of established personal identity (Castex, 1996). Such losses are both environmental, focusing on changes taking place outside of the individual, and internal, relating to cognitive adjustments and to the psychocultural challenges of the new life (Kagan, 1995-1996). Challenges to self-image and personal identity include feelings of confusion, inadequacy, insecurity, and hopelessness, all of which contribute to the weakening of the individual's sense of self-worth. Depression, which often develops following immigration, can be seen as a reaction to these losses. The social isolation, disruption of family and social ties, and the lack of available services in their native language exacerbate the difficulties of immigrants from the former Soviet Union. Moreover, even rapid acculturation can increase isolation and maladjustment, because the rapid acceptance of new values and belief systems leads to increasing separation from the group of origin and thus weakens the support from that group (Goldstein, 1984).

Adjusting to life in the United States can be overwhelming. Given the limited choices in the former Soviet Union, these immigrants are often confused by the numerous choices available in the United States. At the same time, they are resentful of the absence of basic benefits that had been provided to them by the Soviet government. Despite the fact that the majority of former Soviet immigrants are highly educated and sophisticated, they are unprepared for the absence of such services as housing, child care, employment, and free medical and dental care that they had received at home. Moreover, Russian immigrants tend to be extremely resistant to using traditional mental health services, preferring instead to use medical and social services, which had been provided free of charge in their former country (Kagan, 1998).

"Double Denial"

The majority of former Soviets do not recognize various mental health and substance abuse problems as requiring special consideration and treatment. In line with their historical experience, most view drug abuse as a moral problem that produces embarrassment and shame for family members, whereas alcohol abuse is accepted as "natural," particularly for men. "I am not crazy," and "I am not an alcoholic!" are the typical responses among such individuals.

Due to the tendency of immigrants from the former Soviet Union to cover up their addiction and related family issues, denial of alcohol- and drug-related problems provides a challenge for clinicians. Most clients seek help for family, medical, or concrete services, not for their substance abuse problems. Because many Russian-speaking clinicians in the United States are themselves unfamiliar with the signs, symptoms, and interventions related to substance abuse, it is very difficult for them to identify these problems in their clients. Additionally, these clinicians tend to hold the same cultural values as their clients. The resulting "double denial" means that immigrant substance abusers and their family members are often undiagnosed and untreated until a crisis occurs or until they reach the late stage of their addictions.

To address the lack of substance abuse information and education in the Russian-speaking community, aggressive outreach and prevention efforts must be provided through community-based organizations and centers. Training should emphasize the signs and symptoms of alcohol and drug abuse, the value of 12-step programs such as AA and Al-Anon and other community resources, and the impact of substance abuse on the family. These training workshops should be provided to social service, health, and mental health professionals from the former Soviet Union, as well as to the Russian-speaking community at large. Training for service providers also should include sensitivity to confidentiality and privacy, terms unfamiliar to former Soviet citizens.

Issues of Trust

Clinicians need to be aware of and sensitive to the punitive treatment and political tactics used in the former Soviet Union. It is important to consider the client's distrust toward psychiatric and substance abuse treatment facilities. The traditional American treatment methods, based on self-disclosure, trust, and group support, are culturally foreign for substance abusers from CIS. The concept of confidentiality is viewed by many such clients with skepticism and misunderstanding. For example, it is not unusual for a client to say, "I know this is confidential, you explained that to me, but please, don't share what I am about to tell you with anyone."

Former Soviets grew up accustomed to having their privacy violated by the secret police, the KGB, and other authority figures. As indicated earlier, public humiliation and the use of punishment as a form of treatment was common. Consequently, self-disclosure and revealing personal information in front of strangers, a standard in group practice and in 12-step programs, are very threatening to former Soviet immigrants. It usually takes much time and great skill to establish rapport and trust with these substance abusers, and clinicians should be prepared to expect such dynamics. It is therefore essential for clinicians to establish basic trust with clients prior to addressing their substance abuse problems.

Importance of Psychoeducation

An important aspect of treatment with former Soviets is the use of psycho-education. Because education is highly valued in Russia, substance-abusing clients from the former Soviet Union may be initially more open to such an approach than to other forms of treatment. Teaching substance-abusing clients from the former Soviet Union about how substance abuse may affect people's health and interpersonal relationships may be initially less threatening than other methods of initiating the treatment process.

Psychoeducation can be used in order to introduce the client to the treatment models used in the United States, such as the biopsychosocial disease concept and the use of 12-step self-help groups. Education regarding the value of group treatment can be used to help Russian-speaking immigrants understand the value of the mutual process of sharing personal information and expressing feelings in front of strangers.

Psychoeducation with family members should include detailed explanations of such concepts as codependency and other family dynamics, confidentiality, client's rights, and voluntary participation in treatment.

Understanding Spirituality

It takes time for clients from the former USSR to understand the concept of spirituality and to identify their beliefs and how they may utilize them in their recovery process. Acknowledging and practicing a faith or belief in extremely difficult due to the influence of the atheist propaganda promoted by the Soviet totalitarian regime, which attempted to keep people of many different religions and spiritual beliefs from openly practicing their traditions. These experiences, ingrained from the Communist era, contribute to the tremendous resistance of Russian-speaking immigrants to accepting and following the principles of the 12-step programs that are an integral part of many substance abuse treatment programs in the United States. For instance, the term "higher power" may be misinterpreted as being associated with "big brother" governmental agencies. Nonetheless, there is a great hunger for spirituality among the former Soviets. Exploring historical, familial, spiritual, and religious beliefs and practices prior to the Soviet totalitarian takeover can thus be an important tool for healing and recovery for these clients.

Family Dynamics

As with other populations, substance abuse in the Russian immigrant community is strongly associated with family problems, including physical violence. As in many other families, substance abuse among families from the CIS interferes with the establishment of boundaries between family members and distorts the roles and responsibilities within the family structure. It also serves to regulate issues of intimacy and distance in family relationships (Steinglass, 1985). In addition, life in a totalitarian state leads to adherence to collectivism and interdependence; distrust of outsiders; and extremely close family ties. Although such dynamics may be adaptive in a totalitarian regime, they become maladaptive in a society such as the United States with its focus on individualistic, capitalist ideology. For example, close family ties, essential for survival in a pervasively hostile, paternalistic, oppressive environment, can become dysfunctional and interfere with the process of assimilation once the family relocates to the United States (Halberstadt, 1992). Because families in transition have a tendency to become enmeshed and protective of their members, such dynamics further reinforce the controlling and enabling behaviors characteristic of substance abusing families.

Twelve-step programs such as Al-Anon are completely foreign to Russian immigrant family members, and therefore they will usually refuse to participate in such groups. They have a strong reluctance to reveal and discuss family problems in an open forum, and many feel distrustful of other group members. Thus it is important to create specially tailored, culturally sensitive discussion groups for family members, usually wives or mothers of substance abusers. Such groups should provide a safe, secure, and nonthreatening environment and be run in their native language by a trained clinician, not by a peer.

Children of substance-abusing former Soviet families may be the victims of physical abuse and may frequently develop typical survival roles. They may feel hurt, abandoned, lonely, rejected, and confused. Whereas some may take on the role of the caretaker and do extremely well in school, others may have learning problems and resort to acting out (Kagan, 1997a).

Alex, a 16-year-old boy, was referred by the family court following a robbery attempt. His family consisted of his mother, Mrs. A; his 18-year-old brother; and his stepfather, Mr. A. The family had immigrated from Russia 5 years previously and was living in an apartment in a large city. Mr. A was now a successful businessman, and Mrs. A worked as a dog groomer. Due to hyperactivity and learning problems, Alex attended a special education class in a public school. He experienced behavioral outbursts and had difficulty communicating with his stepfather. During a joint session with Alex and his mother, it became apparent that Mr. A, an undiagnosed alcoholic, had been constantly berating and abusing his wife and children, especially Alex. The verbal and physical abuse was taken as a norm within the family. Although severely beaten at times when she tried to protect Alex, Mrs. A denied any family problems and claimed that her husband was just a little too rough on the boy.

It was only following an episode in which Mr. A, who was severely drunk, threatened his wife with a knife and her older son called the police that Mrs. A admitted that there were some problems in her family. She agreed that her husband was probably an alcoholic, but she felt that nothing could be done about it.

Shortly afterward, Alex took a BB gun and began to shoot people on the street from his apartment window. Once again, the police were called. Alex was placed in a special school for emotionally disturbed children and prescribed medication. At this point, the whole family was seen together. Confronted by her oldest son and concerned about Alex's behavior, the mother agreed to participate in a Russian-language parents' group. Mr. A agreed that he would "do something" about his drinking, although he denied that it caused his family any trouble. He viewed his hard drinking as "normal" and appropriate behavior for any Russian man. He refused to attend a Russian-speaking AA group. However, following a couple of individual and family sessions, he stopped his physical abuse of his stepson and wife.

Slowly, the family began its recovery process. The healing process took much longer due to the cultural acceptance of heavy drinking and Mrs. A's feelings that she had to protect her husband from outsiders.

Gender Role and Domestic Violence

Due to limited control of their environment, it was not unusual for men in the former Soviet Union to displace their rage and powerlessness toward their family members. The institutionalization of domestic violence is reflected in the Russian joke that if a husband does not beat his wife then he does not love her. Moreover, the typical pattern for a Russian wife is to let her substance-abusing husband set the rules, follow his lead, withdraw from friends, and deny any existing problems in the family (Kagan, 1997b).

Although data regarding spousal abuse among immigrants from the former Soviet Union are difficult to obtain, it is a common occurrence that has to be carefully assessed. It is not unusual for both substance abuse and violence to become more problematic when a couple has to face the full range of resettlement and acculturation difficulties, in addition to preexisting marital complications.

> The Z family consisted of a husband, wife, and their 10-year-old son, who emigrated from the Ukraine 4 months prior to their first visit with a Russian-speaking therapist. Mr. Z, who was an English teacher prior to immigration, was finally offered a job interview. However, he got lost on his way and missed the interview. Subsequently, he got severely drunk and became violent during a fight with his wife. After a neighbor called the police, the couple agreed to seek help at a mental health center with a Russian-speaking clinician.
>
> During the assessment, it became evident that Mr. Z had a 10-year history of alcoholic drinking. He frequently abused his wife verbally and beat her when intoxicated, believing that his wife was unfaithful even though she kept denying this. Mrs. Z had made an attempt to separate from her husband by moving in with her parents but returned after a short time. She claimed that Mr. Z was a very nice person while he was "normal," meaning sober, and she always forgave him because he apologized and told her he loved her. Mrs. Z appeared to have low self-esteem and was dependent on her husband for validation and for her emotional well-being, in spite of his constant abusive behavior. While in the Ukraine, Mr. Z's drinking patterns included periods of calm, which provided some stability and structure for the family. However, after immigrating to the United States, his drinking became more chronic and the violence more frequent.

Treatment of Substance-Abusing Women

Although recent social developments in Russia indicate that the use of alcohol, cigarettes, and illicit drugs and prostitution have increased among women in the former Soviet republics (Specter, 1997a), there are no data regarding the prevalence of substance abuse among Russian-speaking immigrant women. Given the Communist ideology, which idealized feminine traits that emphasized enabling, caretaking, and codependent behaviors, it is not unusual for a Russian wife to accompany her husband in his drinking binges in efforts to control or curtail the amount of his intake of alcohol and thus develop a problem herself. Moreover, some women turn to substance use as a coping mechanism in order to medicate themselves from their overwhelming feelings of helplessness and grief (Kagan, 1995-1996).

Few, if any, Russian-speaking substance-abusing women seek treatment on their own, and even those referred by family or authority figures face tremendous obstacles in finding appropriate treatment. Few Russian-speaking female clinicians are knowledgeable about substance abuse treatment, and most substance abuse programs, even those that are culturally sensitive, are designed for men. In order to provide treatment for the substance-abusing Russian-speaking woman, outreach workers must be able to identify such women. Then culturally sensitive programming and treatment objectives can be established specifically for this group. Although very little data on treatment outcome of culturally sensitive programs for either men or women are available, in general, women have more successful outcomes when they receive gender-specific treatment for at least several months.

Helping women to develop assertiveness skills and to establish healthier relationships is important to the recovery process for all substance-abusing women (Straussner & Zelvin, 1997). Teaching women from the former Soviet Union how to identify what they need and how to communicate this to others (in Russian and English) without hurting themselves through substance abuse can be an important stepping stone in the recovery process of Russian-speaking women and their families (FADA, 1998).

CONCLUSION

Bruised and battered after many years of totalitarian regimes under Lenin, Stalin, Khrushchev, Brezhnev, and other leaders, the Soviets have kept their souls buoyant with the ever-present bottle of vodka as a symbol of friendship, community, and hospitality. Most immigrants from the former Soviet Union move to the United States with the hope for a new and better life. Some of them are ready to accept new challenges and to stop old coping behaviors such as "escaping through the bottle." Those who are not capable of overcoming their problems with alcohol or drugs, and who have been in denial for a long time need specific, culturally sensitive treatment approaches. The correlation between substance abuse problems and immigration, as related to adjustment, resettlement, and acculturation, must be taken into consideration. Services such as education, aggressive outreach, early identification of at-risk populations, and early intervention with family members play a critical role in working with Russian immigrant substance abusers.

It is important to offer community-based services that provide information and education about signs and symptoms of the substance abuse and dependence and referral information for treatment. It is also important to involve Russian-speaking mental health professionals who can culturally integrate Russian substance abusers and their families to American services and treatment facilities.

REFERENCES

Anderson, D. J. (1992, August 4). Hazelden report: Russia hopes to adapt Western treatment methods. *Star Tribune,* p. 8E.

Benn, A. (Ed.). (1997). *Insight guides: Russia.* Boston: Houghton Mifflin.

Castex, G. M. (1992). Soviet refugee children: The dynamic of migration and school. *Social Work Education, 14*(3), 141–152.

Castex, G. M. (1996). Immigrant children in the United States. In N. K. Phillips & S. L. A. Straussner (Eds.), *Children in the urban environment: Linking social policy and clinical practice* (pp. 43–60). Springfield, IL: Thomas.

Davis, R. B. (1994). Drug and alcohol use in the former Soviet Union. *International Journal of Addictions, 19*(3), 303–309.

Gibbons, B. (1992, February). Alcohol, the legal drug. *National Geographic,* pp. 3–35.

Goldstein, E. (1984). "Homo sovieticus" in transition: Psychoanalysis and problems of social adjustment. *Journal of the American Academy of Psychoanalysis, 12*(1), 115–126.

Halberstadt, A. (1994). The Soviet Jewish family: A cultural perspective. Immigration and resettlement issues facing Jewish émigrés from the former Soviet Union. *Grand Rounds, 1,* 2–12.

Kagan, H. (1992, September). *America and Russia: Recovery options at work.* Paper presented at the Sixth National Annual Great Lakes Conference on Addictions, Indianapolis, IN.

Kagan, H. (1994, October). *Alcoholism, domestic violence, and substance abuse in the Russian community.* Paper presented at the Third National Conference on Refugee Resettlement, Washington, DC.

Kagan, H. (1995-1996). Alcoholism and physical abusive interactions between adult parents and their children. Jewish Board of Family and Children Services. *Grand Rounds, 3.*

Kagan, H. (1996, October). *Distress or dysfunction?* Paper presented at the UJA Conference "Between Two Worlds: Understanding Émigré Mental Health Needs," New York City.

Kagan, H. (1997a, May). *The unique experience of the family oriented treatment program for Russian substance abusers.* Paper presented at the annual National Association of Social Workers Alcoholism Institute Conference, Fordham University, New York City.

Kagan, H. (1997b, August). *Women, ethnicity and substance abuse: Irish, African and Russian-American perspectives.* Paper presented at the "Matinee on Broadway" Conference, Liberty Management Group, New York.

Kagan, H. (1998, February). *Russian émigré's malajustment and substance abuse as a social problem.* Paper presented at the First International "Partnership 2000" Conference, Jerusalem.

Kissin, M. (1991, December). *Culturally sensitive interviewing in the psychological assessment of Russian refugees.* Paper presented at the National Conference on Health and Mental Health of Soviet Refugees, Chicago.

Marlin, O. (1994). Special issues in the analytic treatment of immigrants and refugees. *Issues in Psychoanalytic Psychology, 16*(1), 7–16.

Moore, R. (Ed.). (1989). *Fodor's 90 Soviet Union.* New York: Random House.

Mupedziswa, R. (1997). Social work with refugees. In M. A. Hokenstad & J. Midgley (Eds.), *Issues in international social work* (pp. 110–124). Washington, DC: National Association of Social Workers.

Segal, B. M. (1986). The Soviet heavy-drinking culture and the American heavy-drinking subculture. *Alcohol and culture: Comparative perspectives from Europe and America* (pp. 149–160). New York: New York Academy of Sciences.

Segal, B. M. (1987). *Russian drinking: Use and abuse of alcohol in pre-Revolutionary Russia.* New Brunswick, NJ: Rutgers University Center of Alcohol Studies.

Segal, B. M. (1990). *The drunken society: Alcohol abuse and alcoholism in the Soviet Union.* New York: Hippocrene Books.

Shafer, K. (1994). *A study of the effectiveness of alcohol and drug abuse training for professionals in Russia and the Ukraine.* Unpublished doctoral dissertation, Barry University, Miami, FL.

Smith, H. (1991). *The new Russians.* New York: Avon Books.

Specter, M. (1997a, November 9). A drug plague boils out of Russia's kitchens. *The New York Times,* Sec. 4, p. 5.

Specter, M. (1997b, November 4). At a western outpost of Russia, AIDS spreads "like a forest fire." *The New York Times,* pp. A1, A10.

Steinglass, P. (1979). Stability/instability in the alcoholic marriage: The interrelationship between course of alcoholism, family processing and marital outcome. *Family Process, 24*(3), 365–375.

Straussner, S. L. A., & Zelvin, E. (Eds.). (1997). *Gender and addiction: Men and women in treatment.* Northvale, NJ: Jason Aronson.

U.S. Department of Justice (1997, November). *Immigration in Fiscal Year 1996* [Online]. Available: http://www.ins.usdoj.gov/stats/annual/fy96/1007.html

U.S. Immigration and Naturalization Service. (1997). *Table 5. Immigrants Admitted by Region and Selected Country of Birth: Fiscal Year 1994–96.* Washington, DC: Author.

Weaning newcomers from fear and the bottle. (1993, December 7). *The Jerusalem Post,* International ed., p. 10.

Yandow, V. W. (1992, November–December). Substance abuse treatment in Russia and Hungary. *Addiction and Recovery,* pp. 42–45.

V

Working with Clients of Middle Eastern Background

The two chapters in this section, one on Arab Americans and the other on Jews, focus on a small minority of the population in the United States, yet one that is often in the news and increasingly seen in treatment settings. Nonetheless, their relationship to the use and abuse of alcohol and other drugs has rarely been addressed.

Research on Jewish substance abusers is minimal and totally nonexistent for those of Arab background. Arabs and Arab Americans are often stereotyped as dangerous or radical, whereas Jews are usually lumped together as part of the mainstream "White" group. However, in order to better serve these clients, we need to move beyond both stereotypes and further explore the unique substance use patterns and treatment needs of these two groups that have a long historical connection. The following two chapters attempt to do just that.

14

Substance Use among Arabs and Arab Americans

Nuha Abudabbeh
Andrew Hamid

Arabs and Arab Americans have been described as a hetero-geneous group reflecting a multicultural, multiracial, and multiethnic mosaic population (Abudabbeh & Nydell, 1993). Because the term "Arab" is based on the person's language and culture and does not reflect an individual's ethnic origin, there is much diversity among Arabs. This diversity is reflected in the use and abuse of various substances. Although people of Arabic background may have certain restrictions placed on them regarding the use of alcohol and other drugs, they are not necessarily abstinent from these substances, nor have they escaped the phenomenon of substance abuse. The purpose of this chapter is to provide an understanding of Arab culture and how its teachings affect the use and abuse of alcohol and other drugs among Arabs and Arab Americans.

A HISTORICAL PERSPECTIVE

Several historical factors have significantly influenced how Arabs define and view themselves in today's world. These include the growth of Islam and the process of colonization.

275

The Rise of Islam

The period between the 7th and 10th centuries A.D. witnessed the emergence of one of the most profound and influential historical changes in the Arab world: the growth and spread of the religion of Islam.

In the early 7th century in Mecca, a town in western Arabia, the prophet Muhammad called upon the people of the Arabian Peninsula to submit to the will of God as expressed in a book called the Qu'ran. Uniting the tribes of Arabia in the name of Islam, Muhammad guided them in their conquest of the surrounding countries. By the end of the century, this newly founded empire, called the Caliphate, extended from central Asia in the east to Spain in the west. This era saw the spread of both Islam and the Arabic language and the building of an urban civilization (Hourani, 1970).

The Arab world experienced its second significant historical period during the 15th and 16th centuries as it fell under the domination of the Ottoman Empire. This era also is considered the last great expression of the universality of Islam.

The Impact of Colonization

During the 19th century, as European countries vied for hegemony in the Middle East and North African regions, Muslim states were forced to adopt new systems of government and laws to face the new developing realities. An unstable socioeconomic balance, caused by inequitable trade alliances with Europe, culminated in Egypt and Tunis (and eventually Morocco and Libya) falling under European control.

Islam's legal practices were preserved, but new thought emerged to rationalize the strength of Europe and to proselytize the merit of adopting European ideas without being untrue to Islamic beliefs and culture. A new class of Arab "intelligentsia" was created—one that was convinced of the need to adopt European ideas to improve living conditions in their countries. Their ideas provided the foundation for the crystallization of the 19th-century Arab nationalism.

The partition of Palestine in 1948 and the creation of the state of Israel ignited a political reaction that led to the fall of most of the old regimes in Arab countries. The new regimes were committed to a nationalism that aspired to the close union of all Arab countries, independence from the superpowers, and social reform in the direction of greater equality. These ideas were embodied throughout the 1960s in the personality of Egyptian President Gamal Abdel Nasser. The defeat of Syria, Egypt, and Jordan in the 1967 Arab–Israeli war halted the advance of these goals and led to a period of disunity and increasing dependence by Arab countries on either of the two superpowers. On a grassroots level, however, contact among the people increased, transmitted through the written, visual, and oral media, as well as through the rapid economic growth in some Arab countries, such as Saudi Arabia and Kuwait, which attracted immigration from other Arab countries.

In the 1980s, the Arab world witnessed the reemergence and strong expression of Islamic feelings and loyalties. This resurgence filled an identity vacuum for the uprooted urban population, providing a solid base for their lives and filling a need for their own traditions and customs as opposed to adopting those of the Western world. The 1991 Gulf War, which provoked conflict among the Arabs, was the most recent of historical events to affect Arabs and Arab Americans vis-à-vis the world and Arab identity. This splintering of nations led to a weakened sense of Arab nationalism. One hundred and fifty million Arabs now live in 22 Arab countries: Algeria, Bahrain, Djibouti, Egypt, Iran, Iraq, Jordan, Kuwait, Lebanon, Libya, Mauritania, Morocco, Oman, Palestine, Qatar, Saudi Arabia, Somalia, Sudan, Syria, Tunisia, United Arab Emirates, and Yemen.

LANGUAGE AND RELIGIONS IN ARAB COUNTRIES

Learning about Arab people necessitates an understanding of their significant religious influences and the role that language plays in unifying this heterogenous culture.

Language

Currently, 130 million people speak Arabic. Arabic was named as the sixth official language of the United Nations and is ranked as the fourth most widely spoken (tied with Bengali) language in the world. Hourani (1970) described the significance of language to Arabs by stating that they saw language not only as their greatest artistic expression but also as a unified voice.

The Arabic language is extremely difficult and complex grammatically, its structure lending itself to rhyme and rhythm. Although many other people feel an affection for their native language, the feeling of the Arab people for their language is much more intense. The Arabic language is one the greatest Arab cultural treasures and achievements (Nydell, 1987). Many English words have been borrowed from Arabic and can be recognized as those beginning with *al*, for example, *algebra, alkali,* and *alcove.* Even the word *alcohol* is Arabic in origin. Spoken Arabic is as varied as the different parts of the Arab world. Classical Arabic and written Arabic are used for formal speech, broadcasting, and writing and are the same in all Arab countries, and decorative calligraphy is one of the highest artistic expressions of Arab culture.

The Qur'an was the first book to be written in Arabic, and the advent of Islam changed the way people looked at language. One of the most important linguistic expressions in the Arab culture, however, has always been poetry. Arabic poetry, an elaborate and formal language through which the personality of the poet is portrayed, remains today in all of its varied forms a significant part of Arab culture and a powerful medium of expression.

Arabs use many beautiful elaborate greetings and blessings for different occasions. There are at least 30 situations that call for predetermined expressions; all are predictable and do not differ from one Arab country to the other. There are expressions for marriage, death, engaging in a task, returning from a trip, getting a haircut, coming out of a shower, and buying a new dress. Each of these required statements elicits a specific response (Nydell, 1987).

Religion

Although not all Arabs are followers of the same religion, their religious beliefs are a major cornerstone of Arab life, exerting a profound influence on their values, attitudes, norms, and behavior. Eighty percent of Arabs follow the religion of Islam and are therefore referred to as Muslims (Barakat, 1993). Ten percent are Christians, and the remaining 10% are composed of other religions, including 10,000 Arab Jews who live in Morocco, Tunisia, Egypt, Syria, and Iraq (Shabbas & Al-Qazzaz, 1989). The majority of Arab Americans are Christians; only 33% of Arab Americans are Muslim. The following discussion elaborates on the effects of Islam and Christianity on Arabs and Arab Americans.

Islam

The essence of Islam, as preached by the prophet Muhammad, was transmitted through the Qur'an, the laws of society, which were further elaborated on by adding the Prophet's own traditional sayings (*hadith*) and practices (*sunna*). A fourth dimension was added by integrating certain pre-Islamic traditions and other existing societal norms and customs. "Islamic law (also known as *Shari'a*, or personal law) is considered inherently incompatible with a secular democracy because it determines religious, social, and political standards that Muslims must follow" (Almeida, 1996).

The Qur'an does not contain explicit doctrines or instructions: basically, it provides guidance by implication. The *hadith* and *sunna,* on the other hand, contain specific commands on such issues as marriage and the division of property and also address such daily habits as how often the believer should worship God and how all people should treat each other. Based on the general guidance of the Qur'an and following interpretation by Islamic scholars, five basic obligations of Muslims emerged in the form of the "pillars of Islam." These pillars consist of: (1) oral testimony that there is no God but one God and that Muhammad is His prophet, (2) ritual prayer practiced five times a day with certain words and certain postures of the body, (3) giving a certain portion of one's income for specified alms or charity, (4) keeping a strict regime of no liquid or food from sunrise to sundown for the whole month of Ramadan, and (5) holy pilgrimage to Mecca (*hajj*) once in a lifetime at a specific time of the year. The *hajj* also involves a variety of ritual acts and ends in a festivity celebrated by the whole community. To these specific acts, a general injunction was added, the *jihad.* The universal meaning of the *jihad* is the exercise of strenuous intellectual, physical, and spiritual efforts by every Muslim for the good of all. The more particular meaning of *jihad* is fighting for Islam, but Muslims are discouraged in this if they are incapable of first exercising the greater universal meaning of *jihad* (Shabbas & Al-Qazzaz, 1989).

Muslims belong to one of two sects: Shiite or Sunni. This division is of political origin, stemming back to disagreements over the leadership of Islam upon the death of Muhammad in 632 A.D. The Sunnis adhered to Muhammad, while the Shiites wanted the prophet's cousin's son-in-law to succeed. The Shiites were in the minority. Today, 90% of Muslims are Sunni, although the majority of Muslims in Iraq, Lebanon, and Bahrain are Shiites. Regardless of sect, they practice all the pillars of the faith and disagree only on the historical developments of Islamic leadership.

Christianity

Approximately 14 million Arabs follow the Christian faith. The Arab country with the largest Christian population is Lebanon, in which Christians make up almost one half the population. In all other Arab countries, Christians remain in the minority, with the highest percentage in Sudan, followed by Syria, Egypt, Jordan, and Palestine. The largest Christian congregation in the Middle East is the Coptic Orthodox Church, numbering nearly 6 million believers, most of them in Egypt. Other denominations include Greek Catholics (2.3 million), Greek Orthodox (1 million), Moronites (600,000–800,000), and Druze (400,000–600,000; Shabbas & Al-Qazzaz, 1989). Smaller Christian denominations, each with fewer than 200,000 members, are Syrian Orthodox (Syria), Nestorians (Iraq), Chaldean (Iraq), Coptic Catholic (Egypt), and Armenian Orthodox (Palestine, Jordan, Syria, and Lebanon).

Although Christians compose only 10% of the overall Arab population, they are described as having played a disproportionate part in the political activities of post-World War II Arab countries, especially in the nationalist movement in the Middle East and in the Palestinian movement (Carmichael, 1977). Often Christians would impress outsiders as more "Arab" than Muslim Arabs in their Arab nationalist position. Among Arab Americans it is not uncommon to find Arab Christians holding traditional and conventional attitudes toward a variety of issues identical with those held by Muslim Arab Americans.

THE ROLE OF THE FAMILY

If the Qur'an is the soul of Islam, then the family can be described as the body. Whereas pre-Islamic Arabs found their strength in tribes, Islam emphasized the extension beyond the tribe, focusing on a unified sense of belonging to Islam, known as *umma*. The collective consciousness of all those within the *umma* of Islam takes precedence over one's identity as an individual.

Within the *umma,* families are given importance as units within which men are given specific duties toward their wives, wives are instructed how to treat their husbands, and children are advised to honor their mothers. In the *hadith,* Muhammad asserts that "Paradise is under the feet of mothers." Both men and women are expected to contribute to the support and maintenance of the family unit according to traditional codes of family and honor and to view the good of the family as above the fulfillment of individual wishes. Women are responsible for the rearing of children (Abudabbeh, 1996).

Today there are many signs of strain on the family system, resulting from industrialization, urbanization, war and conflict, and Westernization. Despite these pressures, the family remains the main system of support throughout the Arab world and for Arabs living elsewhere. The family constitutes the dominant social institution through which persons inherit their religion, social class, and identity (Fernea, 1985).

Despite moves toward a more Westernized nuclear family, the extended family remains very important. Family dynamics involve a great deal of self-sacrifice; they also provide a collective form of happiness through vicarious enjoyment of the happiness of others. Satisfaction is based on the happiness of all the members of the family in contrast to that of an individual. Whatever befalls one member of the family can bring either honor or shame to the whole family.

Another important feature of the Arab family is its style of communication, which is described by both Sharabi (1988) and Barakat (1985) as hierarchical, creating vertical as opposed to horizontal communication that is based on authority. Consequently, styles of communication evolved between parents and children in which parents use anger and punishment and the children respond with crying, self-censorship, covering up, or deception (Barakat, 1985).

Marriage

In this section we focus on the Islamic regulations governing marriage because the majority of Arabs are Muslim, a fact that establishes an undeniable Islamic influence on all Arab societies. Islam considers marriage an important duty of every Muslim and a safeguard of chastity. Having moved away from the pre-Islamic tribalistic emphasis on kinship and blood relation, Arabs regard marriage as central to the growth and stability of the basic units of society. Marriage (*nikah*) is recognized as a religious, sacred ceremony. In Islamic law, it is a contract that legalizes intercourse and the procreation of children. A Muslim man is allowed to marry a non-Muslim woman as long as she belongs to the people of the Book, meaning either Jewish or Christian. Women, however, are not allowed to marry non-Muslims (Esposito, 1982).

Marriage is seen as a family affair in which partners are chosen by one's family; it is not based on the Western concept of romantic love. Despite some changes in this regard, such arrangements remain the rule, and romantic marriage is an exception. Although the girl's opinion is supposed to be respected in accepting or rejecting a certain suitor, this is seldom practiced. Some Sunni sects allow the inclusion of clauses in the marriage contract that give women the power to terminate the marriage. Yet, despite these laws and ongoing changes in family laws in some Arab countries, in general women continue to be disadvantaged due to the long-standing traditional pre-Islamic and persisting post-Islamic attitudes toward their role in society.

Practices such as endogamy, that is, marriage within the same blood lineage such as between cousins, still occur among the more traditional and conventional Arab societies (Barakat, 1985). The reasoning behind this custom is rooted in tribal, pre-Islamic tradition by which marriage to close kin assured the kind of security and economic benefit needed to enhance the stakes of the tribe and ensure its position.

Muslim law allows for women to be contracted for marriage by their guardians (in most countries, their fathers). This is the case at all age levels unless they have been married before. Several Arab countries such as Tunisia, however, have enacted laws more favorable to women in this respect, allowing women of major age to draw their own marriage contract. The minimum age for marriage for a Muslim girl in most Arab countries is 15; for boys, it is 18. Studies indicate that the higher the education level of the woman, the more likely it is that she will marry at an older age (Barakat, 1985). The *mahr* is a dowry given by the bridegroom to the bride, but it is often presented to the father of the bride. Pre-Islam, the *mahr* was the price of the bride given to the bride's family. In Islam, the custom of the *mahr* departed from treating women as a chattel to be sold and was given to provide some financial security for the woman in the event of a divorce. In modern Arab societies, the *mahr* is mostly symbolic, but in traditional communities, where old and new notions of marriage still clash, it remains an issue.

Although polygamy is rare in modern Arab society, traditional Islamic law allows men four wives. Although the Qur'an qualifies the multiplicity of wives by stating that a man should not marry more than one unless he is able to treat them equally, the choice is left to him to determine how many women he marries. In recent years, some Arab countries (e.g., Tunisia) have forbidden the practice of polygamy, whereas others (e.g., Iraq) have required that a husband obtain a court's permission before taking a second wife. In still others (e.g., Lebanon and Morocco), a wife can insist on a clause in a premarital contract giving her the option of divorcing her husband in the event he decides to take a second wife (Beck & Keddie, 1978).

Most Arab Christians belong to denominations that do not allow divorce. Among Muslims, it is permitted under certain legal stipulations. Muhammad is reported to have said, "Of all permitted things, divorce is the most abominable to God." Barakat (1985) describes the divorce rate as having risen in Arab countries, attributing it to the pressures of modern life. Studies show that most breakups of Arab couples occur during the "engagement" (which in Islam is usually a binding contract) period or during the first 2 years of marriage (Barakat, 1985). This probably is related to the nature of these marriages, inasmuch as they are arranged. It may be that what Western couples are able to discover in each other before marriage is only possible for Arab couples to discover after "engagement" or during the early period of marriage.

In an event of a divorce, a woman retains custody of her children for only a limited time; they are then placed with the father or the closest male relative guardian. The mother relinquishes custody when the children reach a certain age, which varies according to the Muslim sect. For example, under Sunni Hanafi Muslim law, the mother's custody continues until the son is 7 and the daughter is 9 (the age of puberty); whereas under Shiite law, custody of a son reverts to the father at the age of 2 (the age of weaning) and of a daughter, at the age of 7. In recent decades, some of these custody laws have been amended to accommodate the best interests of the child.

Children

Children are raised to perpetuate the customs and traditions of the family. Because children reflect on the family, they are expected to behave respectfully and in no way shame the family by undesirable or unacceptable behavior. Although these trends are changing, Arab children are expected to maintain close ties with their families even after marriage and are not encouraged to separate from their parents. Children who shame their parents are likely to be disowned by the family. Whereas sons carry the responsibility of perpetuating the family name, both in esteem and generativity, the role of daughters and daughters-in-law includes taking care of aging parents.

ARAB AMERICANS

The Arab American population in the United States is currently estimated to be nearly 3 million. The largest concentration of Arabs in the United States can be found in Dearborn, Michigan, because of the automobile manufacturing opportunities found at the Ford Motor Company, which is headquartered there. Significant numbers of Arab Americans also live in the New York–New Jersey area, in Southern California, and in Washington, DC.

The migration of Arabs to the United States occurred in two distinct waves. The first wave, which came between 1890 and 1940, consisted mostly of merchants and farmers who emigrated for economic reasons from regions that were then part of the Ottoman Empire. Ninety percent of this first-wave immigrant population was Christian and originated in the regions known today as Syria and Lebanon. These Arab immigrants differed from other immigrants in that most chose to work as peddlers, were independent in lifestyle, and were relatively more affluent, earning up to $1,000 per year, in contrast to other immigrants who worked in mines and factories and earned an average of $600 per year (Zogby, 1990). They also seem to have assimilated into their new country with considerable ease.

The second wave of Arab migration began after World War II and continues today. Unlike their predecessors, this group consists mostly of people with college degrees or those who had come to earn them. It also differed in that it came from all over the Arab world. This second wave has been dominated by Palestinians, Egyptians, Syrians, and Iraqis. Their reasons for emigration varied from political change (socialism in Egypt) and civil war (Lebanon) to seeking a better life (Yemen, Morocco, Tunisia). Unlike the first wave of immigrants, which was composed mainly of Christians, the second wave was composed of both Christians and Muslims.

Those immigrants who arrived during the second wave came with an "Arab identity" that was absent among the first group of immigrants. With the crystallization of an Arab identity also came the expression and the continuation of Arab traditions and customs in the United States. The previous trend of easy assimilation began to change into a separateness built on political ideology that centered on the Arab–Israeli conflict and a cultural separateness based on rejecting Western norms and customs.

SUBSTANCE USE AMONG ARABS

According to Islamic law, the consumption of alcohol is forbidden. References to alcohol use in the Qur'an are clear in extolling Islam's condemnation of such indulgence. The Qur'an warns that in both drinking and gambling, there "is heinous sin and uses for men, but the sin in them is more heinous than the usefulness" (Arberry, 1967). In some traditional Arab countries, such as Saudi Arabia and Libya, in which absolutely no alcohol is allowed, it is not sold, nor are the citizens allowed to consume it. In other countries, such as Jordan or most of the North African Arab countries, alcohol is sold and consumed; however, during the holy month of Ramadan, the consumption of alcohol is discontinued. The consequences for indulging in alcohol use vary depending on the country and its adherence to Islamic teachings. In Saudi Arabia, for example, punishments such as flogging or imprisonment are strong possibilities. In Arab countries that are less devoutly to Muslim, one's tendency to consume alcohol is curbed more by social pressure than by state law.

There is no specific reference to other mood-altering substances in Islam or in the Qu'ran. Historically, it is believed that it was Arab traders who introduced opium to the world, particularly to Indian and Southeast Asian countries. Currently, different Arab countries are known for the growth and use of different substances. For example, Egypt, Lebanon, and Morocco are known for their use of hashish; Yemen for its use of Qat, a mood-altering drug similar to hashish. The extent of the substance abuse problem in the Arab world is difficult to assess because there are no published statistics. Anecdotally, there has been mention of substance abuse in different Arab countries under differing social and political conditions. For example, prior to the Intifada, the uprising in the West Bank of Palestinians against Israel in 1991, there was an epidemic of marijuana use among Gaza refugee camp residents. During the 17-year civil war in Lebanon, there was considerable use of heroin among the younger generation. More recently, Egyptian psychiatrists have been reporting heroin addiction as a social and medical problem in Egypt. In Morocco, cocaine became a drug of choice among privileged classes (Okasha, 1985).

ARAB AMERICANS AND SUBSTANCE ABUSE PROBLEMS

Little is known regarding substance abuse among Arab Americans. At the NAIM Foundation, a clinic that provides social, health, and educational services for Arabs in the Washington, D.C., area, there were only five clients with substance abuse problems out of the 2,000 clients seen since 1987. None of the calls received on the telephone counseling service were related to substance abuse (Abudabbeh, 1996). A survey of those who contacted ACCESS, the Arab Community Center Economic and Social Services, in Dearborn, Michigan, suggests that substance abuse, specifically alcohol abuse, was rare (Aswad & Gray, 1990). It is likely that the low incidence of alcohol abuse can be attributed to the influence of Islam, coupled with the possibility that Arab Americans who encounter difficulty with alcohol and other drugs may not seek help or may seek professional help at non-Arab agencies. By and large, it is assumed that those who use American health professionals are those who are English-speaking, are more educated, and are more Westernized. Specialized centers for Arabic-speaking individuals are most probably meeting the needs of those whose English is limited or who are less Westernized and thus less likely to have substance abuse problems than the younger, more Westernized Arab Americans.

Unlike other religions, which sanction the ceremonial and social use of alcohol, Islam condemns its use. As such, many Muslims who abuse alcohol and other drugs experience an automatic sense of guilt and shame and are oftentimes viewed as having strayed morally. Efforts to cope with these feelings are likely to be met with continued and heavier drug use and a withdrawal from family and community. The loss of family and detachment from *umma* can perpetuate a cycle of alienation and self-destruction.

Arab American adolescents who participate in drug experimentation, including cigarette use, with their other American friends are likely to encounter strong disapproval from parents. Parents often respond by blaming the influence of American friends and reminding their teenagers of Islam's condemnation of such behavior. Various forms of punishment may result.

TREATMENT OF ARAB AMERICANS

The likelihood of an Arab family resorting to outside help for the use of alcohol or drugs is very small. The emphasis on family as the source of support and the concept of the *umma* in Islam discourage Arabs from seeking professional help for their emotional problems (Abudabbeh, 1994). Another deterrent to approaching an outsider with regard to a substance abuse problem is the fear of others outside the family knowing about such unacceptable behaviors. The significance of family in Arab American culture may support the wisdom of utilizing family therapy as an approach to ameliorating a substance abuse problem. However, in addition to the threat of revealing treasured family values and traditions, this therapeutic intervention may also be seen as interfering with the authority of the father and the accepted cultural and religious norms.

Theologically and culturally speaking, the use of alcohol and other drugs is viewed among Arab Americans as a departure from religious and family values. Muslim Arabs are likely to view such behavior as a weakness, thus subscribing to a moral understanding of substance abuse, the consequent response to which is punishment. Because this response is incompatible with a rehabilitative agenda, it may become necessary to reeducate Arab American families about alternate theoretical perspectives on drug abuse. A view other than a perspective of morality and sin would aid in reducing guilt and shame.

There is a paucity of research examining how substance-abusing Arab Americans respond to particular modalities of treatment. It makes conceptual sense that Arab-Americans might be amenable to the *Twelve Steps and Twelve Traditions* of Alcoholics Anonymous (AA), because many of its facets are compatible with an Islamic approach to life: AA's spiritual nature and the notion of a higher power can be attractive to both Muslim and Christian Arabs who rely on a God to ease their distress. Through their familiarity with the prescriptions of Islamic law, traditional Muslims may find similarity in the sequential and guiding nature of the 12 steps. The collective consciousness of *umma* may be experienced through the solidarity of AA members bonded together by a common struggle. Participation in 12-step programs would become more helpful for the Arab American only after overcoming initial reluctance to disclosing personal troubles.

Despite these similarities between a 12-step approach and Islamic theology, one study of a substance abuse treatment center in Saudi Arabia (Abdel-Mawgoud, Fateem, & Al-Sharif, 1995) reported that a treatment approach that primarily utilized a 12-step approach was not as effective as one that was more comprehensive. The comprehensive program in this study included individual, group, and family therapy and incorporated religious services, biofeedback, and self-help groups, along with community meetings, pharmacological treatment, and psychoeducation. It is also important to note that dietary and daily praying practices among devout Muslims may prevent them from participating in residential treatment that does not accommodate their practices.

Practitioners attempting to utilize empowerment approaches to substance abuse treatment may be challenged in working with Arab American women who have been socialized to assume a position of subservience. Efforts to emphasize a focus on her own recovery and to make decisions that foster her own growth may be completely foreign to many Arab American women. Depending on her level of Islamic devotion, the most effective treatment agenda may be one that encourages the Arab American woman to reconcile the features of Islam that are important to her with areas of her life in which she may wish to assert greater self-determination.

The following cases illustrate some of the cultural issues that influence the treatment of Arab Americans.

Zaid, a 24-year-old Catholic Lebanese American man, was brought to an outpatient alcoholism treatment program by his parents, who were alarmed and embarrassed by his frequent alcohol binges and consequent behavior. Zaid was engaged to be married to a woman whom his parents had selected for him.

In treatment, Zaid reported that he was not particularly fond of this woman but felt pressured to marry her because of his parents' efforts in selecting the "right family" for him to marry into. Although his parents disapproved of his occasional drinking, they anticipated that he would "settle down" with the responsibilities of marriage.

As the wedding day approached, Zaid's drinking episodes increased in frequency, and he began to show up drunk at his fiancée's home. His future in-laws were outraged and became concerned about their daughter's future. His parents were embarrassed and concerned that their family name would be marred by the culturally unbecoming behavior of their son.

After one drinking episode, Zaid's disrespectful behavior toward his fiancée's father led to the wedding being called off by his in-laws. Shocked and infuriated by Zaid's conduct, his parents were torn between banishing him from the household and committing him to treatment. Fearing that further scandal would arise from "disowning" him, his parents decided to pursue treatment for him.

In attempting to understand the functions of Zaid's drinking, the clinician needed to understand his desire to assert his independence in a family system that was built around certain cultural norms and expectations, a particular one being obedience to parents. As a Catholic Arab, Zaid was raised to view marriage as permanent, and thus the clinician needed to consider the panic and anxiety that resulted from the perceived irreversibility of this sacrament.

During his stay in treatment, it became apparent that Zaid's drinking was a means of dealing with the dilemma of acquiescing to his parent's wishes versus asserting his own choices. Having been socialized to be an obedient son and being unable to directly challenge his parent's plan, Zaid found a way to sabotage his marriage by making himself into an unattractive and undeserving son-in-law.

The clinician needed to appreciate the parents' sense of obligation to find a good family for Zaid to marry into and their reaction to the threat of scandal should their family name be marred by alcohol overindulgence and consequent misconduct. A central focus of alcohol treatment for Zaid involved family counseling to help them understand the role of cultural expectations and family pressures in exacerbating his drinking. In working with this family, the clinician had to be sensitive to the family's reluctance to disclosing family problems.

Farida, a 19-year-old Egyptian American woman, was referred to treatment by her probation officer. She had been arrested and convicted for possession of crack.

As she discussed her 2-year involvement with crack, she stated that she fled the "prison walls" of her parents' home after being "fed up with my father's dictatorship." Farida's father was an Islamic scholar and respected interpreter of the Qur'an at the community *masjid* (house of worship). Attempting to raise their children in a keenly Islamic tradition, Farida's parents instructed her to live by the Qur'an. Her parents were tremendously disappointed by the many ways in which she had failed to abide by the cultural and religious expectations of Islam.

In her middle teens, her American friends at school introduced her to cigarettes. When her parents discovered her cigarette use, they prohibited her from extracurricular contact with school friends. In her efforts to rebel and assert her own independence, she graduated to marijuana use with her American boyfriend. Upon learning of this development, her parents threatened to withdraw her from school, and she responded by moving in with her boyfriend. In this relationship, she began using crack, and after 3 months was arrested for possession of an illicit substance.

In a functional analysis of Farida's drug use, it became important for the clinician to understand her desire to be the Islamic woman that *she* wanted to be while living with the restrictions of her parents. Farida felt stifled by the doctrines of Islam and restricted from being who she wanted to be. She initially found that cigarette use gave her the liberated status of her American friends. As she tried to forge her identity, she later found acceptance through her drug-using boyfriend. Individual counseling combined with a women's group focused on getting Farida to realize that freedom and a self-defined sense of identity can be accomplished in ways less destructive than through drug use.

CONCLUSION

Working with Arab American individuals and families who encounter difficulty with substance use requires an understanding of the factors that guide the attitudes and behavior of this population. From the information provided in this chapter, it is hoped that practitioners working with Arab clients would appreciate the importance of inquiring into such factors as country of origin, religion and sect, degree of Arab identity and *umma,* and perception of the role of the family. It is also hoped that an understanding of the social ecology of Arab family and community life would foster sensitivity to the personal shame and social ostracism that an Arab substance abuser is likely to experience.

REFERENCES

Abdel-Mawgoud, M., Fateem, L., & Al-Sharif, A. I. (1995) Development of a comprehensive treatment program for chemical dependency at Al Amal Hospital, Dammam. *Journal of Substance Abuse Treatment, 12*(5), 369–376.
Abudabbeh, N. (1994). Treatment of post-traumatic stress disorder in the Arab American community. In M. B. Williams & J. F. Sommer, Jr. (Eds.), *Handbook of post traumatic therapy* (pp. 252–263). Westport, CT: Greenwood Press.

Abudabbeh, N. (1996). Arab families. In M. McGoldrick, J. Giordano, & J. K. Pearce (Eds.), *Ethnicity and family therapy* (pp. 333–346). New York: Guilford Press.

Abudabbeh, N., & Nydell, M. (1993). Transcultural counseling and Arab Americans. In J. McFadden (Ed.), *Transcultural counseling: Bilateral and international perspectives* (pp. 261–284). Alexandria, VA: American Counseling Association.

Almeida, R. (1996). Hindu, Christian, and Muslim families. In M. McGoldrick, J. Giordano, & J. K. Pearce (Eds.), *Ethnicity and family therapy* (2nd ed., pp. 395–423). New York: Guilford Press.

Arberry, A. J. (1967). *The Koran interpreted* (2nd ed.). New York: Macmillan.

Aswad, B., & Gray, N. A. (1990, October). *Challenges to the Arab American family and to ACCESS, a local community center.* Paper presented at the annual conference of NAIM, Washington, DC.

Barakat, H. (1985). Arab families. In E. Fernea (Ed.*), Women and the family in the Middle East: New voices of change* (pp. 27–84). Austin: University of Texas Press.

Barakat, H. (1993). *The Arab world: Society, culture and state.* Berkeley: University of California Press.

Beck, L., & Keddie, N. (Eds.). (1978). *Women in the Muslim world.* Cambridge, MA: Harvard University Press.

Carmichael, J. (1977). *Arabs today.* New York: Anchor Books.

Esposito, J. L. (1982). *Women in Muslim family law.* Syracuse, NY: Syracuse University Press.

Fernea, E. (Ed.). (1985*). Women and the family in the Middle East.* Austin: University of Texas Press.

Hourani, A. (1970). *Arabic thought in the liberal age: 1798–1939.* London: Oxford University Press.

Nydell, M. K. (1987). *Understanding Arabs: A guide for Westerners.* Yarmouth, ME: Intercultural Press.

Okasha, A. (1985). Young people and the struggle against drug abuse in Arab countries. *Bulletin Narcotica, 37*(2–3), 67–73.

Shabbas, A., & Al-Qazzaz, A. (Eds.). (1989). *Arab world notebook.* Berkeley, CA: Najda.

Sharabi, H. (1988). *Neopatriarchy: A theory of distorted change in Arab society.* New York: Oxford University Press.

Zogby, J. (1990). *Arab Americans today.* Washington, DC: Arab American Institute.

15

Jewish Substance Abusers

Existing but Invisible

Shulamith Lala Ashenberg Straussner

> Jews are a minority both in numbers (constituting only
> 2.5% of the American population and 1/3 of 1 percent of
> the world population) as well as in the nature of the hatred
> directed against them and the oppression they have
> experienced. . . . Moreover, although America is 83% white,
> it is 95% Christian, making Judaism a more uncommon
> phenomenon than non-whiteness.
> —BRODY (1997, p. 11)

Although few in numbers, Jews are highly visible in American society—yet, paradoxically, they remain ignored in all the recent literature focusing on substance abuse among various ethnocultural minorities. Despite their invisibility in this area, concern regarding alcohol and drug problems among Jews can be found both historically and in more recent times, both in the United States and in Israel. This chapter provides a brief history of Jews as it relates to their cultural beliefs and values and addresses the issue of substance abuse among Jews in the United States and in Israel. Treatment implications for dealing with Jewish substance abusers are identified.

JEWISH IDENTITY AND DEMOGRAPHICS

Although Judaism typically has been defined as a religious category, surveys of Jews found that 90% define themselves as being a "member of a cultural or ethnic group" (Council of Jewish Federation [CJF], 1991). Thus it is more appropriate to view Jews as an ethnocultural group or even as an "ethnoreligious" (Zenner, 1985) or "cultural-religious minority group" (Soifer, 1991, p. 157), not simply as a religious group. Although the majority of Jews in the world today are of European descent, recent genetic studies point to a common Middle Eastern historic lineage (World Jewish Congress, 1998b).

There are approximately 13.5 million Jews in the world, with close to 6 million living in the United States (World Jewish Congress, 1998b). Jews make up fewer than 3% of the U.S. population (compared with more than 4% Asian, more than 10% Hispanic, and 12% Black). Although Jewish communities can be found in every state, close to 60% of the Jewish population in the United States lives in five communities: New York, Los Angeles, Miami, Chicago, and Philadelphia (CJF, 1991).

Compared with the general population, Jews in the United States are overrepresented among those over age 65, and, due to a low birth rate, underrepresented among the young (CJF, 1991). Moreover, because of a very high rate of intermarriage during the past 20 years, many children have only one Jewish parent. According to Wertheimer (1993), "more than half the Jews who married between 1985 and 1990 wedded a partner who was not Jewish" (p. 59). Such a high rate of intermarriage has raised concern regarding the future survival of Jews in the United States; it also may change their children's predisposition to various genetic disorders, including alcohol dependence.

As the so-called people of the Book, Jewish men always have had one of the highest literacy rates in the Middle East and Europe. Similarly, American Jews have a very high level of educational achievement, with one of the highest proportions of college graduates among all ethnic groups (CJF, 1991; Horowitz, 1993; Steinberg, 1981). This is particularly true for Jewish American women, who are believed to be the most highly educated of all women in the world (Antler, 1997; National Commission on American Jewish Women, 1995): 48% of American Jewish women have a college or advanced degree, compared with 26% of other White females in the United States ("A Women's Place?," 1995). Jews are overrepresented among such professions as doctors, lawyers, accountants, architects, academics, and mental health practitioners (Hertzberg, 1989). Nonetheless, it is important to remember that not all Jews are highly educated or economically successful. The 1990 National Jewish Population Survey found that 19% of Jewish households were defined as low income and that half of that number were living below the poverty line (CJF, 1991). The connection between substance abuse and socioeconomic class among Jews in the United

States is unknown, although, as is discussed later, some data are available regarding such a correlation in Israel.

Diversity within the Jewish Population

Most American Jews are now three or four generations removed from their immigrant origins; however, more than one-half million are foreign born, with many of the most recent Jewish immigrants arriving from the former Soviet Union. Among the foreign-born Jews residing in the United States during the 1980s were 160,000 from the former USSR; 80,000 from Western Europe; 70,000 from other Eastern European countries; 65,000 from Israel; 45,000 from Canada; 40,000 from Latin America; and 45,000 from other countries, such as South Africa and Australia (CJF, 1991).

In addition to country of birth, Jews are also diverse racially, with 3.5% of Jews identifying themselves as Black (CJF, 1991). Included in this group are those of Ethiopian origins, African-American Jews by Choice (converts to Judaism) and their children, biracial children of Jewish and Black parents, and Black children adopted by Jewish families.

Three percent of Jews are Hispanic (CJF, 1991), many of whom are Sephardic Jews from Latin America. Over 8% of the American Jewish population consider themselves Sephardic. The Sephardim trace their roots to Jews expelled from Spain and Portugal in 1492 who settled in Greece, Turkey, and the Balkans; in North African countries such as Morocco; and in the Middle East—Egypt, Syria, Iraq, and Iran. Some Sephardic Jews trace their origin to ancestors who arrived in North, Central, and South America during colonial times (Hertzberg, 1989). The majority of American Jews, however, are Ashkenazi, that is, of German or Eastern European background. Many of this group have been directly or indirectly affected by the Holocaust, which still has a tremendous psychic impact on Jews everywhere even more than 50 years later. According to recent research findings, not only Holocaust survivors but also their children show physiological and psychological changes related to this trauma (Danieli, 1998; Yehuda, Schmedler, Giller, & Siever, 1998). The correlation between the impact of the Holocaust and substance abuse among Jews in the United States has yet to be investigated, although such connection has been noted among Ashkenazi Jews in Israel (Wislicki, 1967).

Religious Affiliation

Although the great majority of American Jews are not religious and only about 40% are formally affiliated with a temple or synagogue (Wertheimer, 1993), most maintain some Jewish traditions, such as observing major Jewish holidays—for example, Rosh Hashana, the Jewish New Year; Yom Kippur, the Day of Atonement; Passover, "The Festival of Freedom"; and Hanukkah, "The Festival of Lights." Most Jews have their sons circumcised, and many Jewish children undergo the bar or bat mitzvah ritual. Those who are religiously affiliated tend to belong to one of four main religious groupings. The groups, from least to most liberal, are:

1. *The Orthodox.* Composing only 10% of Jews in the United States but growing rapidly (Wertheimer, 1993), the Orthodox preserve all the traditional religious beliefs and practices, including rigid separation of men and women and arranged marriages. Intermarriage, or even marriage with non-Orthodox Jews, is forbidden and can lead to excommunication from the community.

Various subgroups within the Orthodox umbrella include:

a. The ultra-Orthodox, known as Hasidim, who are led by a "rebbe," or teacher—an inherited dynastic position originating in Eastern Europe. Many of the ultra-Orthodox men are recognizable by their traditional 17th-century Eastern European clothing, their beards, and *peyos*, or sidelocks (Langman, 1995). The best known Hasidic sects are the Satmar and Lubavitcher.

b. The Modern Orthodox, who, while maintaining the traditions and Jewish laws, have adapted to modern ways by wearing contemporary clothes, living among non-Jews, and accepting professional education and careers for women.

2. *The Conservatives.* Conservatives Jews respect most religious laws, such as eating only kosher food, while at the same time adapting to modern times—for example, women sit together with men during religious services and men wear a *kippa,* or head covering, during religious services and meals but not necessarily outside the house. Since 1985, the Conservatives have accepted women rabbis and allow abortion under some circumstances.

3. *The Reconstructionists.* Originating in the 1920s, the Reconstructionists started the tradition of bat mitzvah for girls. Although observant of traditional Jewish practices, they believe in new interpretations of Jewish religious expression, including communal decision making and nonauthoritarian and nonsexist Judaism with equal rights for gay Jews.

4. *The Reform.* Reforms Jews make up the largest denomination in the United States. Started by German Jews, the Reform are considered by

many as focusing more on Jewish culture rather than on traditional Jewish rituals. Services are held in English rather than Hebrew and take place in temples as opposed to synagogues (Conservative or Reconstructionist) or *shuls* (Orthodox). It is common among Reform Jews to have women rabbis and cantors, and gay and lesbian rabbis are generally accepted, as are inter-marriages with non-Jews.

SOCIOCULTURAL DYNAMICS AFFECTING JEWS

According to experts, Judaism is "a way of life reflecting a particular world outlook" (Fast, 1968, p. 326), and many Jews share common cultural dynamics regardless of their country of origin or religious denomination. Jews are seen as having experienced "proportionately more trauma than most, if not all, major cultural groups" (Gannon and Associates, 1994, p. 224). Because the historical suffering and trauma continue to play a role in the Jewish worldview and to influence individual and familial dynamics, it is important for clinicians to have some basic understanding of this history.

Although most people today think of the word "ghetto" as referring to an inner-city, poverty-ridden community, the word, as well as the concept of a ghetto, originated in Venice in 1509. It was in Venice that Jews, escaping from Germany where they were being attacked, sought sanctuary. The Venetians, who up to that point had not allowed Jews to settle there because they were viewed as competitors in seafaring trade, disliked the Germans even more. Therefore, they agreed to allow Jews to settle in a confined area of Venice known as Ghetto Nuovo, or "New Foundry." In 1555, Pope Paul IV decided that the Jews in Rome, who had lived freely there for 2,000 years, should also be confined into a restricted area—a ghetto. And that idea spread throughout Europe, particularly to German and Eastern European countries. Thus what was originally viewed as a sanctuary for Jews became a place of confinement and an easy target during anti-Semitic pogroms, or mass murders, which swept through Europe in almost every century after the Crusades (Fast, 1968; Hertzberg, 1989).

The term "anti-Semitic" was not coined until 1879, when it was used by an anti-Jewish German journalist, Wilhelm Marr. Marr was describing the theory of White Aryan superiority proposed by two Frenchmen, Ernest Renan and Joseph-Arthur Gobineau, who formulated a notion of hierarchy of race. According to them, the White race was superior to darker races, and within the White race there were superior and inferior Whites. Because "White" people looked the same color, the distinction was based on language. Spoken languages were divided into Aryan and Semitic-based languages. At the top of this White pyramid were the "Noble Teutons"—the Germanic Aryans; at the bottom were the Semitic Jews (Fast, 1968).

The term "anti-Semitic" was rapidly disseminated to various European countries, and Anti-Semitic Political Leagues were quickly set up in Hungary, Austria, and Rumania. By 1882 the Anti-Semitic Congress was held in Dresden, Germany, to discuss how to get rid of Jews in their respective countries (Fast, 1968). Not coincidentally, that time saw the beginnings of the largest pogroms in Russia—leading to massive immigration of Jews to the United States; the Dreyfus trial in France; and numerous blood libel murders (in which Jews were falsely accused of killing Christian children and using their blood in making matzo for the Passover holiday) in other parts of Europe. The European persecution of Jews culminated with the Nazi Holocaust, during which 6 million Jews, one third of the Jews in the world, perished.

Anti-Semitism in the United States

Anti-Semitism is intrinsically connected to the arrival of the first Jews in the Americas. Escaping from the Spanish Inquisition, "New Christians," that is, Jews who had converted to Christianity under force, arrived with the Spanish conquistador Hernando Cortés in Mexico in 1519 (Hertzberg, 1989). By 1521 there were so many "New Christians" in Mexico that the Spanish closed the territory to all those who could not show descent from four generations of Catholic ancestors. In 1528, when the Church discovered a "Judaizer," he was soon burned as a heretic in the first auto-da-fé in the Americas; by 1571 the Inquisition was formally established in Mexico City, resulting in deaths of many former Jews and other individuals suspected of being of Jewish descent (Hertzberg, 1989).

The first officially documented Jews to arrive in today's United States were 23 Dutch Jews who landed in the harbor of New Amsterdam, present-day New York City, in 1654. Arriving aboard the boat *Ste. Catherine,* which originated in Recife, Brazil, these refugees were escaping from the Portuguese, who just reconquered Brazil from the tolerant Dutch. Refused permission to dock first in Jamaica and later in Cuba, which was controlled by the Spanish, the ship's captain decided to dock in a Dutch territory, hoping that he would be paid for his expenses for transporting these Dutch Jews. However, the governor of New Amsterdam, Peter Stuyvesant, was not welcoming. He did not want "hateful, poor Jews" in his community. Calling them "repugnant," "deceitful," and "enemies and blasphemers of Christ," Stuyvesant recommended that they be required "to depart" (Hertzberg, 1989, p. 20). However, the shareholders of the Dutch West Indies Company, who employed Stuyvesant, decided to allow these poor Jews to stay under the condition that the well-to-do Jews in Amsterdam pay for their keep (Hertzberg, 1989; Margolis & Marx, 1972). The experiences of these first Jewish settlers in the United States—persecution for being Jews; seeking safety and being dependent on the tolerance of whatever community they found themselves in; and being rescued and cared for by other Jews—have been the prototypical experiences affecting the Jewish community since their dispersion from the Holy Land in the second century A.D.

With the increase of Jewish immigrants in the United States and the rapid growth of the Jewish population at the end of the 19th and early 20th centuries, pervasive institutional anti-Semitism became established. More than 3 million Jews migrated to the United States between 1881 and 1910, most of them from Eastern Europe. So great was the demand of their children for admission to universities and medical schools that a quota system was established that limited the admission of Jews to top schools (Fast, 1968). In addition to experiencing discrimination in education, Jews faced institutional discrimination in many communities in housing, in hotel lodging, in admissions to private clubs, and in high-level positions in industries such as banking, insurance, public utilities, railroads, and corporate head offices (Glazer & Moynihan, 1970). It was only in the 1960s, following the election of the first Catholic president of the United States, John F. Kennedy, and the decreasing power of the old Protestant establishment, that the last pockets of institutional anti-Semitism began to disappear. And not until the 1980s did Jews become fully accepted politically and socially (Hertzberg, 1989), although vestiges of individual and group anti-Semitism still remain. Thus anti-Semitism continues to play an important role in the lives of many Jews. To quote from one author: "I believe that most Jews, even the most assimilated, walk around with a subliminal fear of anti-Semitism the way most women walk around with a subliminal fear of rape" (Beck, 1991, p. 22).

Jewish Cultural Values

Because of their history of constant adversity, Jews developed certain values and attitudes that have allowed them to survive under a variety of difficult circumstances. Although the values discussed herein should not be used to stereotype a client and although each client needs to be seen as an individual with his or her own value system, they are offered in the hope that clinicians will find them helpful in understanding clients of Jewish background.

Focus on Family and Children

An essential component of Jewish survival has been the focus on the family—"be fruitful and multiply" is a major Jewish edict. Thus Jews have always emphasized marriage and having children (Rosen & Weltman, 1996). Unmarried Jews tend to be highly devalued, which affects their self-esteem. For example, in his 1979 description of going home for the Jewish high holidays, the author David Sax describes how during holiday services his parents' acquaintances offer them their "condolences" for having an unmarried adult son. Having an unmarried adult child is a much more common phenomenon today; due to their focus on obtaining higher education, Jews tend to marry later than other Americans (Kosmin, 1994). Nevertheless, having an unmarried adult child is still a source of shame and guilt for many Jewish parents. The issue of marriage is also a factor for Jewish gay men and lesbians, especially among the Orthodox, who still consider homosexuality sinful.

Arranged marriages still exist among some Orthodox Jewish families, and among most, if not all, ultra-Orthodox. This is an important dynamic for families with a substance-abusing member because a history of such a disorder in a family makes all family members less marriageable, thereby reinforcing the need for secrecy and denial. For example, I was involved in a brief treatment with the family of an ultra-Orthodox cocaine-abusing man. Due to the extreme need for secrecy, the four sessions and a follow-up interview 2 months later were held over the phone without my ever knowing the family's last name and with payment made through a third party, who had made the initial referral.

Among heterosexual Jewish couples, given the generally high level of education of both partners and a very high proportion of working women it is not unusual to find competition between men and women, and a high level of stress and conflict between home and work life (National Commission on American Jewish Women, 1995). Moreover, Jewish American families tend to be very child centered. Success and failure has often been validated by children, who are expected to bring *nachas*, or pleasure, to parents ("my son/daughter, the doctor") and to the extended family (Rosen & Weltman, 1996). This expectation puts great pressure on children to succeed. Although many Jewish children do succeed and make their parents proud, such success is often tinged with high levels of anxiety—making them vulnerable to anxiety and depressive disorders and to increased use and abuse of sedative and antianxiety medications (Blume, Dropkin, & Sokolow, 1980). Such pressure to succeed is particularly traumatizing for those children who, because of learning disability or other physiological or psychological reasons, are unable to excel academically or in other ways, such as artistically. During adolescence, their low sense of self-esteem may put these children at high risk for abuse of alcohol or, more commonly, marijuana and other drugs.

Importance of Self-Sufficiency and Money

During their diaspora in Europe, Jews were "forbidden by the Catholic Church either to own farmland or to engage in basic industry of that time, agriculture, [therefore they] had to turn to commerce and finance" (Fast, 1968, p. 165). Consequently, moneylending and the selling of goods became an important skill and a source of communal strength, providing means of survival in times of trouble. Having money or valuable goods allowed the Jews to trade for food or to escape from danger. Lack of money or poverty in general put one in life-threatening danger. Thus, unlike the Christian notions of poverty as a blessing (Catholic) or as damnation (Protestant), for Jews poverty was something to ameliorate. Therefore, Jews, in general, tend to work hard to earn a living, and workaholism is frequently seen among Jewish adults. Today, poverty is culturally acceptable only among those who devote their time to study or among the elderly. For these "deserving poor," Jewish communal funding is frequently available; not so for substance abusers.

Emphasis on Education

Among Jews, education has been valued for itself and as a way out of poverty. As pointed out by Weiner (1991), "It is often said within Jewish homes that a person can lose everything, but what's inside the head cannot be taken away" (p. 125). Overall, the American Jewish population, as indicated previously, has a very high level of educational achievement, with a high rate of literacy. The focus on education is often evident in clinical treatment, in which the use of self-help literature and a high regard for expert opinion is commonly seen among Jewish clients.

Importance of Verbalization of Feelings

In general, Jews tend to be easily motivated toward psychological treatment and will seek treatment earlier than other ethnic groups (Devore & Schlesinger, 1996; Rosen & Weltman, 1996). Moreover, Jewish men and women are highly visible in the treatment field—an area that emphasizes verbal ability, articulation of feelings, and cognitive understanding. However, at times, talking and expressing feelings may serve as a substitute for making needed changes: Thus, although some Jews may love to analyze things and "talk the talk," they may not necessarily "walk the walk."

Concern about Physical Health

The cliché of the suffering Jewish mother who clutches her heart when she does not get her way is, like all stereotypes, an exaggeration built around a grain of truth. As discussed previously, suffering is part of Jewish history, and hypochondriasis or somatization are not uncommon among many Jewish clients in treatment. As pointed out by Devore and Schlesinger (1996), Jews

> have a long history of extensive concern with matters of health, a concern attributed to "the sense of precariousness" and fear concerning survival related to centuries of dispersal and persecution . . . these cultural themes manifest themselves in a volatile, emotional response to pain accompanied by a concern about how the illness will affect the future. Medical specialists of all sorts are highly valued and their advice is sought extensively. (pp. 308–309)

However, although doctors are respected, they are not revered (Gannon and Associates, 1994); given their own general high level of education, many Jews are not shy about challenging credentials or seeking other experts if they disagree with a particular diagnosis or recommendation. By and large, many educated Jews feel the need to get the "best" of help and are often willing to pay for the "best" treatment.

Value of Humor

As with many groups that experienced trauma, Jews have used laughter as a way of sublimating psychological pain and coping with their inability to control the external environment. According to Benton (1988), Jews living in Eastern Europe and czarist Russia during the 19th century invented the political joke as a way of subtly criticizing their oppressors. More recently, Jewish comedians have become well known for their use of bittersweet humor to mock life's travails. This ability to laugh at one's own misery and pain is an important cultural strength that should be used in treatment.

Value of Charity

Tikkun olam, or repairing the world, is one of the most important *mitzvah*, or Jewish deeds. This cultural emphasis on helping others is one of the factors accounting for the extensive network of Jewish charitable and medical institutions and may account for the overrepresentation of Jews in the helping professions. It is a value that can be used to reinforce involvement in 12-step groups and "twelve stepping," or helping other substance abusers as a way of helping oneself.

Role of Women

In the United States, Jewish women have been stereotyped as "JAPs"— "Jewish American princesses" who are manipulative, bossy, anxious, vulgar, ambitious, and focused on money (Beck, 1991). According to Beck (1991), such views seem to be based on an exaggerated reflection of the Jewish cultural values discussed previously, compounded by anti-Semitism and misogyny.

As indicated previously, Jews place a high value on marriage, and unmarried Jews are devalued. Such devaluation is particularly common for women, whose role is to maintain the home (Rosen & Weltman, 1996). Moreover, although married Jewish women are seen as powerful within the family and many are highly educated and professionally successful, traditional status is still based on the men they marry. A poor scholar is acceptable, but an alcoholic or a gambler who is a poor provider for the family is not. This is vividly reflected in the old Jewish proverb, "The innkeeper loves the drunkard, but not for a son-in law." Moreover, because having children is a crucial value in Jewish families, Jewish couples are more likely to adopt a child when unable to have their own than other people in the United States (Kosmin, 1994). Clinical observations point to a high rate of substance abuse problems among some of the adopted males.

SUBSTANCE ABUSE AMONG JEWS IN THE UNITED STATES

A comprehensive review of published literature revealed a paucity of studies of substance abuse among the American Jewish population and no national prevalence data. Much of the existing literature, most of it more than 20 years old, focuses on the historically lower rate of alcoholism among Jewish men as compared with other ethnic groups (Bailey, Haberman, & Alksne, 1965; Bales, 1946; Blume, Dropkin, & Sokolow, 1980; Daum & Lavenhar, 1986; Flanzer, 1979; Glad, 1947; Knupfer & Room, 1967; Perkins, 1985; Schmidt & Popham, 1976; Snyder, 1958/1978; Spiegel, 1986; Zimberg, 1977, 1986). Despite limited research data, anecdotal and clinical observations point to the fact that addiction to alcohol and other drugs can be found among all members of the Jewish community "from the ultra-assimilated to the ultra-orthodox" (Hass, 1991, p. 32). A comprehensive study of the Jewish population of greater New York in 1991 found that 10,100 Jewish households (2% of all Jewish households studied) sought "assistance for alcohol or drug problems" and that 600 households sought assistance for "gambling problems" (Horowitz, 1993, p. 116). Extrapolating from this study, it can be assumed that a minimum of 120,000 Jewish households in the United States have an acknowledged substance abuse problem, with probably three to four times as many having an undiagnosed or misdiagnosed alcohol and/or other drug disorder.

The existence of substance abuse in the Jewish community, as well as its unique nature, is also reflected in the rapid growth of non-12-step organized groups and programs aimed exclusively at this population. The New York-based group called Jewish Alcoholics, Chemically Dependent Persons and Significant Others (JACS), a self-help group currently under the auspices of the Jewish Board of Family and Children's Services, was established in 1980 and has a mailing list of over 3,000 people (M. Udal, personal communication, April 1999). Approximately 30 similar groups exist in various parts of the United States (Dinnerstein, 1993), including JACS in Philadelphia and Boston, L'Chaim and AJIRA (Addicted Jews in Recovery), located, respectively, in southern and northern California, and SLICHA, an acronym for St. Louis Information Committee and Hotline on Alcoholism and the Hebrew word for forgiveness, in St. Louis, Missouri.

Despite the existence of such groups and the fact that a number of synagogues have opened their doors to 12-step self-help groups such as Alcoholics Anonymous (AA) and Pills/Drugs Anonymous, substance abuse problems in the Jewish community are generally denied, and this issue does not appear to be of high priority for funding. For example, a standing committee on Addictions in the Jewish Community, first established as the Task Force on Alcoholism in 1978 and funded by the Federation of Jewish Philanthropies of New York (Trainin, 1986), was defunded and disbanded in 1996. Thus to be a Jewish alcohol and/or drug abuser means having a problem that continues to be highly stigmatized and denied by the Jewish community.

Alcohol Problems among Jews

According to available data, Jews appear to have a lower rate of alcoholism or alcohol dependence than is found among the general population in the United States. Quoted rates vary from a low of 2% to a high of 8% (Bailey, Haberman, & Alksne, 1965; Bainwol & Gressard, 1985), with the most likely estimates averaging about 3% of the population. Only additional research can provide more accurate current data.

The traditionally low rate of alcohol problems among Jews has been attributed to a variety of factors, including genetic predisposition, sociological and cultural dynamics, and religious values (Glassner & Berg, 1985; Keller, 1970; Monteiro, Klein, & Schuckit, 1991; Snyder, 1958/1978; Snyder, Palgi, Eldar, & Elian, 1982; Zimberg, 1977, 1986). A recent study of Jewish males in Jerusalem found that 35% had "a genetic mutation that may guard against alcoholism" ("A Genetic Mutation," 1998, p. 52). Much of the literature emphasizes the fact that, traditionally, drinking among European Jews has been seen as limited to ritualized and ceremonial occasions, but that drunkenness has not been tolerated: "The Jewish family maintains . . . a permissive drinking culture in which drinking is permitted, but excessive drinking is not" (Glassner & Berg,1985, p. 97). It is possible that as Jews have become more acculturated to mainstream American values, their rates of alcohol abuse and dependence have increased. Such hypotheses can only be confirmed by national epidemiological and other research studies.

Drug Use among Jews

Jews appear to have an interesting paradoxical view regarding drug use: They distrust its use, yet they are frequent users of both prescribed and nonprescribed drugs. For example, in the classic study by Zborowski (1969) of physically ill patients of various ethnic backgrounds, Jewish patients were reluctant to take painkilling medications because they worried about the harmful effects of drugs on their general health and wanted to "understand" the "real source" of their problem. Such views are still commonly held among many Jews today. Nonetheless, unlike alcohol abuse, the use and abuse of both licit and illicit drugs among Jewish adolescents and adults in the United States is high, at times even higher than among their peer groups or the general population. For example, a study of 278 college students found that Jewish male adolescents were more frequent users of marijuana than were Catholic or Protestant students (Eisenman, Grossman, & Goldstein, 1980). Daum and Lavenhar (1986) also found that Jewish students were less likely to be "regular consumers of alcohol alone" but more "likely to be heavy users of other drugs alone" than non-Jewish students (p. 208). An unpublished household telephone survey of illicit drug use among adults in New York State, conducted in 1986 and repeated in 1994, found that the "lifetime use" of illicit drugs among Jewish adults is slightly (but not statistically) greater than in the population at large (see Table 15.1). The primary illicit drug used by Jews was marijuana, followed by cocaine and hallucinogens (the use of heroin was too limited to be included, although clinical observations indicate a growing rate of heroin use during the late 1990s). As was true for all adults in New York State, the rate of illicit lifetime drug use among Jewish adults was higher in 1994 than in 1986 (B. Frank, personal communication, April 1999).

The high use of drugs among the New York Jewish adults confirms an earlier study of patients treated in Hazelden in Minnesota, which found that 10% of their patients treated for cocaine (alone or with other substances) were Jewish—greatly overrepresenting their numbers in the population. In contrast, only 1% were treated for alcohol alone and 3% for a combination of alcohol and drugs other than cocaine ("Study Suggests," 1987). In a recent, as yet unpublished national study of 379 Jewish substance abusers by Blume and Vex (S. Vex, personal communication, August 11, 1999), the authors found that although 55% of their subjects had a primary addiction to alcohol, 45% were addicted to such drugs as cocaine

TABLE 15.1. Rates of Illicit Drug Use During Lifetime among Jewish Adults and All Adults in New York State 1986 versus 1994

	Jewish adults[a]	All adults[a]
Any illicit drug use		
1986	30%	29%
1994	39%	38%
Marijuana		
1986	30%	28%
1994	39%	37%
Cocaine		
1986	11%	9%
1994	13%	12%
Hallucinogens[b]		
1986	6%	4%
1994	8%	8%

Note. Information obtained from Dr. Blanche Frank, Chief, Bureau of Applied Studies, New York State Office of Alcoholism and Substance Abuse Services. Sources: 1986 survey, New York State Division of Substance Abuse Services; 1994 survey, New York State Office of Alcoholism and Substance Abuse Services.

[a]Adults are 18 years and older.

[b]Hallucinogens include LSD, mescaline, psilocybin in the 1986 survey, with the addition of PCP in the 1994 survey.

(11.8%), opiates (11.6%), marijuana (11.3%), tranquilizers (2.4%), sedatives (1.8%), and other drugs. In general, it appears that Jews in the United
States are high users of drugs in addition to, or instead of, alcohol. This is
particularly true for Jewish men.

The use of drugs by American Jewish men is not a new phenomenon.
Although studies of patients hospitalized for alcoholic psychoses during the
early years of the 20th century found that Jews had lower rates of such diagnoses when compared with other White ethnic groups (Snyder, 1958/
1978), Jews were among the frequent users of narcotics (morphine and heroin) and cocaine at that time. For example, Perry Lichtenstein, a physician
in the City Prison in Manhattan, wrote in 1914 that based "upon the
observation and treatment of 1,000 cases within the City Prison . . . the
Hebrew American is very frequently addicted" (Jews followed only the
"Chinese, American and Italian" in frequency of incarcerated addicts;
Lichtenstein, 1914, pp. 962, 964). Moreover, Jews and Italians apparently
dominated the street trade in heroin sales in New York City during this period (Helmer & Vietorisz, 1974).

Multiple Substance Use and Dual Diagnosis

Studies of Jewish substance abusers indicate that although alcohol rates
may be lower than for other groups, they may have higher rates of multiple
substance use—particularly alcohol and prescribed pills such as sedatives,
tranquilizers, and analgesics. A study of participants attending a JACS retreat found that 61% of the men and 78% of the women were dually addicted, a rate much higher than seen among non-Jewish substance abusers
(Trainin, 1986). Blume and Vex (S. Vex, personal communication, August
11, 1999) found a 71% rate of dual addictions, with alcohol (24%), sedatives (11%), and tranquilizers (8%) cited as the most commonly used secondary substances.

Although some authors believed that Jews are more likely than other
groups to use alcohol and other substances for pharmacological or medicinal uses (Spiegel, 1986), as opposed to recreational purposes, Blume,
Dropkin, and Sokolow (1980), in their pioneering study of 100 Jewish
American alcoholics, found a 19% rate of dual diagnosis, a figure not significantly different than that found in the non-Jewish population at that
time. However, the higher rate of dual diagnosis for alcohol-abusing Jewish
men (22%) compared with women (14%) is highly unusual. Most of their
participants, middle- to upper-middle-class individuals living in the community, were diagnosed with depression and anxiety disorders, although
Blume and colleagues (1980) note that among a group of 77 identified Jew-

ish alcoholics hospitalized in a psychiatric unit, 5% (four patients) were dually diagnosed with schizophrenia.

In addition to schizophrenia, depression, and anxiety disorders, Jews are believed to have a high rate of coexisting bipolar disorder, eating disorders, sexual disorders, and gambling problems (Linn, 1986). No data regarding HIV/AIDS among Jewish substance abusers in the United States could be found.

Some of the issues described previously can be seen in the following case study.

Jack is a 36-year-old man brought up in a Conservative upper-middle-class Jewish family in a large city. His maternal grandparents were Holocaust survivors from Poland, and his father grew up in Cuba in a family of German Jews. A bright but poor student, Jack had trouble concentrating in school and was kicked out of three different private schools before graduating from a public high school. He started drinking and smoking marijuana with his friends at age 15 and first used cocaine at a party at age 17. His parents sent him to therapy, but his drug use was never discussed. He dropped out of college after his first year and decided to go into a retail business with the financial support of his parents. Although the business was a success, Jack "felt bored" and had his partner buy him out. At that point he began to attend night clubs, where his drinking and cocaine use escalated. He also began to use quaaludes. In his early 20s he fell in love with a non-Jewish woman, and together they started snorting heroin. They married despite the strong opposition of his parents, who refused to talk to him following the marriage. Three years later, just as he was starting another business, his wife left him. Jack's use of cocaine with heroin ("speedballing") increased and, despite the initial success of his business, he was unable to manage his finances. To make money, he started dealing cocaine to people he knew, but he became increasingly paranoid that the police were after him. Afraid of having a heart attack, he checked himself into a hospital, where he was detoxified from heroin. His parents came to see him, and he agreed to move back home with them. Shortly afterward, he resumed his drug use. Unable to cope with his mood swings, his mother decided to seek treatment for herself. At the recommendation of her therapist, the family arranged for an intervention with a substance abuse expert. Jack refused to go into an inpatient facility but agreed to go to a private methadone clinic. Once on methadone, he stopped using heroin but continued using cocaine, alcohol, and marijuana. At the recommendation of his mother's therapist, his parents asked him to leave their house and stopped supporting him financially. As his business and health deteriorated, Jack agreed to go into a long-term rehabilitation center. He was detoxified from methadone, stopped using alcohol and drugs, and became active in AA. Four years later, Jack was diagnosed as having a manic depressive disorder and put on lithium. Currently, he is drug free, attending AA and individual therapy, working at his own business, and dating a Jewish woman.

Jewish Women and Substance Abuse

The first American movie about a substance-abusing woman was the life story of a Jewish performer, Lillian Roth, dramatized in the movie *I'll Cry Tomorrow* and based on her book of the same name (Roth, Connoly, & Frank, 1954). Roth's recovery included converting to Roman Catholicism and taking an important role in spreading the message of AA. It is interesting to note that Lillian Roth's father, the child of highly religious Russian Jewish immigrants, died a destitute alcoholic without ever being diagnosed or treated for his disorder. A study by Blume and Dropkin (1980) of 42 Jewish alcoholic women found that a very high proportion, 50%, had blood relatives who were alcoholic—a greater percentage than found in the literature among non-Jewish women during the same time frame. Moreover, a very high proportion of these women, 42%, also had histories of drug abuse—most commonly tranquilizers and other sedatives, followed by stimulants and opiates. Only 14% had psychiatric histories, suffering mainly from depression and anxiety disorders. More than one fourth of these women (29%), whose average age was 46.5, were single. Blume and Dropkin also noted that the ratio of alcohol-abusing women to men appeared to be higher among Jews than in other populations, a finding that was reaffirmed in a recent study by Blume and Vex (S. Vex, personal communication, September 1999). Whether this finding is a reflection of the higher socioeconomic class of these women or an indication of some unique dynamics of Jewish American women must be explored further. Such a high ratio of substance-abusing Jewish women to men does not exist in Israel (Weiss, 1991).

SUBSTANCE ABUSE ISSUES IN ISRAEL

Although only 65,000 American Jews are listed as being born in Israel, it is believed that 350,000 Israelis and their descendants are currently residing in the United States (World Jewish Congress, 1998a), with many more Jews moving between Israel and the United States for various lengths of time. Moreover, it is not uncommon for Jewish parents to send their substance-abusing children to Israel in the hope that a stay in that country will make them "better." Thus it is important to have some understanding of Israeli society and of the issues related to substance abuse in that population. Before discussing the issue of substance abuse in Israel, we need to understand the dynamics of Israel, particularly the tremendous cultural diversity within that small country.

Although 80%, 4.8 million, of Israelis are Jewish, one fifth of the population is made up of Muslim and Christian Arabs and Druse (Harris, 1998). In addition, several hundred Vietnamese "boat people" were given shelter in Israel, and a growing number of Black Israelites, a group of African Americans from Chicago and Philadelphia, have migrated to Israel and are fighting for citizenship status. The following discussion focuses exclusively on Israeli Jews, who themselves originated in 80 different countries.

Until the recent immigration of Jews from the former Soviet Union, the majority of Israeli Jews were "Oriental" or of Arabic background whose families originated in North Africa and Middle Eastern countries (in recent years, the term "Oriental" has been subsumed under the label "Sephardic"). It is the Jews of Moroccan and Yemenite background who tended to have the lowest socioeconomic and political status in Israel—and the highest rate of both alcohol and other drug abuse (Hes, 1970; Snyder et al., 1982).

Politically and economically, the Ashkenazi Jews are the most successful of all Israelis. Since the 1980s, the Ashkenazi population has increased through the addition of almost 1 million immigrants from the former Soviet Union (Sontag, 1999). The rapid growth of this population has led to numerous absorption and acculturation problems, including a large increase in alcohol and other drug problems that are discussed subsequently.

Another recent group of immigrants has been Ethiopian Jews, with over 60,000 arriving since 1980. The Ethiopian acculturation process had to address not only the racial difference but also the cultural shock of moving almost overnight from primitive, clan-based farming communities to a modern, highly educated, Western, mainly urban society. The culture shock, combined with the trauma of evacuation that resulted in numerous separations of family members, has led to one of the highest rates of suicide in Israeli society, as well as to high risk for alcohol and other drugs (Cohen, 1999). The abuse of alcohol, particularly beer, by the Ethiopians has been explained by its close resemblance in taste to that of the native, non-alcoholic drink *tale* (Weiss, 1993a). Of particular concern is the heavy drinking of beer by pregnant Ethiopian women; this group has been the target of special prevention efforts in their native language, Amharic (S. Weiss, personal communication, February 1994). The immigration of the Ethiopians also raised concern regarding AIDS, with about 2% of Ethiopians testing positive for HIV—an issue that was previously unaddressed in Israel (Auslander & Ben-Shahar, 1998). Israel has close to 2,000 people infected with the HIV virus ("50-Percent Rise in Israeli AIDS Cases," 1998); it is believed that up to 25% may be drug related—mostly among Sephardic Jews and immigrants from the former Soviet Union (R. Isralowitz, personal communication, July 1998).

Like the Jews in the United States, the Jews in Israel have been traumatized by the Holocaust. They also have been struggling with a 50-year-old war with their Arab neighbors. These experiences have been used to explain the so-called Israeli "national character," consisting of a basic pessimism combined with hopefulness and stubbornness, a general suspiciousness of outsiders, and a urge for self-reliance (Elon, 1971; Gannon and Associates, 1994). Informality is the norm in Israel, with power and social distance deemphasized—first names are used in almost all encounters, including therapeutic ones (Gannon and Associates, 1994).

Substance Abuse Problems in Israel

Unlike the general denial of substance abuse problems in the American Jewish community, concern about substance abuse in the Israeli Jewish community is a frequent news topic.

The estimated rate of alcohol problems among Israeli Jews, 3% of the population (Bar, Elder, & Weiss, 1990; Weiss, 1993b), is similar to that believed to exist among Jews in the United States. However, there has been a documented rise in alcohol consumption among young Israelis (Barnea, Rahav, & Teichman, 1992), attributed to the growing acceptance of pub drinking among young people and to the stress resulting from the struggles with the Palestinians and the ongoing fighting in Lebanon (J. Gleser, personal communication, March 1994). In addition, there has been a very high rate of alcohol problems among the more recent Russian-speaking immigrants (R. Isralowitz, personal communication, July 1999; see also Weiss, 1993a). Still, a 1993 survey of alcohol consumption around the world placed Israel near the bottom, 45th out of the 51 countries listed, with an annual consumption of only 1.0 quarts of alcohol per capita (compared with 7.2 quarts per capita in the United States; "The Tipplers and the Temperate," 1995).

According to the Israeli government, drug use by young people doubled from 4.8% to 9.2% between 1992 and 1995 ("Understanding Alcohol and Other Drugs," 1997). The most common substances used in Israel are hashish and a snorted, highly potent, Middle East heroin called "Coke Parsi," or Persian "coke." A growing number of immigrants from the former Soviet Union, many of whom are non-Jewish, are injecting heroin (R. Isralowitz, personal communication, July 1999).

Recently, there has been a growing use of cocaine, LSD, and amphetamines ("Understanding Alcohol and Other Drugs," 1997), mainly among middle and professional classes of Askenazi background. Furthermore, there is a high incidence of abuse of two commonly prescribed medications—Rohypnol (known as Hypnodol), a sleeping medication, and Fitton, a central nervous system stimulant (J. Gleser, personal communication, March 1994).

Treatment Approaches in Israel

Israeli treatment approaches consist of a combination of traditional U.S.-based disease-model approaches, an increasing emphasis on a European-based harm-reduction approach, and some unique Israeli interventions that emphasize family and community. The latter include mobile treatment units that make regular stops in small towns and villages, in-home, family-monitored detoxification from drugs under close medical and social work supervision, and the "adoption" of drug addicts by families in some of the Orthodox kibbutzim.

Most of the treatment in Israel is not based on 12-step programs, and a 1989 survey identified only 150 AA members in all of Israel. According to Weiss (1990), AA's emphasis on the subjective individuality of spiritual beliefs—"God as we understood Him"—makes AA unacceptable to Orthodox Jews in Israel. However, the popularity of 12-step groups has increased in the past decade.

TREATMENT OF JEWISH SUBSTANCE ABUSERS

Whether in Israel or in the United States, the tremendous power and role of the family for most Jewish substance abusers has to be recognized and utilized in treatment. As was seen in the case of Jack, it is not uncommon for Jewish parents and spouses to enable the use of alcohol and other drugs by a loved one due to their lack of knowledge regarding the dynamics of addictions and their sense of guilt and responsibility toward a family member. Therefore, it is important to educate families as to the nature of addiction to alcohol and other drugs. The use of bibliotherapy, or the recommendation of appropriate literature, is usually of great value. For those clients who have lost contact with their families, helping them to reconnect with their family members can be an important aspect of long-term recovery.

Despite the generally high level of acculturation among American

Jews, clinicians must understand individual clients' reactions to what it means for them to be Jewish in the United States and must be sensitive to the impact of anti-Semitism and of the Holocaust on a particular client. Moreover, they need to be able to assess and to understand the difference between observant or religious Jews and cultural Jews and to tailor referrals accordingly. Observant Jews are unlikely to go to an inpatient treatment facility that cannot meet their dietary needs for kosher food or make accommodation for their daily prayers and observance of Shabbat, whereas a nonreligious Jew may feel uncomfortable if referred to a religious, or even a spiritually focused, setting. Except for those who are dually diagnosed with a severe mental illness, Jewish individuals are much more likely to prefer to receive services from a private practitioner or to attend a treatment facility that is in the private rather than the public sector (Bainwol & Gressard, 1985). The issues of shame and stigma must be fully explored and addressed during treatment.

Although many Jews actively participate in traditional 12-step programs (Master, 1989), many may feel uncomfortable going to a meeting that is held in a church and may find it particularly objectionable to be in meetings that start or end with the Lord's Prayer, which is viewed as a Christian prayer. Thus it is important that Jewish clients be offered alternatives. Such clients may find it more helpful to attend 12-step groups that meet in a synagogue or to be informed about special programs geared exclusively to substance-abusing Jews and their family members. Information regarding various Jewish self-help groups can be obtained online (www.jacsweb.org/networks/index.html).

Many Jewish substance abusers have found books such as Olitzky and Copans's (1991) *Twelve Jewish Steps of Recovery: A Guide to Turning from Alcoholism and Other Addictions*, as well as the numerous publications by Rabbi Abraham Twerski, an Orthodox psychiatrist specializing in addiction treatment, to be particularly meaningful in meeting their spiritual needs within a Jewish context. Some clients, particularly those who are more cognitively oriented, may find treatment groups such as Rational Recovery more acceptable than traditional 12-step programs.

Given the generally high level of education that Jews have, clinicians should not be surprised by clients questioning their credentials and training and should be nondefensive in offering their qualifications, when appropriate. In general, it is more helpful to begin treatment by focusing on cognitive understanding of substance abuse and only later to move to affective or emotional interventions. As indicated previously, some Jewish clients may be quick to learn the proper "talk," without necessarily making the changes needed to achieve and maintain recovery.

When working with substance-abusing Jewish women, it is important to identify and address any conflict and guilt in their struggle to balance home and work life. Although most women suffer if they have lost their children due to substance abuse, for a Jewish woman such loss is doubly stigmatizing—both as a woman and as a Jew. Moreover, it is important to assess for sexual abuse and domestic violence, an area that has been getting increasing recognition in the Jewish community.

Dual Diagnosis

As indicated previously, Jewish substance abusers often suffer from coexisting mental disorders. Thus it is important to assess for coexisting diagnoses by obtaining a comprehensive history of psychiatric symptoms and a thorough listing of all medications used. Clients and their families need to be educated regarding cross-addiction and cross-tolerance of substances and prescribed medications. In addition, it is crucial to assess for eating disorders among women and problem gambling among men. It is also important to assess for sexual dysfunction, as well as compulsive spending, among both men and women.

Countertransference

Clinicians working with Jewish clients need to be attuned to both their positive and negative countertransference. Some may overidealize a verbal, intelligent Jewish client and expect more than the client is capable of. Others may find it difficult to empathize with clients who seemingly have had a caring family, good education, and so forth, and yet are unable to obtain and maintain recovery. Although Orthodox Jews are unlikely to attend a mainstream treatment program, when they do, they often encounter clinicians who may not be empathic to their unique needs and who may have a difficult time understanding how a religious person can lie and have shameful sexual experiences—just like many other substance abusers. Such lack of empathy can add to the client's existing shame and guilt and make it more difficult to engage the client in the recovery process.

Jewish clinicians need to be open to exploring their own Jewish identity and to pay attention to their countertransferential reactions to both Jewish and non-Jewish clients based on their own cultural and familial values. They need to be attuned to the possibility that they may overvalue clients who are verbal and who are family oriented and be less accepting of clients who may not be very child focused. Moreover, given their cultural emphasis, Jewish clinicians may be less tolerant of clients who do not value education or of women who are dependent on men and nonassertive on their own behalf. Finally, it is important to appreciate that although the Jewish clinician may identify with the struggles of his or her African American client as a minority individual, the client may not necessarily reciprocate such identification.

CONCLUSION

As pointed out by Kaye/Kantrowitz (1991), clinicians need to move beyond the myth "about the close, happy Jewish family, that Jewish men don't drink or beat their wives or sexually abuse their daughters" (p. 11). Despite the relative invisibility and general denial of substance abuse problems in the Jewish community, alcohol and drug abuse are a problem for many Jewish men and women and their families. Careful assessment of substance abuse and their sequelae must be done by all clinicians, and appropriate referrals and intervention strategies must be undertaken. Most important, we need more research data in order to get a greater understanding of the full scope of substance abuse problems and the best treatment strategies for Jewish substance abusers and their family members.

REFERENCES

Antler, J. (1997). *The journey home: Jewish women and the American century*. New York: The Free Press.

Auslander, G., & Ben-Shahar, I. (1998). Social work practice in health care. In F. M. Loewenberg (Ed.), *Meeting the challenges of a changing society: Fifty years of social work in Israel* (pp. 98–143). Jerusalem: Magness Press, The Hebrew University.

Bailey, H. B., Haberman, P. W., & Alksne, H. (1965). The epidemiology of alcoholism in an urban residential area. *Quarterly Journal for the Study of Alcohol, 26*, 19–40.

Bainwol, S., & Gressard, C. F. (1985). The incidence of Jewish alcoholism: A review of the literature. *Journal of Drug Education, 15*(3), 217–223.

Bales, R. F. (1946). Cultural difference in rates of alcoholism. *Quarterly Journal of Studies on Alcohol, 6,* 480–499.

Bar, H., Elder, P., & Weiss, S. (1990). Three national surveys on nonritual-alcohol drinking practices of the Israeli Jewish adult population in the '80s: What are the trends? *Israeli Journal of Psychiatry and Related Sciences, 27*(1), 57–63.

Barnea, Z., Rahav, G., & Teichman, M. (1992). Alcohol consumption among Israeli youth—1989: Epidemiology and demographics. *British Journal of Addiction, 87*(2), 295–302.

Beck, E. T. (1991). Therapy's double dilemma: Anti-Semitism and misogyny. In R. J.

Siegel & E. Cole (Eds.), *Jewish women in therapy: Seen but not heard* (pp. 19–30). New York: Harrington Park Press.

Benton, G. (1988). The origins of the political joke. In C. Powell & G. E. C. Paton (Eds.), *Humour in society: Resistance and control* (pp. 33–55). New York: St. Martin's Press.

Blume, S. B., & Dropkin, D. (1980). The Jewish alcoholic: An unrecognized minority. In A. Blaine (Ed.), *Alcoholism and the Jewish community* (pp. 123–133). New York: Federation of Jewish Philanthropies.

Blume, S. B., Dropkin, D., & Sokolow, L. (1980). The Jewish alcoholic: A descriptive study. *Alcohol Health and Research World, 4,* 21–26.

Brody, L. (1997). *Daughters of kings: Growing up as a Jewish woman in America.* Boston: Faber & Faber.

Cohen, A. Y. (1999, January 11). School dropout rate double for Ethiopians. *The Jerusalem Post,* p. 5.

Council of Jewish Federations. (1991). *Highlights of the CJF 1990 National Jewish Population Survey.* New York: Author.

Danieli, Y. (Ed.). (1998). *Intergenerational handbook: Multigenerational legacies of trauma.* New York: Plenum Press.

Daum, M., & Lavenhar, M. A. (1986). Religiosity and drug use: A study of Jewish and Gentile college students. In S. J. Levy & S. B. Blume (Eds.), *Addiction in the Jewish community* (pp. 323–336). New York: Federation of Jewish Philanthropies.

Devore, W., & Schlesinger, E. (1996). *Ethnic-sensitive social work practice* (4th ed.). Boston: Allyn & Bacon.

Dinnerstein, J. (1993). *The Jewish recovery movement in the United States: A study survey.* Unpublished paper.

Eisenman, R., Grossman, J. C., & Goldstein, R. (1980). Undergraduate marijuana use as related to internal sensation, novelty seeking and openness to experience. *Journal of Clinical Psychology, 36*(4), 1013–1019.

Elon, A. (1971) *The Israelis.* New York: Penguin.

Fast, H. (1968). *The Jews: Story of a people.* New York: Dell.

50-percent rise in Israeli AIDS cases. (1998, September 14). *The Jerusalem Report,* p. 8.

Flanzer, J. P. (1979). Alcohol use among Jewish adolescents: A 1977 sample. In M. Galanter (Ed.), *Currents in alcoholism* (pp. 257–268). New York: Grune & Statton.

Gannon, M. J., and Associates. (1994). *Understanding global cultures: Metaphorical journeys through 17 countries.* Thousand Oaks, CA: Sage.

A genetic mutation. (1998, October, 26). *The Jerusalem Report,* p. 52.

Glad, D. D. (1947). Attitudes and experiences of American-Jewish and American-Irish male youth as related to differences in adult rates of inebriety. *Quarterly Journal of Studies on Alcohol, 8,* 406–472.

Glassner, B., & Berg, B. (1985). Jewish Americans and alcohol: Processes of avoidance and definition. In L. Bennett & G. Ames (Eds.), *The American experience with alcohol: Contrasting cultural perspective* (pp. 93–107). New York: Plenum Press.

Glazer, N., & Moynihan, D. P. (1970). *Beyond the melting pot: The Negroes, Puerto Ricans, Jews, Italians, and Irish of New York City* (2nd ed.). Cambridge, MA: MIT Press.

Harris, D. (1998, November 16). Population passes 6m. *The Jerusalem Post, International Edition,* p. 4.

Hass, N. (1991, January 28). Hooked Hasidim. *New York Magazine,* pp. 32–37.

Helmer, J., & Vietorisz, T. (1974). *Drug use, the labor market, and class conflict.* Washington, DC: Drug Abuse Council.

Hertzberg, A. (1989). *The Jews in America: Four centuries of an uneasy encounter: A history.* New York: Simon & Schuster.

Hes, J.P. (1970). Drinking in a Yemenite rural settlement in Israel. *British Journal of Addictions, 65,* 293–296.

Horowitz, B. (1993). *1991 New York Jewish Population Study.* New York: United Jewish Appeal and Federation of Jewish Philanthropies.

Kaye/Kantrowitz, M. (1991). The issue is power: Some notes on Jewish women and therapy. In R. J. Siegel & E. Cole (Eds.), *Jewish women in therapy: Seen but not heard* (pp. 7–18). New York: Harrington Park Press.

Keller, M. (1970). The great Jewish drink mystery. *British Journal of Addictions, 64,* 287–296.

Knupfer, G., & Room, R. (1967). Drinking patterns and attitudes of Irish, Jewish and White Protestant American men. *Quarterly Journal of Studies on Alcohol, 28,* 676–699.

Kosmin, B. A. (1994, August 12–18). A new angle on the intermarriage rate: Jews have a unique set of attitudes on moral and family issues. *The Jewish Week,* p. 6.

Langman, P. F. (1995). Including Jews in multiculturalism. *Journal of Multicultural Counseling and Development, 23,* 222–236.

Lichtenstein, P. (1914). Narcotic addictions: Based on observation and treatment of one thousand cases. *New York Medical Journal, 14,* 962–966.

Linn, L. (1986). Jews and pathological gambling. In S. J. Levy & S. B. Blume (Eds.), *Addiction in the Jewish community* (pp. 337–358). New York: Federation of Jewish Philanthropies.

Margolis, M. L., & Marx, A. (1972). *A history of the Jewish people.* New York: Atheneum.

Master, L. (1989). Jewish experiences of Alcoholics Anonymous. *Smith College Studies in Social Work, 59*(2), 185–199.

Monteiro, M. G., Klein, J. L., & Schuckit, M. A. (1991). High levels of sensitivity to alcohol in young adult Jewish men: A pilot study. *Journal of Studies on Alcohol, 52*(5), 464–469.

National Commission on American Jewish Women. (1995). *Voices for change: Future directions for American Jewish women.* Waltham, MA: Brandeis University.

Olitzky, K. M., & Copans, S.A. (1991). *Twelve Jewish steps of recovery: A guide to turning from alcoholism and other addictions.* Woodstock, VT: Jewish Lights.

Perkins, H. W. (1985). Religious traditions, parents, and peers as determinants of alcohol and drug use among college students. *Review of Religious Research, 27*(1), 15–29.

Rosen, E. J., & Weltman, S. F. (1996). Jewish families: An overview. In M. McGoldrick, J. Giordano, & J. K. Pearce (Eds.), *Ethnicity and family therapy* (2nd ed., pp. 611–630). New York: Guilford Press.

Roth, L., Connoly, M., & Frank, G. (1954). *I'll cry tomorrow*. New York: Frederick Fell.

Sax, D. B. (1979, September 27). A holiday at home: A widening gulf. *The New York Times*, p. 42.

Schmidt, W., & Popham, R. (1976). Impressions of Jewish alcoholics. *Quarterly Journal of Studies on Alcohol, 37*, 931–939.

Snyder, C. R. (1978). *Alcohol and the Jews: A cultural study of drinking and sobriety*. Carbondale: Southern Illinois University Press. (Original work published 1958)

Snyder, C. R., Palgi, P., Eldar, P., & Elian, B. (1982). Alcoholism among Jews in Israel: A pilot study: I. Research rationale and a look at the ethnic factor. *Journal of Studies on Alcohol, 43*(7), 623–654.

Soifer, S. (1991). Infusing content about Jews and about anti-Semitism into the curricula. *Journal of Social Work Education, 27*, 156–167.

Sontag, D. (1999, February 21). Memo from Jerusalem. *The New York Times*, p. 8.

Spiegel, M. C. (1986). Profile of the alcoholic Jew. In S. J. Levy & S. B. Blume (Eds.), *Addiction in the Jewish community* (pp. 45–61). New York: Federation of Philanthropies.

Steinberg, S. (1981). *The ethnic myth: Race, ethnicity, and class in America*. New York: Atheneum.

Study suggests differences in cocaine and alcohol abusers. (1987, December). *Hazelden Update, 6*(2), 8.

The Tipplers and the temperate: Drinking around the world. (1995, January 1). *The New York Times*, p. B1.

Trainin, I. N. (1986). Alcoholism in the Jewish community. In S. J. Levy & S. B. Blume (Eds.), *Addiction in the Jewish community* (pp. 15–27). New York: Federation of Jewish Philanthropies.

Understanding alcohol and other drugs: A multimedia resource [CD-ROM]. New York: Facts on File.

Weiner, K. (1991). Anti-Semitism in the therapy room. In R. J. Siegel & E. Cole (Eds.), *Jewish women in therapy: Seen but not heard* (pp. 119–126). New York: Harrington Park Press.

Weiss, S. (1990). Characteristics of the Alcoholics Anonymous movement in Israel. *British Journal of Addiction, 85*, 1351–1354.

Weiss, S. (1991). Adult women's drinking in Israel: A review of the literature. *Alcohol and Alcoholism, 26*(3), 277–283.

Weiss, S. (1993a). Non-ritual alcohol use among Israeli Jews. *Jewish Journal of Sociology, 35*(1), 49–55.

Weiss, S. (1993b). Point of view: Alcoholic physicians in Israel. *Israeli Journal of Psychiatry and Related Science, 30*(2), 116–118.

Wertheimer, J. (1993). *A people divided: Judaism in contemporary America*. New York: Basic Books.

Wislicki, L. (1967). Alcoholism and drug addiction in Israel. *British Journal of Addictions, 12*, 367–373.

A woman's place? (1995, November 4–10). *The Jewish Week*, p. 3.

World Jewish Congress. (1998a, October). Israelis abroad. *Dateline World Jewry*, p. 7.

World Jewish Congress. (1998b, October). Jewish world. *Dateline World Jewry*, p. 3.

Yehuda, R., Schmedler, J., Giller, E., & Siever, L. (1998). Relationship between PTSD characteristics of Holocaust survivors and their adult offspring. *American Journal of Psychiatry, 155*, 935–940.

Zborowski, M. (1969). *People in pain.* San Francisco: Jossey-Bass.

Zenner, W. P. (1985). Jewishness in America: Ascription and choice. *Ethnic and Racial Studies, 8*, 117–133.

Zimberg, S. (1977). Sociopsychiatric perspectives on Jewish alcohol abuse: Implications for the prevention of alcoholism. *American Journal of Drug and Alcohol Abuse, 4*(4), 571–579.

Zimberg, S. (1986). Alcoholism among Jews. In S. J. Levy & S. B. Blume (Eds.), *Addiction in the Jewish community* (pp. 75–85). New York: Federation of Jewish Philanthropies.

VI

Working with Clients of Asian Background

Despite the growing awareness that the "model minority," as Asians have been frequently characterized, has its own problems. Asian substance abusers are frequently underrepresented in treatment settings. Yet substance abuse problems, both among the newer Asian immigrants and those whose families have been here for generations, are not uncommon.

The existing literature often lumps the various Asians together, ignoring the wide cultural distinctions among the different Asian groups—differences in terms of language, religion, gender roles, and reasons for immigrating to the United States. Whereas some Asians, such as the Cambodians and some Chinese, may be refugees from terror and trauma, others, such as Indians, Koreans, and Japanese, may have migrated to seek greater economic opportunities, and still others may have moved because of family ties. The following five chapters attempt to explore to what degree these differences influence the use and abuse of substances and what the implications of these dynamics are for treatment.

16

Substance Abuse Treatment Issues with Cambodian Americans

Mary Ann Bromley
S. K. Chhem Sip

The decade of the 1980s saw an unprecedented number of refugees from Southeast Asia entering the United States. The United States census reported more than 1 million Southeast Asians, who came to the United States as refugees, living here in 1990. Approximately 150,000 of these refugees were Cambodian. Whereas more than half of the Southeast Asian population settled in California and Texas (Tran & Matsuoka, 1995), many of the Cambodians resettled in Massachusetts, Pennsylvania, Virginia, New York, and Rhode Island (Le, 1993). There are vast differences in the degree to which different Asian groups are acculturated with regard to the White Anglo-American mainstream society (Kitano & Daniels, 1988). In general, Cambodian Americans, who began arriving in the United States in substantial numbers in 1981, are among the least acculturated of the Asian American groups.

Many of the Cambodians who came here during the 1980s spoke little or no English and, because of language and cultural barriers in particular, have had a difficult adjustment in the United States (Bromley & Olsen, 1994). In addition, in examining the life experiences of these refugees, it is apparent that almost all of them have been affected by numerous hazardous events and that the traumatic war experiences and the Pol Pot reign of terror shattered the entire Cambodian society: "Children, as well as adults, witnessed and were often forced to participate in brutal displays of mass beatings, dismemberments, and burnings of live victims of the Khmer Rouge. Those who survived to make it to the work camps had to face more beatings, starvation, dehydration, and excessively long and arduous work days" (Bromley, 1987, p. 237; see also Hood & Ablin, 1987; Karnow, 1984; Kinzie, 1987; Wain, 1981).

These alarming experiences have been cited as contributing to the Cambodian refugees' vulnerable state—the breakdown of their traditional coping mechanisms and the overall status of their mental health (Bromley, 1987; Kinzie, 1987). They are also important variables when considering substance abuse risk factors for many Cambodians and Cambodian Americans (Amodeo, Robb, Peou, & Tran, 1996). This chapter explores the historic and cultural background of Cambodians in the United States, their patterns of substance use and abuse, and practice implications for substance abuse treatment.

HISTORICAL BACKGROUND
OF CAMBODIAN AMERICANS

There is considerable ethnic diversity in cultural norms, customs, language, religion, history, and the process of urbanization among the major Southeast Asian refugee groups of Laotians, Hmong, Vietnamese, and Cambodians (Bromley, 1987). For example, a large number of the Hmong refugees tend to be animists and/or Christians, whereas Laotians and Cambodians tend to be Buddhists, although some are Christian and a small number of Cambodians are Muslim. The Vietnamese who came to the United States as refugees tend to be either Buddhist or Catholic. In addition, there are a number of ethnic Chinese, particularly from Cambodia and Vietnam, of various religions who also came to the United States as refugees. Many Laotians and Vietnamese came primarily from urban areas, whereas many of the Hmong and Cambodians who came to the United States as refugees came from more rural areas. The Vietnamese, Hmong, Laotian, and Cambodian languages are all separate and distinct. And, although many Americans born in the United States refer to "the Vietnam War," for the people in Southeast Asia, there were widely separate experiences of this war, as well as its trauma and aftermath.

The Cambodian people, whose language and culture is known as Khmer, come from a largely agrarian country that is situated in Southeast Asia and bordered by Vietnam, Laos, Thailand, and the Gulf of Thailand.

The name Khmer comes from Kambuja, a name designating the descendants of Kambu, the founder of the country (Garry, 1980). The great Khmer Empire was one of the most powerful states in Southeast Asia in the 13th century. Roughly 97% of ethnic Khmer people are believed to be Theravada Buddhists (McKenzie-Pollock, 1996). There are also a very small number of Moslem and Christian Cambodians. Traditional Khmer society and family is largely hierarchical, with male heads of household usually having authority over most decision making that takes place outside the family unit. Prior to the American involvement in Southeast Asia during the Vietnam conflict, most of the Cambodian people had little or no exposure to Western cultures.

The Cambodian Agony, a book published in 1987, begins with the statement "Cambodia has risen from the ashes, but the embers still smolder" (Hood & Ablin, 1987, p. xv). Little did we realize that in 1997 the ashes would be rekindled, the embers would continue to smolder, and old battles would flare in Cambodia.

During the era of the American involvement in the war in Southeast Asia (1959–1979), Prince Sihanouk's Royal Kingdom of Cambodia fell in 1970. The next 5 years saw a full-scale civil war in Cambodia, accompanied by massive United States bombing of Cambodia that was aimed at stopping the flow of supplies and personnel from North Vietnam to South Vietnam during the Vietnam conflict. According to Hood and Ablin (1987), more than 539,000 tons of bombs were dropped on Cambodia, more than three times the amount of explosives that had been dropped on Japan during World War II.

The United States Congress ended the bombing in Cambodia on August 15, 1973. This was also the year in which the Khmer Rouge made its first major attempts to reshape Cambodian life. The name Khmer Rouge (Red) was coined by Prince Sihanouk to designate the Cambodian Communists led by Pol Pot (Garry, 1980). In April 1975, just 2 months after the fall of Saigon in South Vietnam, the Khmer Rouge, in control of the Cambodian government, declared Year Zero and began a 4-year reign of terror that would leave between 1 million and 3 million Cambodians dead. Democratic Kampuchea, the name the Khmer Rouge chose for Cambodia, was a radical effort aimed at the social transformation of the country, which had been a monarchy under Prince Sihanouk, into a communist state. Within hours of their victory march into the capital city of Phnom Penh, the Khmer Rouge began the forced exodus of its 3 million residents.

The Khmer Rouge established social categories that determined not just the quality of one's life but often if one lived at all (Hood & Ablin, 1987). Buddhist monks were defrocked, tortured, and killed by Khmer

Rouge soldiers as part of Pol Pot's efforts to enforce systematic thought control and to rid the country of all religious and intellectual influences. Most of the 70,000 to 100,000 ordained Buddhist monks died during Pol Pot's regime. Medical care was virtually abolished. All but 55 Cambodian doctors are thought to have died during his rule (Hood & Ablin, 1987).

> Children were separated from their parents, put into children's camps, and made to inform on their parents. People were put in forced labor camps and made to work long hours. With the dismantling of the old social order, the once relatively prosperous country went into collapse, and famine and disease became endemic. Conditions in the labor camp became even more nightmarish. The Khmer Rouge maintained control by mass public torture, execution, and disembowelment of all dissidents or suspected dissidents. Family members, neighbors, and coworkers were forced to watch without showing emotion; any outpouring of emotion was punished by similar brutality. (McKenzie-Pollock, 1996, p. 309)

On December 25, 1978, Vietnam launched a full-scale invasion of Cambodia. Within 3 weeks, the Vietnamese army captured Phnom Penh and secured all of Cambodia except for some of the regions bordering on Thailand. Following this Vietnamese invasion, millions of Cambodians left the communes in which they had been held captive by Pol Pot's soldiers and fled the country for neighboring Thailand. This flight to Thailand was perilous, and many Cambodian refugees witnessed or were themselves victims of land mines; rape, capture, and torture by enemy soldiers; illness and death from malaria and other diseases; and a whole host of other horrors. Cambodian refugees lived in constant fear of capture or death during their journey through the jungles and across the border in Thailand. Upon arrival into Thailand, refugees from Cambodia were kept in barren camps surrounded by barbed wire, where they waited for years, in most cases, for the resettlement process that would take them from Thailand to the United States and other resettlement countries. With an accumulation of overwhelming physical and emotional scars, Cambodian refugees and immigrants arrived in the United States in large numbers during the 1980s and continued to arrive in much smaller numbers during the 1990s.

TRADITIONAL CAMBODIAN CULTURAL VALUES

As pointed out by Ebihara (1987), "pre-1975 Cambodian society as a whole could be roughly divided into three broad classes: an upper stratum of royalty and high government officials; a 'middle class' of white-collar workers, professionals, minor bureaucrats, etc.; and a lower class of peasants, artisans, and urban proletarians" (p. 20). People from the villages generally would speak of themselves as "poor country folk" in contrast to people from the city and those with nonagricultural occupations, such as schoolteachers. Ebihara (1987) goes on to state: "Although villagers recognized degrees of relative wealth among themselves, there also existed simultaneously a general ethic of fundamental egalitarianism . . . material wealth in and of itself was not the basis for high status among fellow villagers. Rather, individuals were given special respect or prestige on the basis of qualities such as age, religiosity, and especially 'good character' " (pp. 20–21). Although women in traditional Cambodian society were often subservient to their husbands, gender roles, especially in the rural parts of the country, were not absolutely rigid and women would undertake a host of tasks related to raising crops and animals, as well as marketing them and their handicrafts, to make ends meet (Ebihara, 1987).

As mentioned earlier, roughly 97% of ethnic Khmer people are Theravada Buddhists (McKenzie-Pollock, 1996). For Cambodians, Buddhist beliefs are not just a part of their religion, they are also an important part of individual, family, and community life. According to Ebihara (1987), for most Cambodians, the Buddhist temple serves as a moral, social, and educational center. Buddhists believe that every person goes through a cycle of reincarnations and that the number of meritorious deeds performed in this lifetime will affect one's position in the next life. Ebihara states, "Villagers strove to earn merit in a number of ways: by becoming a monk (a path open, however, only to males); by giving offerings of food, money, goods, and services to the monks and temple; by attending ritual observances at the temple; and importantly, by following Buddhist norms of conduct in one's daily life, particularly the major injunctions against killing living creatures, lying, theft, immoral sexual relations, and alcoholic beverages" (p. 21).

With the advent of Democratic Kampuchea under Pol Pot, Buddhist temples were destroyed and monks were killed. Religion was replaced by secular norms and state codes of conduct, and changes were geared toward the dissolution of certain basic institutions, such as the family, village, and temple, that would have competed with the state for people's loyalties (Ebihara, 1987). Traditional family structure, loyalties, and activities were reshaped or suppressed by a variety of means. For example, Ebihara (1987) points out that children past the age of about 7 were separated from their families, housed separately in dormitory-like arrangements, and mobilized into youth labor teams. Young people were a special target for indoctrination into revolutionary ideology. In many ways, this process of indoctrinating the Cambodian youth was reminiscent of Hitler's youth movement.

State control over what had once been parental or individual preroga-tive was manifest also in another critical sphere: marriage (Ebihara, 1987). In traditional Khmer society, a young woman was presumably free to ac-cept or reject a marriage proposal brought by a go-between from a young man and his parents to her parents. In practice, however, the parents of both the young man and young woman often exerted control over a child's marriage. However, in Pol Pot's Democratic Kampuchea, "the state, through local officials, replaced parents in the negotiation and regulation of marriages . . . [and] forced marriages occurred when soldiers or disabled veterans were allowed to marry any woman of their choosing. Ordinary men and women were sometimes arbitrarily married off to one another in hasty mass weddings" (Ebihara, 1987, pp. 29–30). With the takeover by the Vietnamese in January 1979, some of the basic elements of traditional (pre-1975) Khmer culture were resurrected under the policies of the Peo-ple's Republic of Kampuchea, including the reconstitution of the family as a social unit. However, because many women had been forced into horren-dous marriages under the Pol Pot regime, many families now experienced divorces rather than reunions of spouses (Ebihara, 1987).

SUBSTANCES USED IN CAMBODIA

Some of the Buddhist norms of conduct cited herein, such as the dictates against alcoholic beverages, continued to be valued by the Khmer Rouge, who viewed drinking as an "aspect of delinquency" (Ebihara, 1987, p. 34). Moreover, during the Pol Pot reign of terror from 1975 to 1979, it was nearly impossible for the ordinary Cambodian to access alcohol and other drugs. However, with the downfall of this regime, access to both legal and black market supplies opened up. After having undergone years of over-whelming loss, devastation, and stress, many Khmer have turned to alcohol and other drugs as a means of coping with their residual traumas.

Currently, alcohol, either homemade or factory produced, is sold ev-erywhere in Cambodia. In every town, including isolated villages, one can find people with substance abuse problems, particularly related to alcohol consumption. In addition, prostitution, illegal drug use, and the spread of the HIV virus are on the rise. In 1992, the United Nations Transitional Au-thority in Cambodia (UNTAC) was established, and more than 18,000 United Nations peacekeeping forces from various countries have been sent to Cambodia at a cost of over 2 billion dollars. Concurrent with the arrival of the peacekeeping forces, the demand for prostitutes, alcohol, and other drugs has increased to unprecedented levels.

Some authors have suggested that there is a predominant belief in the Cambodian community that "alcohol is a harmless substance unless the individual using it is engaged in behavior that disgraces the family. Further, alcohol is seen as helpful for dealing with sadness and forgetting painful memories" (Amodeo et al., 1996, p. 405; see also D'Avanzo & Frye, 1992; Morgan, Wingard, & Felice, 1984). Amodeo, Robb, Peou, and Tran (1997) also point out that many Cambodians use alcohol as a basic ingredient in many traditional home remedies. Alcohol is viewed as having healing properties and is often used to self-medicate as a means of providing temporary relief from feelings of sadness, loneliness, and grief. Herbal medicines with a small amount of alcohol as a base have also been used by pregnant Cambodian women. The women believe that this mixture will increase their blood flow and return their body to a youthful state (Amodeo et al., 1997).

Given the enormity of the social problems with which this country must currently contend (for example, unexploded land mines that have greatly reduced the land available for farming and that have been responsible for losses of limbs in an inordinate number of people), it is predicted that the alcohol and other drug problems in Cambodia will get much worse before formalized prevention and treatment programs are available in any numbers to cope with the issue. Currently in Cambodia, family members will oftentimes keep the person with an alcohol- or drug-related problem hidden within the family for fear of the shame that the problem might bring upon the family. This puts additional emotional, as well as financial, stress on the other family members, who must "cover" for the person with the problem. A family member might also seek help and support from the Buddhist monk. Individual self-discipline and abstinence are the most common approaches to dealing with alcohol- and drug-related problems. In severe cases, the individual might move into the temple for a brief period of time for spiritual support and guidance through the process of developing this self-discipline and as a support for sobriety.

SUBSTANCES USED IN THE UNITED STATES

There is a lack of research data on tobacco, alcohol, and other drug use among Cambodian Americans. Although a 1996 article on adapting mainstream substance abuse interventions for Southeast Asian clients states that "alcohol and other drug abuse (AODA) is an increasing problem for this client population" (Amodeo et al., 1996, p. 403), the literature reviewed in this publication, with the exception of one study, is based on anecdotal information. As stated by Kim, McLeod, and Shantzis (1992), "Most information pertaining to AOD use among Asian Americans comes from isolated, ad hoc, non-random, snowball (referral) surveys conducted either by individual researchers or State agencies" (p. 210). In addition, research studies that have looked at prevalence rates of substance abuse within Asian American groups have generally included only Chinese, Japanese, Korean, Pacific Islander, and Filipino Americans. Very little has been written about AOD use among Southeast Asians in the United States, and even less has been written about AOD use among Cambodian Americans.

Kuramoto (1995) identified only two studies that focused on alcohol and other drug use among Southeast Asian respondents. In the first study cited by Kuramoto (Yee & Thu, 1987), household interviews were used to sample adult Southeast Asian refugees, mainly Vietnamese, in Texas. This study found that approximately one half of the respondents reported that they used alcohol and/or smoked tobacco to cope with stressful situations or personal problems (Kuramoto, 1995). The second study looked at substance abuse among youth involved in the Job Corps in San Diego (Morgan, Wingard, & Felice, 1984). Southeast Asian youth in this study had the "lowest level of drinking (use in the last six months) compared with Whites, African Americans, and Hispanics. Sixty-six percent of Indo-Chinese males and 43 percent of Indo-Chinese females drank, compared with an average of 87 percent for males and 88 percent for females in the other groups. The Indo-Chinese youth who drank reported very low levels of other drug use: None had used cocaine, and only 3 percent reported using marijuana" (Kuramoto, 1995, pp. 114–115). Given the date and location of this study, it is highly unlikely that Cambodian American youth were included in this sample of Southeast Asian youth.

A survey of key community informants in California by Hatanaka, Morales, and Kaseyama (1991) suggested that the problems of acculturation and posttraumatic stress placed recent Southeast Asian refugees and immigrants at risk for substance abuse. Southeast Asian males were considered particularly at risk due to peer and social pressures. A California drug abuse needs assessment that used community forums as a mechanism to obtain data reported that alcohol and tobacco were the two most prevalent substances abused by Cambodians. Crack cocaine and methamphetamine ("ice") were also reported as major problems (Sasao, 1991). Kuramoto (1995), in discussing this needs assessment, states that "The high-risk groups included low-income Cambodians of all ages and genders. The

AOD-related problems in the community included family or marital conflict, juvenile delinquency, gang activity, and peer pressure" (p. 133).

CONCEPTUAL APPROACHES TO UNDERSTANDING CAMBODIAN USE OF ALCOHOL AND OTHER DRUGS

Some of the major hypotheses with regard to AOD use among Asian Americans can be grouped along three conceptual approaches: cultural content approaches; cultural interaction approaches; and cultural risk-factor approaches (Kim, McLeod, & Shantzis, 1992). These approaches are discussed in this section.

Cultural Content Approaches

Alcohol and other drug use is governed by cultural norms and values. For traditional Cambodians, these cultural norms and values include very controlled coping styles, such as suppressing emotions, suffering silently, and acting pleasantly toward others regardless of one's true feelings. "Sublimating direct expressions of negative feelings such as fear, anger, grief, or hostility, might result in physical illness, such as a severe headache, backache, or stomach disorder. This, for the Khmer, is the culturally acceptable response to stress" (Bromley, 1987, p. 237).

According to Khmer culture, sadness is to be kept within the heart, and for centuries the Khmer people have been accustomed to linking physical with emotional functioning. In addition, with the paucity of Western medicine in Cambodia, it was not unusual to use alcohol, along with traditional herbs and drugs, for medicinal purposes. The use of alcohol and other drugs was usually done in moderation because drugs and alcohol were not readily available or affordable in the countryside. However, upon arrival in the United States, and suffering from the cumulative effects of the losses from war, persecution, and escape, coupled with adjustment and adaptation problems, many Cambodian refugees turned to alcohol to "medicate" themselves from the impact of these horrifying experiences. They found alcohol to be much more available and affordable in the United States, and it is theorized that this situation, along with the Cambodian traditional coping styles and coping mechanisms, has contributed greatly to the scope of AOD abuse problems of Cambodian Americans today.

Cultural Interaction Approaches

Cultural interaction approaches attempt to explain AOD problems "based on the different processes through which individuals in an ethnic/racial culture adapt to the larger WAAM [White Anglo American Mainstream] culture" (Kim, McLeod, & Shantzis, 1992, p. 218). The leading cultural interaction approaches described by Kim and colleagues (1992) are as follows:

1. *Acculturation theory.* This theory assumes that the degree of acculturation is a significant predictor of AOD use. According to this theory, Cambodians who are recent refugees and immigrants are most likely to drink and use other drugs in a manner similar to native Cambodian alcohol and drug users. As Cambodians acculturate to the mainstream society, their AOD use will become more similar to that of the mainstream society.

2. *Orthogonal or multidimensional cultural identification theory.* According to this theory, a person's cultural identification does not rest along a single continuum, and higher cultural identification is related to more positive psychosocial characteristics such as better self-esteem and stronger socialization skills (Oetting & Beauvais, 1990). There are a number of independent dimensions of cultural identification, and increasing cultural identification does not require decreasing identification with another culture. Oetting & Beauvais (1990) suggest that strongly bicultural youth have the highest self-esteem and the strongest socialization links, whereas youth who have a low level of identification with either culture (native or host) would be expected to show low self-esteem and weak links to family and school. This theory suggests that Cambodians who are fully bicultural, as well as Cambodians who are strongly tied to either the traditional Khmer culture or the American mainstream culture, will have higher self-esteem and better socialization links—two very important factors in reducing AOD abuse. However, Cambodians who are not bicultural and at the same time do not identify strongly with either traditional Khmer culture or mainstream American culture are at greater risk of AOD abuse in this society. Cambodian American adolescents are particularly susceptible to feeling a lack of strong cultural identification in that they may have had very little identification with their traditional Khmer culture either in Cambodia or in the United States, and many do not feel accepted by the American mainstream because of prejudice, discrimination, and racism.

3. *Cultural conflict theory.* According to this theory, cultural conflicts, such as generational gaps and conflicts within families, can contribute to family instability, which can in turn contribute to AOD problems. Peer group pressure among youth, role conflicts between parents and children,

and feelings of alienation and identity conflict also add to cultural conflicts and AOD-related problems. Kim, McLeod, and Shantzis (1992) point out that "new immigrant youth also lose respect for their parents and begin to identify more with peer clusters. An extreme example of such peer involvement is the Asian youth gangs, whose delinquent behaviors are on the rise in some major metropolitan areas of this country" (p. 221). Such dynamics certainly apply to Cambodian parents and their children.

Cultural Risk-Factor Approaches

Extensive work has been done on identifying AOD high-risk factors (see, e.g., Cooper, 1983; Hawkins, Lishner, & Catalano, 1985; Hawkins & Weise, 1985; Jessor, Chase, & Donovan, 1980; Kandal, 1982; Kaplan, 1980; Kim, 1981; Maddahian, Newcomb, & Bentler, 1988; Murray & Perry, 1985). Identified AOD high-risk factors that are believed to be shared cross-culturally include low self-esteem, stress, negative peer pressure, excessive rebelliousness, lack of value attachment to school, poor student–teacher relations, low religiosity, perception of a lack of cohesive family relationships, and negative social attitudes (Kim et al., 1992). In addition, a number of other potential high-risk factors are particularly pertinent to Asian Americans. These factors may be applicable to Cambodian Americans as well and include the following:

1. *Feelings of personal failure.* Many ethnic Cambodians families who were forced to flee their country and who came here as refugees had been successful in their own country prior to the Pol Pot reign of terror and the Vietnamese invasion. Now, both men and women may work long hours in menial jobs just to make ends meet. In addition, they may feel that their children no longer respect them, given their "failure" to provide adequately for their family. Additionally, if the children are having problems in school or in society, this may also be viewed as a personal failure on the part of the parents.

2. *Problems of role reversal.* As pointed out by Kim, McLeod, and Shantzis (1992), "In families in which the parents do not speak English, children who do may be forced to accept certain adult responsibilities—e.g. spokesperson for the family. This is a clear role reversal for the father in his traditional role as the source of authority in the family" (p. 223). Such role reversal can contribute to a loss of respect of children for their parents and other elders, which in turn contributes to cultural alienation of the children and cultural conflict within the family.

3. *Emotional stress and feelings of alienation.* Most Cambodian

Americans came to the United States as refugees. In other words, their migration to this country was forced rather than by choice. This factor exacerbates all the other stressors mentioned previously. In addition, the current antirefugee and anti-immigrant sentiment in the United States can contribute to a Cambodian American's feelings of alienation from the mainstream American culture.

4. *Economic stress resulting from immigration.* Many recently arrived Asian immigrants are supporting not only their immediate family but also their extended family members in their native country (Kim et al., 1992). This is certainly true for many Cambodian Americans. In addition, many are extremely worried about the health and safety of their relatives in Cambodia due to increased political instability, the dangers posed by the extensive networks of hidden land mines, and the extreme poverty in many areas of the country. Such economic obligations and personal concerns place additional pressures on the family. These pressures, in turn, limit the parents' involvement in their children's lives. Moreover, because of their parents' long working hours and low wages, many children are unsupervised and live in marginal conditions (Kim et al., 1992). As a result of such economic stresses, Zane and Sasao (1990) put refugees and recent immigrants in a higher AOD risk category than other Asian groups.

IMPLICATIONS FOR TREATMENT

Treatment approaches must begin with the client's current situation and require a multifaceted approach based on a comprehensive assessment of the client's risk factors and an understanding of his or her unique cultural adaptational dynamics and place along the cultural transition continuum. All three approaches to understanding and explaining alcohol and other drug abuse—cultural content, cultural interaction, and cultural risk factors—are applicable to understanding and working with Cambodians in the United States. Successful AOD treatment usually requires an overall approach that is acceptable to the client and his or her family and that does not violate traditional Cambodian beliefs, customs, and values.

Several authors have provided the following practical suggestions that can be used to guide clinical interventions with substance-abusing Cambodian Americans (Bromley, 1987, 1988; Bromley & Olsen, 1994; Green, 1995; Ishisaka, Nguyen, & Okimoto, 1985; Muecke, 1983).

1. Conduct a thorough assessment that identifies the relative contribution of the traditional Khmer culture to the client's current functioning. For

example, Bromley and Olsen (1994) have developed a cross-cultural family assessment scale that measures such factors as understanding of Cambodian language and culture; degree of isolation from both mainstream culture and the Cambodian community; level of English comprehension; understanding of American customs; ability of family to access services; level of depression; and current alcohol or other drug use. Most standardized assessment instruments, such as depression scales and AOD use scales, need modification in order to accurately reflect Cambodian norms, values, and experiences.

2. Many Cambodian families with a substance-abusing member come for help because of crises such as domestic violence, child abuse or neglect, legal difficulties, and/or financial emergencies. Therefore, in order to engage the family and establish a relationship, it may be necessary to focus first on crisis resolution and the provision of case management and concrete services before addressing the substance abuse issue. Meeting basic human needs such as food and shelter must be a first priority; AOD treatment will usually not be accepted by the Cambodian family without addressing simultaneously what the family perceives to be the most pressing issues.

3. Learn enough about Cambodian culture to permit interaction that respects the person's sense of propriety in interpersonal relationships.

4. Avoid approaches that rely heavily on the expression of emotions. The ability to suppress emotions and to suffer silently in order to maintain dignity are highly valued in Khmer society.

5. Emphasize Cambodian family and community strengths and adaptive coping skills, such as the ability to rely on family and ethnic community support, strong individual and group survival skills, acceptance of one's fate and one's responsibilities, and a deep sense of family and community loyalty. For those individuals who have maintained their Cambodian culture and faith or who are interested in restoring their traditional support systems, the guidance and support of the Khmer Buddhist monks, the use of the Khmer Buddhist Temple as a place for culturally sensitive convalescence and recovery, and interventions from other traditional helpers such as Kru Khmer healers can enhance AOD treatment. It is important to keep in mind that many Cambodian Americans are uncomfortable with mainstream helping systems such as mental health centers, drug and alcohol treatment centers, Alcoholics Anonymous (AA), and so forth, and will avoid using them.

6. Provide opportunities for the client and his or her family to discuss their unique perspectives and values in the context of their experiences and their AOD-related issues. For example, ask the client and/or family mem-

bers how they or other Cambodians they have known have dealt with problems in the past, especially in Cambodia, during their escape, and during their stay in refugee camps. Help the clients assess the usefulness of these strategies in coping with their current situation.

7. Carefully describe all possible treatment approaches, along with the rationale for recommending a particular treatment approach.

8. Accept definitions of successful interventions that are meaningful to the members of the Cambodian American community. This may mean supporting the client who opts to stay at the Khmer Buddhist Temple instead of checking into a mainstream treatment program. It may also mean encouraging a client who may not be comfortable with attending AA meetings to attend group gatherings at the Temple that are led by a monk who may only indirectly address the AOD issues but who reminds the gathering about the meaning of life and helps to guide them on their path to enlightenment.

Treatment Approaches and Case Examples

Treatment should begin with an assessment of the presenting problems and issues; a cross-cultural assessment of the client's status in regard to acculturation and/or adaptation to the U. S. mainstream norms, customs, values, and religions; a screening for alcohol and other drug use, taking into account Cambodian beliefs, customs, and values with regard to AOD use and abuse; and finally, the use of a culturally appropriate case management approach to help the client and family to resolve presenting crises and to meet basic needs.

In order for intervention to be effective and for a clinician to establish a rapport with a more traditional Cambodian American family, both counseling and case management services must be, at minimum, cofacilitated by a Khmer-speaking case manager. The following case vignette is illustrative of this approach.

> Mr. and Mrs. K came to the United States from Cambodia in 1986 and were resettled in California. Both have a history of heavy alcohol abuse in this country, although alcohol abuse was never a problem for them in Cambodia or during their stay in refugee camps in Thailand. Their two daughters, aged 8 and 3, and two sons, aged 6 and 1, had been in foster care for the previous 8 months due to child neglect. The children were often left in the care of the 8-year-old while their parents were drinking. Neighbors often reported that the children were out in the street playing at all hours of the night and were improperly clothed for the weather. The family's problems were well known in the Cam-

bodian community. In order to regain custody of their children, Mr. and Mrs. K were ordered to participate in an alcohol treatment program and to abstain from drinking. Both parents stated that they very much wanted their children back home with them.

Mr. K actively followed through with treatment for his alcoholism at a local substance abuse treatment clinic with a Khmer-speaking alcoholism counselor and was clean and sober for about 6 months. However, Mrs. K had great difficulty maintaining her sobriety and refused inpatient treatment. Mrs. K showed up at a recent 9:30 a.m. children's services case conference with alcohol on her breath. Also present at the conference, in addition to the children's services worker from the state agency and Mr. K, were a Khmer-speaking family caseworker, a Khmer-speaking substance abuse counselor, and a non-Khmer-speaking clinical social worker. All of the practitioners had worked with the K family over an extended period of time and were somewhat trusted and respected by Mr. and Mrs. K (because these three workers were also working cooperatively with the state child welfare department, there was some erosion of trust).

After exchanging greetings, the clinical social worker began the meeting by gently commenting in English to both Mr. and Mrs. K about the smell of alcohol on Mrs. K's breath. The social worker spoke to them directly but with indirect eye contact, and their family caseworker translated the comment into Khmer. At first, they both denied that Mrs. K had been drinking. The substance abuse counselor then added in Khmer that she too noticed the smell. Mrs. K responded that she had used some Cambodian medicines that morning that may have contained alcohol. The clinical social worker then turned her attention to Mr. K, gently reminded him of the importance of helping his wife overcome this difficulty that they were having, and asked him if his wife might be drinking again. Mr. K did not respond or make eye contact; Mrs. K stayed silent. The Khmer substance abuse counselor then spoke softly but firmly about the difficulty of getting and remaining sober. Neither Mr. nor Mrs. K responded, but their silence was understood as an indirect acknowledgment of the importance of what the counselor said. The rest of the meeting then focused on how best to help Mr. and Mrs. K. The clinical social worker, with the assistance of the family caseworker and substance abuse counselor, developed a new case plan with Mr. and Mrs. K that would focus on a more traditional approach to treatment for the couple. It was agreed that the Khmer family caseworker would make weekly supportive home visits to Mr. and Mrs. K and provide transportation and support for Mrs. K to attend a weekly women's group at the Khmer Buddhist temple, where discussions about being a good person and other teachings of Buddha, such as the ideal way of living and the ways of attaining enlightenment, are a part of other rituals that include chanting and the offering of food to the monks.

Confrontation is a common approach to helping people who are in denial with regard to a substance abuse problem. In Cambodian culture, however, confrontation is usually avoided because of the danger of loss of face, both for the sender and the receiver of the message. As pointed out by Amodeo and colleagues (1996), "With Cambodian and Vietnamese clients, it is imperative to avoid aggressive approaches, which tend to result in loss of face" (p. 406). Nonetheless, substance abuse issues cannot by ignored or overlooked. Therefore, as exemplified in the case study, the best approach is to be direct but in the most nonconfrontational way possible. It is important to note that is was the non-Khmer worker who brought up Mrs. K's drinking. Cambodian clients are oftentimes more accepting of the non-Khmer worker's direct approach, especially if they already have a trusting relationship. Such directness of approach may not be tolerated if used by the Khmer worker. The need to translate the words from English to Khmer allowed the Khmer workers a less direct, more culturally acceptable approach to addressing the topic of Mrs. K's drinking. The utilization of such a team approach offered the opportunity to appropriately challenge both Mr. and Mrs. K with regard to her drinking.

The presenting problem in the next case vignette is domestic violence. Mrs. L had requested help and was able to acknowledge Mr. L's problems with substance abuse and issues related to posttraumatic stress. This case illustrates the difficulty of engaging a client with a dual diagnosis in substance abuse treatment.

Mr. L, aged 36, lived with his wife, Mrs. L, and their daughter, aged 13, and two sons, aged 10 and 14, in Rhode Island. Mr. L came alone to the United States from Cambodia in 1979 shortly after his father was killed by Pol Pot soldiers and his mother died from starvation. Mr. L had been forced into one of Pol Pot's youth camps at age 12. He learned as a young boy how to be an armed guerrilla soldier, and he was forced to kill and commit other acts of violence if he wanted to survive under the Khmer Rouge regime. Mr. L came to live with his uncle in California and began drinking while still a freshman in high school. He dropped out of school in the 11th grade at the age of 17. At age 19 he moved to Rhode Island with several other Cambodian youths and met and married Mrs. L shortly afterward.

Since moving to Rhode Island, he held a number of different low-skilled jobs but was never able to maintain steady employment. Mr. L was primarily a binge drinker and had a history of violence toward Mrs. L when drunk. Mrs. L called the police to the apartment on several occasions; however, she always regretted her action the following day, and in the past she bailed him out of jail and dropped the charges.

However, following his most recent assault, because of a change in state law with regard to domestic violence, the police would not drop the charges at Mrs. L's request. Consequently, Mr. L served 5 days in jail and was ordered to receive treatment for his domestic violence. He was also referred to an outpatient substance abuse treatment center; however, he did not call for an appointment there.

One morning, Mrs. L arrived at the Cambodian Community Services Center stating that Mr. L was drunk and passed out in their car outside. After establishing that the children were safely at school, the social worker reviewed the events of the morning and of the previous evening. Mrs. L agreed with the worker's assessment that she and the children were not safe with Mr. L in the house. She asked the worker to try to convince Mr. L to enter an inpatient alcohol detoxification and treatment facility. While the clinician was on the phone checking on treatment vacancies, Mr. L walked into the office. After much discussion, Mr. L agreed to enter treatment, and arrangements were made to have a male Khmer counselor transport him to the detoxification facility. Once they arrived there, however, Mr. L changed his mind, stating that the facility, which had no Khmer-speaking staff and no other Cambodian clients, reminded him too much of a prison.

Mr. L went home and continued his drinking and abusive behavior for another 3 months, at which time the children were placed in foster care because of the risk to their safety. Mrs. L then forced him, with the help of a Cambodian domestic violence counselor, to move out of the apartment so that she could begin the process of family reunification with her children. With no place else to go, Mr. L went to the Khmer Buddhist Temple and asked the monks if he could temporarily stay with them. They agreed to take him with the condition that he abstain from drinking. Mr. L remained at the temple, clean and sober, for approximately 4 months, then he moved back home and obtained employment. Although he had periodic relapses, he managed to avoid his previous pattern of domestic violence and was able to return to sobriety following each relapse. Mr. L never acknowledged the need for professional help for his alcohol dependence, domestic violence, or any other problem, such as posttraumatic stress.

Unfortunately, the preceding case is not an unusual one. Assessment of Mr. L indicated that, in addition to his alcohol dependence and violent behavior, Mr. L was suffering from posttraumatic stress disorder brought on by his experiences in Cambodia. Memories of the confined quarters and forced indoctrination of the youth camp flooded back to him as soon as he saw the stark public detoxification center.

It is important that treatment providers have a good understanding of the Cambodian client's past experiences, as well as his or her current situation, before embarking on a treatment plan. Although detoxification and rehabilitation in a facility specializing in drug and alcohol treatment may be the most sound approach under most circumstances, Mr. L's unique experiences in terms of how he survived the Cambodian holocaust made such an approach to treatment unacceptable to him. In addition, part of his way of coping had been to keep inside the horrors of his past, which is a typical survival strategy for Cambodians who suffered under Pol Pot. Mr. L, like many other Cambodian holocaust survivors, had learned to persevere in spite of the pain. Clinicians must be prepared to accept and respect their Cambodian client's need to suffer silently and allow the posttraumatic stress to go untreated, by Western standards, if this is the client's wish. Moreover, although the Cambodian client's plan for substance abuse treatment may not be the most effective from a Western perspective, it may be the only feasible treatment approach that the client will accept.

Substance-abusing Cambodian adolescent clients and their families can sometimes present clinicians with a number of challenges, as the following case vignette illustrates.

> The V family came to the United States from Cambodia in 1991. They were sponsored by relatives in a moderately sized Massachusetts city, where they found a small Khmer community of approximately 2,000 people. Sok V, aged 14, began drinking, smoking pot, and hanging out with a gang of other Cambodian youths during the previous year. He missed school regularly and had no extracurricular activities other than hanging out with his gang. Both Mr. and Mrs. V worked long hours to support the family. They were very disappointed in Sok and concerned about the negative influence he might have on his younger brother, whom they describe as a "good boy."
>
> Sok was arrested with his friends for petty larceny at a local store. The youth officer involved with the case told Mr. & Mrs. V through an interpreter that they must get help for Sok. He informed them that the gang that their son had been hanging with was well known to the police because of their delinquent and sometimes criminal acts. The Vs did not know what to do to help their son and felt ashamed because of the disgrace he brought to the family. At that point, they were more concerned about his gang membership and lack of school attendance than about his drinking and drug use.

This is again a case situation that, unfortunately, is all too familiar to those who work with Cambodian youths and their families. Although a language barrier is not an issue for Sok, he would probably feel isolated in any program that did not involve other Cambodian youths. Such isolation and cultural alienation is oftentimes what impels youths (in this case a

Cambodian youth) to join a gang. Therefore, in order for intervention to be effective in such a case situation, it is important to develop indigenous programs for Cambodian American youths and their families that addresses all of their problems, including substance abuse issues.

In addition, Mr. and Mrs. V would face both a language and a cultural barrier if their son was referred to a mainstream youth program with no Khmer-speaking workers. They may blame American culture for their son's behavior problems and would thus be reluctant to trust a youth program outside the Cambodian community. Even with youth and family programs that hire Cambodian interpreters when needed, Mr. and Mrs. V would feel reluctant to engage in a non-Cambodian approach to their son's problems. However, if the youth program is linked to a Cambodian social services or community center, Cambodian parents would be more trustful and willing to allow their children to participate in such a program. Such a program could also provide programming to help parents better understand what life is like for their more Americanized children. Programs aimed at helping older children to better understand and accept the values, norms, and experiences of their more traditional parents are also helpful.

Cross-Cultural Interventions in the Cambodian Community

James Green (1995) suggests the use of a help-seeking behavioral model for providing human services in ethnocultural communities. This model has a great deal of applicability to providing AOD treatment with the more traditional Cambodian American families. Such a model, according to Green (1995), consists of the following components:

1. *The individual's definition and understanding of an experience as a problem.* Green (1995) points out that presenting problems of clients may be either general or specific, such as a vague feeling of pain, a loss of appetite, loss of a job, a death in the family, or violence. How these conditions are interpreted is a significant part of the experience for the client. He states: "I take it for granted that until shown otherwise, ethnic or minority clients have a view of the world that is not the same as that of the help provider, a view that is a mix of idiosyncratic and community elements" (p. 58). Cambodian Americans who may be perceived by others as having a problem with alcohol or other drugs may have a definition and understanding of the problem that is likely to be vastly different from the definition and understanding arrived at by a mainstream American substance abuse counselor. Thus the treatment approach must take into account both Cambodian and American mainstream community norms and the individual's

perception of his or her own situation (Bromley, 1987). The successful clinician will begin with the Cambodian client's evaluation of the problem and will be patient and gentle in suggesting the role that alcohol and other drugs might play in his or her problems.

2. *The person's semantic evaluation of a problem.* Language is the storage medium of an individual's cultural knowledge, and if we truly want to know where a client is "coming from," then we must reasonably begin with the semantic dimensions of the client's explanatory model (Green, 1995). "To start with the client's emotions . . . presumes that the worker already understands, exactly like a native, the sensibilities and meanings those emotions express. But if one is not a native in the client's culture, then such a presumption is dubious and exploration of emotions may be superficial at best" (Green, 1995, p. 64). In order to gain an understanding of the Cambodian American's semantic evaluation of the problem, a clinician must have more than a superficial understanding of both Khmer language and culture. Thus, it is important for non-Khmer clinicians to work with a Khmer-speaking case manager or cocounselor. If this is not possible, a Khmer-speaking interpreter can help, but the clinician should understand that there are limitations to understanding the person's semantic evaluation of the problem when the meaning is conveyed through an interpreter.

3. *Indigenous strategies of problem intervention.* There is an enormous range of help-seeking activity in all cultures (Green, 1995). In almost every Cambodian American community, healers and herbalists such as the Kru Khmer are available as an indigenous source of help. Kru Khmer healers are generally not known outside the ethnic Cambodian neighborhood; however, the mainstream clinician can access a Khu Khmer, if needed and desired by a client, by linking the client first to the closest Cambodian community-based social services agency. These agencies generally know how to connect the client to the appropriate indigenous healer. In addition, the Khmer Buddhist Temple, which is traditionally a place where Cambodians can go for help with personal, family, and community problems, has been a place of refuge, support, and help for many persons who are troubled by alcohol and other drugs, as seen in the case of Mr. L.

4. *Culturally based criteria of problem resolution.* The difficulty of relating specific treatment to outcomes is compounded when there are cultural differences. Green (1995) points out that sometimes clinicians rely on common, everyday explanations for cultural differences and then make superficial, even stereotypic, judgments about clients based on these explanations. Reliance on ethnographic trivia can lead to the truth in the cliché that a little knowledge is a dangerous thing. Anecdotal information oftentimes becomes a primary and misleading source of knowledge. One way of re-

solving this difficulty is to learn how people solve problems within their own communities and what to them are reasonable outcomes (Green, 1995). Canda and Yellow Bird (1997) suggest that, in order to discover and focus on individual and community strengths and resources, "clinicians must become involved in the forces of strength and resiliency within the culture" (p. 248). This may necessitate that, in working with a substance-abusing Cambodian client, the non-Khmer clinician accompany the client to a meeting at the Khmer Buddhist Temple in order to get a better understanding of the client's community. Change is stress-inducing enough without further exacerbating the community's problems by having helpers who have very limited (or no) awareness of the customs, traditions, and languages of these communities (Canda & Yellow Bird, 1997).

CONCLUSION

In order to help Cambodian American clients work on their AOD-related problems, clinicians must search for and test innovative ways to bridge mainstream American and traditional Cambodian norms, values, and customs. Whatever approach is used, it must be culturally sensitive to the client's unique ways of communicating, coping, and problem solving and must also function in this society. This is not an easy task. If substance abuse clinicians are to be successful in developing AOD prevention and treatment programs that are culturally relevant and sensitive to the needs of the Cambodian American community, they must be willing to work side by side with the representatives, helpers, and indigenous leaders of the Cambodian American community and must be willing to accept the community's definition, understanding, and evaluation of the problem, along with their suggestions for indigenous strategies for problem resolution.

REFERENCES

Ablin, D. A., & Hood, M. (1987). The path to Cambodia's present. In D. Ablin & M. Hood (Eds.), *The Cambodian agony* (pp. xv–lvi). Armonk, NY: M. E. Sharpe.

Amodeo, M., Robb, N., Peou, S., & Tran, H. (1996). Adapting mainstream substance-abuse interventions for Southeast Asian clients. *Families in Society, 77*(7), 403–412.

Amodeo, M., Robb, N., Peou, S., & Tran, H. (1997). Alcohol and other drug problems among Southeast Asians: Patterns of use and approaches to assessment and intervention. *Alcoholism Treatment Quarterly, 15*(3), 63–77.

Bromley, M. A. (1987). New beginnings for Cambodian refugees—or further disruptions. *Social Work, 32*(3), 236–239.

Bromley, M. A. (1988). Identity as a central adjustment issue of the Southeast Asian unaccompanied refugee minor. *Child and Youth Care Quarterly, 17*(2), 104–114.

Bromley, M. A., & Olsen, L. J. (1994). Early intervention services for Southeast Asian children. *Social Work in Education, 16*(4), 251–256.

Canda, E., & Yellow Bird, M. (1997). Another view: Cultural strengths are crucial. *Families in Society, 78*(3), 248.

Cooper, S. E. (1983). Surveys on studies on alcoholism. *International Journal of the Addictions, 18*(7), 971–985.

D'Avanzo, C. E., & Frye, B. (1992). Stress and self-medication in Cambodian refugee women. *Addictions Nursing Network, 4*(2), 59–60.

Ebihara, M. (1987). Revolution and reformulation in Kampuchean village culture. In D. A. Ablin & M. Hood (Eds.), *The Cambodian agony* (pp. 16–61). Armonk, NY: M. E. Sharpe.

Garry, R. (1980). Cambodia. In E. Tepper (Ed.), *Southeast Asian exodus: From tradition to resettlement* (pp. 33–53). Ottawa: Canadian Asian Studies Association.

Green, J. (1995). *Cultural awareness in the human services* (2nd ed.). Boston: Allyn & Bacon.

Hatanaka, H., Morales, R., & Kaseyama, N. (1991). *Asian Pacific alcohol peer consultation and training project.* Los Angeles: Special Services for Groups.

Hawkins, D. J., Lishner, D. M., & Catalano, R. F. (1985). Childhood predictors of adolescent substance abuse. In C. L. Jones & R. J. Battjes (Eds.), *Etiology of adolescent substance abuse* (DHHS Publication No. ADM 87–1335, pp. 134–148). Washington, DC: U.S. Government Printing Office.

Hawkins, D. J., & Weise, G. J. (1985). The social development model: An integrated approach to delinquency prevention. *Journal of Primary Prevention, 6*(2), 73–97.

Ishisaka, H. A., Nguyen, Q. T., & Okimoto, J. T. (1985). The role of culture in the mental health treatment of Indochinese refugees. In T. C. Owan (Ed.), *Southeast Asian mental health: Treatment, prevention, services, training, and research* (pp. 41–63). Rockville, MD: National Institute of Mental Health.

Jessor, R., Chase, J. A., & Donovan, J. E. (1980). Psychosocial correlates of marijuana use and problem drinking in a national sample of adolescents. *American Journal of Public Health, 70,* 604–613.

Kandal, D. (1982). Epidemiological and psychological perspectives on adolescent drug use. *Journal of the American Academy of Child Psychiatry, 21*(4), 328–347.

Kaplan, H. B. (1980). Self-esteem and self-derogation theory of drug abuse. In K. Sayers & H. W. Pearson (Eds.), *Theories of drug abuse* (pp. 87–96). Rockville, MD: National Institute on Drug Abuse.

Karnow, S. (1984). *Vietnam: A history.* New York: Penguin.

Kim, S. (1981). Student attitudinal inventory for program outcome evaluation of adolescent drug abuse. *Journal of Primary Prevention, 2,* 91–100.

Kim, S., McLeod, J. H., & Shantzis, C. (1992). Cultural competence for evaluators working with Asian-American communities: Some practical considerations. In M. A. Orlandi, R. Weston, & L. G. Epstein (Eds.), *Cultural competence for evaluators: A guide for alcohol and other drug abuse prevention practitioners working with ethnic/racial communities* (pp. 203–260). Rockville, MD: U.S. Department of Health and Human Services, Public Health Service, Alcohol, Drug Abuse, and Mental Health Administration, Office for Substance Abuse Prevention, Division of Community Prevention and Training.

Kinzie, J. D. (1987). The "concentration camp syndrome" among Cambodian refugees. In D. A. Ablin & M. Hood (Eds.), *The Cambodian agony* (pp. 332–353). Armonk, NY: M. E. Sharpe.

Kitano, H. H. L., & Daniels, R. (1988). *Asian Americans: Emerging minorities.* Englewood Cliffs, NJ: Prentice-Hall.

Kuramoto, F. (1995). Asian Americans. In J. Philleo, F. Brisbane, & L. G. Epstein (Eds.), *Cultural competence for social workers: A guide for alcohol and other drug abuse prevention professionals working with ethnic/racial communities* (pp. 105–155). Rockville, MD: U.S. Department of Health and Human Services, Public Health Service, Substance Abuse and Mental Health Services Administration, Center for Substance Abuse Prevention.

Le, N. (1993). The case of the Southeast Asian refugees: Policy for a community "at-risk." In *The state of Asian and Pacific America: A public policy report—Policy issues to the year 2020* (pp. 167–188). Los Angeles: LEAP Asian Pacific American Public Policy Institute and UCLA Asian American Studies Center.

Maddahian, E., Newcomb, M. D., & Bentler, P. M. (1988). Risk factors for substance abuse: Ethnic differences among adolescents. *Journal of Substance Abuse, 1*(1), 11–23.

McKenzie-Pollock, L. (1996). Cambodian families. In M. McGoldrick, J. Giordano, & J. K. Pearce (Eds.), *Ethnicity and family therapy* (2nd ed., pp. 307–315). New York: Guilford Press.

Morgan, M., Wingard, D., & Felice, M. (1984). Subcultural differences in alcohol use among youth. *Journal of Adolescent Health Care, 5,* 191–195.

Muecke, M. A. (1983). Caring for Southeast Asian refugee patients in the USA. *American Journal of Public Health, 73,* 431–438.

Murray, D. M., & Perry, C. L. (1985). The prevention of adolescent drug abuse: Implications from etiological, developmental, behavioral, and environmental models. In C. L. Jones & R. J. Battjes (Eds.), *Etiology of adolescent substance abuse* (pp. 201–226). Washington, DC: National Institute on Drug Abuse.

Oetting, E. R., & Beauvais, F. (1990). Orthogonal cultural identification theory: The cultural identification of minority adolescents. *International Journal of Addictions, 25,* 655–685.

Sasao, T. (1991). *Statewide Asian drug service needs assessment: A multimethod approach.* Sacramento: California Department of Alcohol and Drug Programs.

Tran, Q. D., & Matsuoka, J. K. (1995). Asian Americans: Southeast Asians. In R. Edwards (Ed.), *Encyclopedia of social work* (19th ed., pp. 249–255). Washington, DC: National Association of Social Workers.

Wain, B. (1981). *The refused: The agony of Indochina refugees.* Hong Kong: Dow Jones Asia.

Yee, B., & Thu, N. (1987). Correlates of drug use and abuse among Indochinese refugees. *Journal of Psychoactive Drugs, 19,* 77–83.

Zane, N., & Sasao, T. (1990). *Research on drug abuse among Asian Pacific Americans.* Unpublished manuscript, University of California, Santa Barbara.

17

Ethnocultural Background and Substance Abuse Treatment of Chinese Americans

Ting-Fun May Lai

Chinese Americans, with a total population of over one and one-half million people, are the largest and fastest growing Asian group in the United States (U.S. Bureau of the Census, 1995). The rapid growth of the Chinese population has increased both its heterogeneity and the visibility of various social problems.

For many years, the Chinese population in the United States has not been considered as having serious alcohol or drug problems. Yet research data on Chinese drinking and drug use are scarce. This chapter briefly discusses the Chinese historical and cultural heritage and examines the substance problems and treatment of Chinese Americans. Besides reviewing the available studies and literature, I share my own clinical experiences working with alcoholics and drug abusers at an outpatient clinic in New York City's Chinatown.

HISTORICAL BACKGROUND
AND CULTURAL HERITAGE

China is one of the oldest civilizations in the world, with a recorded history of more than 4,600 years. China was governed by about 15 dynasties varying in length of rule from several decades to several centuries. The last dynasty, the Qing, was overthrown by Sun Yat-sen, who founded the Chinese Republic on October 10, 1911. The present government took over the mainland in 1949 and established the People's Republic of China. On July 1, 1997, Hong Kong was officially returned to China and now is a special administrative region of the People's Republic of China.

China is a highly diverse country with many different ethnocultural groups, and its people speak a variety of languages. People from various geographic territories, both urban and rural, have their distinct beliefs, customs, and ways of living. Modernization, cultural influences from Western countries, and different political systems, such as capitalism and communism, further diversify the Chinese population. However, most Chinese do share a common culture and values.

Ethnocultural Populations

The Chinese population, currently estimated to be over 1 billion, makes up about one fifth of the world's population. Han is the largest ethnocultural group of Chinese people. Other major ethnocultural minorities are Manchurian, Mongolian, Moslem, Tibetan, and Miao. Hong Kong and Taiwan have the largest Chinese populations outside of mainland China.

Language

The Chinese language is formed by more than 40,000 characters that were developed from picture writing. Although the majority of Chinese share the same written language, they have their own distinct spoken dialects. Mandarin, or Kuo-Yu, is the national dialect. Other major dialects are: (1) Cantonese and Taishanese from Guangdong province and Hong Kong; (2) Fukienese, Amoy, and Taiwanese from Fujian province and Taiwan; (3) Shanghainese, from Shanghai region and Jiangsu and Zhejiang provinces; and (4) Hakka, from a region extending east to west from Fujian to Guangxi provinces.

Major Religions and Philosophical Beliefs

The Chinese religions and philosophical beliefs offer a useful framework for understanding Chinese spiritual life, philosophy of life, value system, interpersonal relationships, and disease concepts. Among the common beliefs that are held by many Chinese, including Chinese Americans, are the following:

Ancestor Worship

Ancestor worship is based on the belief that the living can communicate with their deceased ancestors and that the deceased still influence their living family members. The rituals of ancestral worship include offering incense and candles to tablets on which ancestors' names are inscribed. During special occasions, such as the New Year, All Soul's Day (ChingMing), and birth and death anniversaries, food, wine, and flowers are offered and paper money is burned. Ancestor worship reinforces commitment to the family and builds strong family ties.

Confucianism

Strictly speaking, Confucianism is more of a philosophy and value system than a religion; it poses no "God" or supernatural symbols for worship, nor does it stresses a personal relationship with supernatural powers. The closest idea of "God" is "Heaven." Confucianism is concerned with elaboration of the proper behavior for social roles, relationships, and social order. It stresses the concept of filial piety and principles of developing virtues and morality. Its goal is to reach the highest standard in personal development, family fulfillment, governing of one's country, and ruling of the world.

Taoism

Taoism is both a philosophy and a religion. As a religion it borrows many features from Buddhism and ancestor worship. Taoism is often identified with alchemy, geomancy, astrology, fortune-telling, witchcraft, and communication with the dead. It also focuses on regulating breathing and dieting in a manner that promotes health. It emphasizes the intuitive and expressive nature of human beings and sees people as living in harmony with nature. Taoism is not concerned with the artificial constructs of society, social order, or regulation. It urges a form of natural spontaneity and emancipation from the restrictions of ritual and other artificial structures.

Buddhism

Buddhism was introduced to China from India in the first century A.D. It provides the Chinese people with an emotional outlet because the gods (Amitabha, Guan Yin, and others) can be petitioned for help against evil and to grant blessings. Buddhism teaches the eternity of life and the idea of reincarnation and that people must purify themselves through meditation, good deeds, and prayers in order to achieve the state of eternal bliss. People's conduct and behavior in this world can influence their eventual existence in the next world.

Attitudes toward Health and Illness

Chinese medical orientation and views of health and illness are based on the concepts of Chinese medicine. Health is viewed as the balance of "Yin" and "Yang" and the harmony of body, mind, and soul. Illness is viewed as the imbalance of Yin and Yang or sometimes as punishment or fate. The attitude toward physical and mental illness is one of denial, tolerance of suffering, and, consequently, delay of treatment. It is not unusual to observe patients who have suffered from a chronic illness for many years and have come to treatment only for an acute medical crisis. Spiritual healing, herbs, and acupuncture are usually the choice of treatment approaches. Only after exhausting all the traditional treatment methods will some Chinese come to a medical clinic or hospital. However, once they do show up at the clinic or hospital doorstep, they expect instant remedy and relief from their symptoms. Extensive and long diagnostic examinations and tests are usually resisted, and many Chinese are fearful of having blood specimens taken from them.

The Traditional Chinese Family and Family Association

In Chinese culture, it is the family, not the individual, that is considered the basic unit of society. The welfare of the family always takes precedence over individual interests. Confucianism is the foundation of the traditional Chinese family; it spells out the organization and relationship of the members within the family.

The traditional family is usually an extended one. Sometimes three or four generations of family members live under the same roof. Family members are ranked according to sex, generation, and order of birth. The oldest male of the family is the head of the household, and his first-born male descendant inherits the lineage. However, the division of inheritance among the sons upon the death of the father does lead to the setting up of separate households. Elderly parents are expected to be cared for by their children.

Marriage is an important matter for Chinese families. Although arranged marriages are disappearing, the family still has a strong influence on an individual's mate selection. Marriage does not mark the creation of a new family but a continuation of the man's family. Clans, or *Zu,* are the extensions of relations through five or more generations based on male descendants of a common ancestor.

The role of Chinese women has been highly prescribed. In traditional Chinese families, married women live with their husbands' families. Women are not included in important family functions such as ancestor worship. Moreover, they are not listed in the family's genealogical book. As pointed out by Lee (1996), traditionally, in accordance with the custom of "thrice obeying," women were expected to obey their fathers in youth, their husbands in marriage, and their sons after their husbands' death. As wives, their value was judged by their ability to produce male heirs and to serve their in-laws. It is obvious how such traditional Chinese values can lead to cultural conflict for some Chinese immigrants in the United States.

HISTORY OF THE CHINESE IN AMERICA

Since the mid-18th century, millions of Chinese have emigrated overseas. Much of the emigration can be traced to events such as political upheaval, natural disasters such as floods and famines, and a population increase in southern China.

The Chinese began arriving in Hawaii as early as 1789 to work as laborers in sugarcane plantations. In 1848, gold was discovered in California, near present-day Sacramento. Thousands of Chinese came to work in the gold mines: By 1860 there were 35,000 Chinese miners, forming the largest non-White minority. In 1865, the first Chinese were hired to build the Western half of the transcontinental railroad. They faced terrible dangers and harsh working conditions, yet their contribution to the building of America's railway system went unacknowledged for a long time. After the railroad was completed, some Chinese laborers became farm or factory workers; others opened laundries or restaurants (Tan, 1987).

The early Chinese immigrants encountered many forms of discrimination. In 1859, Chinese Americans were barred from San Francisco schools. In 1882, the Chinese Exclusion Act was passed. This law forbade Chinese laborers or their families to enter the United States—the only time in history that the United States barred a specific ethnic group from entering the country (Mark & Chih, 1993; Tan, 1987). The policy was initially designed to eliminate competition for American male laborers and to prohibit Asian prostitutes from entering the United States. However, it was enforced so strictly that it discouraged many Chinese wives whose husbands worked in the United States from emigrating. Consequently, the sex ratio of Chinese males to females in the United States was very uneven, with hundreds of males to one female. Even as late as 1890, there were dozens of males to one female (Tan, 1987). Therefore, many of the early Chinese male immigrants were not able to establish natural families and led very lonely lives.

The Exclusion Act was repealed in 1943 as a result of China's alliance with the United States during World War II. In 1946, a new law gave the Chinese, for the first time, the right to become naturalized citizens. The same act provided for the admission of Chinese wives of U.S. citizens on a nonquota basis, whereas immigration of wives and children of permanent residents was still limited to the quota allocated to residents of Asian countries.

The bulk of early Chinese immigrants to the United States came during three stages. The first stage occurred before the passing of the Exclusion Act in 1882. The Chinese who came during this period were mostly illiterate men who worked as laborers. The second stage occurred between 1882 and 1943. The few Chinese immigrants who came during this period engaged mainly in trade or came to study in American schools and colleges. The third stage followed the repeal of the Exclusion Act in 1943. At this time, a great influx of Chinese women and children arrived in the United States.

Soon after the Communists took over China in 1949, large groups of Chinese professionals, scholars, and students began arriving from Hong Kong and Taiwan. Most of these immigrants were originally from mainland China. When the United States normalized relations with the People's Republic of China in the late 1970s, immigration from mainland China also increased. Many of the recent immigrants came to be reunited with their family members who had migrated earlier.

Following the Vietnam War, many Indochinese refugees of ethnic Chinese descent arrived, along with the mass exodus of Vietnamese, Cambodians, and Laotians. More recent immigrants include middle-class and well-to-do Chinese coming from Hong Kong and Taiwan, who are increasingly concerned about the changing political situation (Lee, 1996).

DEMOGRAPHIC PROFILE OF CHINESE AMERICANS

According to the 1990 U.S. Census figures, there were 1,645,472 Chinese Americans, composing 0.7% of the total U.S. population (U.S. Bureau of the Census, 1995). This is actually a conservative figure because of the underenumeration of illegal immigrants and those who were excluded from the census count because of language barriers or other reasons. The 10 states with the highest numbers of Chinese are California (42.8% of all

Chinese in the United States), New York (17.3%), Hawaii (4.2%), Texas (3.8%), New Jersey (3.6%), Massachusetts (3.3%), Illinois (3%), Washington (2.1%), and Maryland and Florida (1.9% each; U.S. Bureau of the Census, 1990).

According to Gaw (1993), Chinese American households comprise four major types: elderly single men, old immigrant couples, new immigrant families, and acculturated suburban families.

The typical elderly single man came to the United States from Guangdong province in his late teens and has lived and worked his whole adult life in Chinatown either in New York City or San Francisco. Typically, he supported himself by working in a Chinese restaurant or laundromat. He might have been married to a Chinese woman but was unable to bring his wife and children to the United States, or he may never have married. He usually lives in poverty, speaks little English, and has little education.

In the old immigrant couple, the man succeeded in bringing over his wife and children. Through hard work and frugal living, some couples managed to send their children to college and on to professional careers and suburban living. They themselves may not speak much English and prefer to live in a Chinatown or other communities with a high Chinese population.

The new immigrant family usually consists of a male immigrant who has a found a steady job and a wife who works in the garment industry. Despite two paychecks, their income is still quite low. They are usually underpaid, with few fringe benefits, and endure long work hours. Some also have debts they accumulated from relocating their families.

The acculturated suburban family may consist of U.S.- or foreign-born parents with a high level of education and successful professional careers or businesses. Sometimes only the mother/wife lives with the children in this country, whereas the father/husband works in Hong Kong or Taiwan. They usually live in an affluent community with a good school district, and the children are highly acculturated into the American lifestyle and values (Gaw, 1993).

Myths, Stereotypes, and Their Implications

Chinese culture and people have been defamed, stereotyped, and seen as mysterious by Westerners for hundreds of years. Miller (1969) indicated that America has two images of China and its people: the favorable images of ancient greatness and wisdom and the unfavorable image of a multitude of perverse and semicivilized subhuman tribes. Both stereotypes are damaging because they do not describe the reality of China and its people and because they ignore individual and intragroup differences.

A more positive image of Chinese Americans developed in the mid-1960s in the wake of nationwide urban riots and amid growing unrest among other minorities. Since then, Chinese Americans have been portrayed as the "model minority" (Mark & Chih, 1993). They are perceived as hard working, intelligent, and good at math and sciences. They are also seen as doing well in school, having good jobs, having strong families with good values, and being free of any social or emotional problems and of experiencing discrimination.

Unfortunately, the model-minority myth not only denies Chinese Americans access to affirmative action programs but also alienates them from other minority groups and the rest of the American people. It evokes resentment and sometimes even hostility, violence, and harassment from other groups. Moreover, this model-minority myth applies to only a small portion of the people, the successful Chinese, and ignores the real gap between the few highly successful and the more typical Chinese American. This myth also provides an excuse for governments and communities to neglect the needs of the Chinese Americans for physical, mental health, and social services. Consequently, those Chinese Americans who need social services, mental health, and substance abuse treatment have a difficult time obtaining the needed services and find their problems and shortcomings especially embarrassing and difficult to accept.

Contemporary Social Problems

The realities of various social problems such as poverty, overcrowded housing, poor working conditions, youth gangs, rising crime, and serious mental illness are threats to the Chinese American's pursuit of a more peaceful, secure, and prosperous life in the United States. This is particularly true for many new immigrants who, because of the political changes and movements in China in the past several decades, have already suffered from severe emotional strain before they arrived in the United States. Much of their energy was consumed in dealing with their losses and separations and in adjusting to a foreign land in which they cannot communicate with people and cannot understand the social system. They also need to cope with practical day-to-day problems such as expensive, rundown, and overcrowded housing, long working hours, low pay, and dead-end jobs. Disappointment resulting from their inability to fulfill their dreams of a better life in this country, together with losing their old support systems, can often drive them into a state of depression, making them feel hopeless and helpless and susceptible to increased drinking and drug abuse.

Families consisting of Chinese immigrant parents who have American-born children often experience communication problems and cultural conflicts. Usually the parents speak very little English, and the children speak little Chinese. Moreover, parents and children may have different value orientations. The parents still hold on to values from their homeland, whereas children are usually more influenced by American culture. Role reversals are common, as parents need to depend on their children's assistance to communicate with the outside world. Because of parents' long working hours, low income, and low-status positions, the children have a difficult time giving them the kind of respect expected by parents in Chinese culture. Another significant dynamic relates to the expression of feelings and emotions. Because traditional Chinese parents do not show the kind of verbal and nonverbal expression of love and affection typical of American culture, the children often feel that they are unloved.

Families descended from immigrants that consist of American-born parents and their children usually speak English at home and are more Westernized in their value orientation. Such families are expected to have adapted better and to have fewer social adjustment problems. However, it is not uncommon for members of these families to have psychological problems caused by subtle racism, identity conflicts, and family problems. These families are susceptible to testing and acting out behaviors by their adolescent children, including alcohol and drug usage.

SUBSTANCE ABUSE AMONG THE CHINESE

In contrast to the patterns of alcohol and narcotics dependence among Westerners, China has had a high prevalence of narcotics use and low to moderate prevalence of alcohol abuse (Singer, 1974).

The Chinese have a long history of narcotics use. Arab traders probably brought opium to China in the 9th century, and it became widely used by the 14th century. Introduction of tobacco smoking in China by the Portuguese during the 17th century gave rise to the smoking of opium. During the 19th century, European trade and colonial interest in China further increased Chinese opium consumption (Singer, 1974). England's opposition to Chinese policies of prohibition of opium led to the Opium War in 1841, and, as a result, the importing of opium was legalized and its cultivation in China was permitted. By the beginning of the 20th century, 8 million people in China were estimated to be using opium (Singer, 1974).

Current Substance Use among Chinese in Mainland China, Hong Kong, and Taiwan

Very little research or data regarding substance abuse are available from mainland China today. Minimal drug problems have been reported prior to 1980. As China became more open to the outside world and the government began loosening its control over the people, informal reports suggested an increase in heroin addiction and in the use of alcohol. Yamamoto, Yeh, and Lee (1986) found that alcohol intake among Chinese in Taiwan increased threefold between 1957 and 1984 and that cases of diagnosed alcoholism increased one hundredfold from the mid-1940s to the mid-1980s.

During the 1970s, an estimated 6–10% of the Chinese adult male population in Hong Kong was addicted to narcotics (Hong Kong Action Committee Against Narcotics, 1993). During the past three decades, many drug users switched to inhaling or injecting heroin instead of smoking opium. According to the data on drug abuse reported to the Hong Kong Central Registry of Drug Abuse in 1993, out of 17,491 drug-abusing individuals, 93% were abusing heroin, 5.4% cannabis, 2.7% cough medicines with codeine, 2% flunitrazepam, 2% triazolam, and 1.7% used physeptone/methadone (Hong Kong Action Committee Against Narcotics, 1993).

Limited data from Taiwan indicate that the substance of choice varies according to different age groups: Elementary school abusers primarily use model glue; a high concentration of young people about 20 years old use amphetamines; those in their mid-20s abuse minor tranquilizers such as secobarbital, amobarbital, and triazolam; and people in their late 30s use heroin and morphine (Lin, 1991). Data from the Taiwan detoxification and treatment centers within the criminal justice system indicate the following rank of preference of substances among offenders: (1) pentazocine, (2) model glue, (3) morphine and heroin, (4) alcohol, and (5) sedative/hypnotics such as secobarbital and triazolam (Lin, 1991).

Patterns of Substance Use among Chinese

The following observations on Chinese drinking behavior are taken from the few existing studies.

1. The Chinese consume much smaller amounts òf alcohol than other ethnic groups (Johnson et al., 1985; Lin & Lin, 1982; Sue & Nakamura, 1984).
2. The Chinese tend to drink alcohol with their meals or at banquets

and social occasions and so are less likely to be involved in excessive drinking (Singer, 1972; Tseng & Hsu, 1969).

3. The Chinese are likely to experience a facial "flushing phenomenon" when they drink alcohol because they lack two major liver enzymes for alcohol metabolism; the resulting discomfort discourages them from heavy drinking (Sue & Nakamura, 1984).

4. Narcotic and gambling addiction may be substituted for alcohol addiction in the Chinese population (Chu, 1972).

According to Singer (1974), the choice of substance and the prevalence patterns among Chinese people is determined by physiological, psychological, and cultural factors.

- *Physiological factors.* The Chinese drinking practice—drinking only at meals—restricts individual consumption and contributes to a low rate of alcoholism, whereas Chinese opiate use practice—through inhalation—is less intoxicating than by injection, causes less physical dependence and fewer adverse effects, has high social acceptability, and leads to widespread use.

- *Psychological factors.* The low prevalence of alcoholism in the Chinese is accounted for by their disapproval of the active and aggressive traits promoted by alcohol. The high prevalence of narcotic consumption in the Chinese is due to cultural sanction of the passive and peaceful traits enhanced by opiate use.

- *Cultural factors.* The Chinese, whose way of life is heavily influenced by Taoism and its emphasis on seeking harmony with the environment, find more satisfaction in drugs such as opium that enable a person to retreat into a state in which conflict with the environment is reduced to a minimum. Also Confucian ideology, with its doctrine of the "golden mean" that calls for moderation in all things and condemns extremism, could be expected to control excessive alcohol intake and discourage the aggressive behavior associated with it.

In 1990 Johnson and Nagoshi reexamined the genetic versus sociocultural influences on alcohol use among Asians. They found the evidence attributing the low use of alcohol to the inhibitory effect of genetic factors, such as the flushing syndrome, to be less convincing than the evidence for the influence of sociocultural factors. This view is also supported by Lee (1987), who reviewed historic Chinese literature and laws as they relate to alcohol consumption. Lee found that there have been periods in Chinese history when alcohol use was very heavy and periods in which its use was extremely low—changes that were unlikely to be due to genetic causes.

ALCOHOL AND DRUG PROBLEMS
AMONG CHINESE AMERICANS

Data on alcohol and drug use among Chinese Americans are limited and often lumped together with those on other Asian populations. Trimble, Padilla, and Bell (1987) attributed the lack of information on Asian substance use to a stereotype held by drug researchers and service providers that Asians do not have substance abuse problems and therefore are in little need of study. In 1998, the Uniform Facility Data Set (UFDS; an annual survey of facilities providing substance abuse treatment conducted by the Substance Abuse and Mental Health Services Administration [SAMHSA]) reported that Asians and Pacific Islanders composed 0.8% of the total population in substance abuse treatment; between 1990 and 1998 the percentages ranged from 0.8% to 1%. Manifestation of alcohol and other drug problems may differ for various Chinese American subgroups according to their socioeconomic and educational backgrounds, religious affiliations, places of birth, immigration histories, and degrees of acculturation (Makimoto, 1998).

Alcohol Problems among Chinese Americans

Despite the limited data, alcoholism does exist among Chinese Americans, particularly among men (Chi, Lubben, & Kitano, 1989). Many drink only on weekends or on days off from work rather than every day. Therefore, their drinking may not have any impact on their job performance. Shame and fear of stigma reinforce denial by the family, and the existence of a drinking problem tends to be covered up by family members. Alcoholics seen at treatment facilities are usually in the advanced stage of their alcoholism.

My colleagues and I at New York City Chinatown Alcoholism Services (CAS) of Hamilton–Madison House, an outpatient treatment facility, have found that most of our patients diagnosed as alcohol dependent have nine or more drinks daily. The majority of patients reported drinking hard liquor only, without food, and that they drink alone. Most of these men are immigrants who only speak Chinese and are employed in restaurants, garment factories, and laundries. When asked about facial flush, some reported that flushing disappeared after a period of steady heavy drinking, whereas others reported continued drinking despite facial flush and physical discomfort. Although it is difficult to verify the substitution assumptions, gambling appears to be a serious problem among these Chinese male alcoholics.

The clinical picture of the patients treated at CAS is similar to that found by Singer and Wong (1973) in their study of 100 male alcoholic patients at the Castle Peak Psychiatric Hospital in Hong Kong. For example, a good number of alcoholics lost one or both parents at an early age or were raised by adopted parents or had an alcoholic father. The age of onset of regular drinking was about age 20, and development of alcoholism occurred at about age 40. Most drank daily, at first drinking with each meal and eventually drinking between meals and even instead of meals. Most alcoholics in these studies did not exhibit drunken or violent behavior but went to sleep after they got drunk.

Drug Use among Chinese Americans

Few surveys have been conducted on the use of other drugs among Chinese and other Asians in the United States. A 1966 study of 137 Chinese male narcotics users admitted to Lexington Hospital, Kentucky, revealed a unique group of Chinese heroin addicts. They were older bachelors employed in laundries and restaurants. The typical addict had been taking heroin, opium, or both for over 20 years and later found the habit to be too expensive and consequently sought treatment (Ball & Lau, 1966).

The Lower Eastside Service Center, a mental health and substance abuse treatment agency of New York City located in Chinatown, had a "lounge" day program that started in the 1960s and served very similar patients to those described by Ball and Lau (1966). The program served about 80 male patients. They had started using opium in China prior to leaving for the United States in their early 20s. After they came to the United States, they used heroin instead of opium. Their treatment included the use of methadone, individual and group counseling, and the provision of lunch, recreation, and social services. By the late 1980s, about 20 patients remained in the program. Many patients lived until age 70 or even 80. The program terminated in 1991 when the last few elderly addicts died.

A Hawaiian study of Chinese, Japanese, and Filipino Americans (McLaughlin, Raymond, Murakami, & Goebert, 1987) found that their levels of use of various licit and illicit drugs were significantly lower than those of native Hawaiians and Caucasians. However, the Chinese (and Japanese) showed higher use of tranquilizers than native Hawaiians.

Observations of drug-abusing patients treated by my colleagues and I at CAS indicate the following:

1. The majority of drug patients are within the age group of 30 to 50.
2. The most common drugs used are heroin and cocaine.
3. The majority of these patients also have some degree of psychiatric problems.
4. Most are unemployed or have unstable job histories.
5. Many have previous histories of drug detoxification or emergency psychiatric hospitalization.

6. Although some are known to have had minor brushes with the law, few have been involved in violent or serious crime.

Substance Abuse among Chinese American Women

Research and clinical data reveal that alcohol abuse is rare among Chinese women. A study of drinking patterns of Chinese, Japanese, and Korean people in California (Sue, Kitano, Hatanaka, & Yeung, 1985) found that compared with Japanese and Korean women, Chinese females had a higher rate of abstinence, with almost 74% reporting being abstinent. However, given the changing attitudes among younger Chinese women in the United States toward their role and function, their increasing opportunities for education and employment, and the added pressure from both work and household responsibilities, we can expect an increasing rate of drinking, leading to drinking problems.

Substance Abuse among Chinese American Youth

Studies on drug use among Asian American youths suggest a lower level of use compared with other ethnocultural groups (Austin, Prendergast, & Lee, 1989). However, a pilot survey done in San Francisco's Chinatown that utilized a sample of 123 youths aged 13 to 19 found high rates of drug use among these Chinese youths. The most frequently used substances were cigarettes, marijuana, beer, hard liquor, and quaaludes. Substances that ranked in moderate to low frequency use were hashish, cocaine, LSD, barbiturates, Valium, and codeine. These youths also reported physical and psychological problems associated with substance use, including (1) becoming sick from drinking alcohol (48%), (2) having a smoker's cough (41.5%), (3) having a bad hangover from alcohol (39.8%), (4) having shortness of breath from smoking (38.2%), and (5) suffering from memory loss due to alcohol and drug use (24.4%). Another study of Chinese youths found that 40% had used marijuana at school, nearly 11% on a regular basis (Wong, 1985).

SUBSTANCE ABUSE TREATMENT IN CHINA, HONG KONG, AND TAIWAN

China

No published material is available about current alcohol and substance abuse treatment in China. Consequently, I conducted informal interviews with several professionals who had recently migrated from China, including two former medical doctors and a traditional herbal doctor.

Although cirrhosis of the liver due to alcohol is not uncommon, none of the respondents were aware of any formal alcohol treatment program in China. Patients with cirrhosis are usually treated at a medical hospital and advised to abstain from drinking. People with drinking problems usually try to recover from their hangovers by going to sleep or taking some herbal tea. Although new drug rehabilitation centers were being established recently in Canton and other major cities to combat an apparently increasing drug problem in China, public information regarding drug use or treatment was not readily available. For the past six years, Daytop International, a well-known drug treatment organization in the United States, has worked with the Yunnan Institute of Drug Abuse of China to develop the first therapeutic community in China. This venture is the beginning of China's changing approach to drug treatment.

Hong Kong

Most of the drug treatment in Hong Kong is targeted at heroin or opium abusers. There are three major types of treatment programs: a compulsory placement program operated by the Correctional Services Department; a voluntary outpatient methadone maintenance program; and a voluntary, 2-year inpatient drug-free rehabilitation program. The approach in the latter program is to place the patients on methadone to block off their craving for heroin or opium and to gradually reduce their daily dosage of methadone until they are completely drug free. Individual and group counseling and activity therapy are provided to all patients. The inpatient treatment is followed up with participation at a self-help association.

Other smaller scale drug-free clinics, residential programs, and halfway houses are operated by religious Christian groups, and there are a few private clinics aimed at upper-class White and Chinese substance abusers. More recently, a small outpatient counseling service was established for the treatment of psychiatric substance abusers (Hong Kong Action Committee Against Narcotics, 1993). An alcoholism outpatient clinic was also established in 1996. Previously, all alcoholic patients were treated at psychiatric hospitals and clinics.

Taiwan

Detoxification centers, outpatient clinics, and inpatient hospital programs are examples of the substance abuse treatment facilities available in Taiwan. There are involuntary programs within the criminal justice system, as well as voluntary programs operated by the government, and private clinics and hospitals. The general approach to treatment is drug free. Importing methadone is prohibited, and it is not used in treating heroin and opium patients. Counseling is generally not as valued by the patients as somatic and medical treatment.

TREATMENT OF CHINESE AMERICANS

As indicated previously, Chinese Americans in the United States have a very low rate of usage of alcohol and drug treatment services. The reasons for their underutilization of services include (1) a lack of knowledge about treatment, (2) the language barrier, (3) a high level of endurance for pain and symptoms, (4) the feeling of shame and stigma involved in using treatment services, (5) a lack of insight and motivation, (6) difficulties in verbalizing problems and feelings, (7) a fear of taking time away from work and family, (8) the family's tolerance of their substance problems, and (9) a lack of health insurance.

An unfortunate obstacle to effective substance abuse treatment services comes from the Chinese communities themselves. The Chinese, in general, hold a moralistic attitude toward alcoholism and drug problems: Individuals having such problems are considered to be a disgrace to the community and unworthy of help. As a result, leaders, as well as members, of these communities often downplay the existence of such problems, and there is little sympathy for alcohol or drug addicts or support for substance abuse services. The development of such services is further hindered by insufficient data justifying the need for services, the lack of funding from the government and private sources, and the lack of enough bilingual and bicultural staff interested in providing such services.

Only a handful of substance abuse treatment facilities in the United States have the capacity to serve both Chinese-speaking (Cantonese and Mandarin) and English-speaking individuals. They are mostly located in Hawaii, California, and New York. Some of the programs are for residential drug-free treatment, some are a part of Asian American mental health programs, and others are a part of mainstream programs with Chinese-speaking staff members. Chinese Americans who speak English and are more assimilated to the mainstream culture are usually seen by at-large treatment providers. Very little has been written about this population.

Chinatown Alcoholism Services (CAS) of Hamilton–Madison House is a unique program in New York City aimed at serving the population of

Chinese substance abusers. Established as a demonstration project in 1983, it was certified as an outpatient alcoholism clinic in 1987. Its services include ambulatory detoxification; individual, family, and group counseling; alcohol and drug education; life skill training; psychiatric evaluation and treatment; medical services provided by a registered nurse; case management and other services, such as translation and escort services. CAS also provides ongoing community education and outreach through a radio hotline, periodic newletters, street fairs, and educational workshops. CAS provides the following unique features:

1. The staff makes home visits and reaches out to homeless Chinese people.
2. It provides crisis intervention, pain reduction, and concrete services before focusing on the patient's insight and motivation for abstinence from substances.
3. It offers patients tangible help to facilitate their recovery, such as escorting them to a hospital for detoxification, providing translation, and assisting them in applying for benefits.
4. It educates patients on their role in treatment and aids them in understanding the treatment process, such as the reasons for gathering personal and family history, for requiring a physical examination, and for Breathalyzer testing and urine screening.
5. It encourages patients to celebrate Chinese festivals, as well as American holidays, in order to help them both to treasure their cultural heritage and to learn to appreciate the American culture.

Most CAS patients come or are forced to come to treatment at the very late stages of their disorder, when their physical health is already quite deteriorated. Many have been abandoned by their families. Most are unemployed and do not have much hope for themselves and their recovery. It is a challenge to engage and keep them in treatment. The following three cases exemplify some of the issues discussed.

Mr. X is a 59-year-old Chinese man. He was an only child, born in a village near Canton. His father left China before he was born and went to the United States for business. He died there when Mr. X was 3, and his mother left him with his paternal grandmother when he was 5. His mother then remarried and had no further contact with him. The family was supported by his paternal grandfather. During the political change in China, the grandparents were persecuted because they owned land. In his late teens Mr. X, who completed only 3 years of schooling, escaped from China by swimming to Hong Kong. He was alone and penniless. He started to work as a laborer and eventually became a sailor. He found his work and life on the ship boring and started to drink for recreation and to relax. He married a Chinese woman, and they had a son. Mr. X continued working as a sailor and visited his wife and son only two or three times a year. By his mid-30s he was drinking heavily: He could consume up to half of a 750ml bottle of whiskey a day, several days per week. He reported no effect of alcohol upon his health or job during that period.

Mr. X immigrated to New York with his wife and son about 20 years ago. At first, he worked in a restaurant as a cook. He was not happy with his work and kept changing jobs. He drank more and more, and by his late 40s drank up to a bottle a day. His teenage son became involved in a gang.

Although Mr. X changed jobs quite often, he was able to support his family until 2 years ago when he fell down and hurt himself after having too much to drink. He was hospitalized and was found to have cirrhosis of the liver and diabetes. Mr. X was very resistant and defensive when he first came to the program: He did not think that he had a drinking problem. After he was convinced by the psychiatrist and the nurse of the impact of his continued drinking on his cirrhosis and diabetes, he bargained with the clinic's staff to cut down his drinking, to switch to beer, or to dilute his drinks. Eventually, he was able to achieve total abstinence due to fear of dying of cirrhosis. His health and relationship with his family improved steadily. Although he continued to struggle with craving and relapse, he was motivated to continue working on his recovery.

Mr. Y is a 31-year-old Chinese man who was born in Hong Kong. His father died when he was 10, and he came to the United States with his mother, with whom he continues to live. Mr. Y had trouble with English and could not concentrate in school. He soon got involved with gangs. He started to drink and experiment with different drugs. He mostly drank beer, up to six to seven cans a day, but he also used marijuana, cocaine, and heroin. He dropped out of school and was unable to secure a steady job. He was involved in several robberies of stores and was eventually arrested and put on probation. About 5 years before entering treatment, he started to have auditory hallucinations. He did not tell anyone about them and tried to use alcohol and drugs as self-medication. He was sent to a hospital after accidentally overdosing on drugs. In the hospital he was thoroughly examined and diagnosed with schizophrenia and polysubstance dependence. He was referred for outpatient treatment at a Chinese mental health clinic that had a substance abuse program. He was relieved to learn that medication and counseling might stabilize his mental illness and was willing to work on his substance abuse problems. He soon learned the danger of taking drugs while he was on antipsychotic medication. Mr. Y was seen for weekly individual counseling by a social worker and was seen monthly by the psychiatrist who monitored his mental status and medication. The nurse provided health and substance abuse education and monitored his blood alcohol level and urine screening.

Ms. Z is a 29-year-old woman who was born in Canton, China. She had a high school education and had held a good job back home. She came to the United States 5 years ago through an arranged marriage to a Chinese man living in the United States. After having met each other once while he was visiting Canton, they kept up a short period of courtship through correspondence and married shortly afterward. She moved to the United States to live with her husband and in-laws. She did not get along with her in-laws, and her relationship with her husband slowly deteriorated. She felt homesick and trapped. She could not find work because she did not speak English and had no skill. Shortly afterward, she found out that she was pregnant. Her relationship with her husband deteriorated further, and he began to abuse her physically. She left him and found a small place to live with the help of a distant relative.

While in China in her late teens, Ms. Z had started to drink wine and beer socially. After she came to the United States, she had used alcohol to soothe herself during her days of extreme homesickness and the stress of adjusting to her husband's family. After she found herself pregnant and alone, she became depressed and suicidal, and her drinking increased. She was unable to care for her newborn infant and was referred to a mental health clinic by a child welfare agency. She was seen by a psychiatrist, put on antidepressant medications, and referred for both substance abuse and psychiatric outpatient services. Her son was placed at a day care center. She found both individual counseling and a women's support group helpful in improving her coping skills. The fear of losing her child to foster care motivated her to begin working on her drinking problem. As her condition improved, she enrolled in an ESL (English as Second Language) class to prepare herself to find a job.

RECOMMENDATIONS FOR TREATMENT OF CHINESE AMERICANS

Professionals working with Chinese American substance abusers and their significant others have found that the most effective way to treat their patients is to combine supportive counseling with somatic treatment (Chin, Lai, & Rouse, 1991). Although a psychiatrist and a nurse can be authoritative and need to present medical facts about the physical damage of alcohol and drug abuse on the body, the substance abuse clinician is most effective when he or she is understanding and problem oriented. The following are some treatment strategies for Chinese Americans.

1. Have patience during the initial stage of engaging the patient in treatment. It usually takes a long time for a Chinese patient to establish trust in the counselor. Refrain from asking too many sensitive questions. Focus on external stress first and demonstrate care by giving tangible help.
2. Take an active role in counseling. Prove your expertise by letting the patient know your quick grasp of his or her problems and your ability to help resolve them.
3. Be willing to work with a patient whose initial goal is not total abstinence. Work with the patient at his or her pace toward total abstinence.
4. Work with the patient's family but use individual counseling rather than couple and family therapy. Joint and family sessions can be arranged when necessary but should be used with caution.
5. Individual counseling is preferred to group counseling. Avoid process and dynamic group approaches. Groups can be used for educational purposes and social activities. Do not push the use of 12-step groups, such as Alcoholics Anonymous (AA) or Al-Anon.
6. Include medical staff, such as doctors and nurses, in the treatment team. Taking the patient's blood pressure, ordering vitamins, and giving advice for minor physical ailments, as well as handling other health-related problems, can increase the patient's trust in the treatment facility.
7. Chinese patients are receptive to pharmacological treatment. Benzodiazepine for alcohol withdrawal and other medication for the treatment of alcoholism, such as disulfiram (Antabuse) and naltrexone (ReVia) are generally welcomed. However, it is important to closely monitor how patients comply with their prescriptions, because due to language problems and other factors many Chinese patients do not follow the medication schedule as prescribed.
8. Respect the patient's need to use culturally relevant alternative care such as acupuncture, to consult with Chinese herbal doctors, and to take Chinese herbal medicine.
9. Finally, it is important to assure patients of confidentiality of treatment. Because many of the patients live in the same community, belong to the same family association, and have wives who work at the same garment factories and children who go to the same schools, anonymity may not be feasible. However, clinicians must be careful not to reveal information about one client to another.

CONCLUSION

Although indirect evidence suggests that the magnitude of alcohol and other drug problems may be greater than what is commonly associated with the "model minority" stereotype, substance abuse problems among Chinese Americans have received insufficient attention from researchers, treatment providers, and prevention specialists. The "flushing syndrome" and low treatment utilization were often used as excuses for not funding Chinese American substance abuse initiatives. Chinese Americans utilize alcohol and drug treatment services at a very low rate, largely due to their tendency to handle problems within the family, as well as lack of Chinese-speaking staff and culturally appropriate services. Much effort is needed to develop further research on Chinese Americans' substance abuse problems. An increased knowledge of the subject can contribute greatly to the development of sound and effective treatment programs.

ACKNOWLEDGMENTS

I am grateful for the help of Una Shih in research and for the invaluable support from my colleagues of the Chinatown Alcoholism Services of Hamilton–Madison House.

REFERENCES

Austin, G. A., Prendergast, M., & Lee, H. (1989, Winter). *Substance abuse among Asian American youth* (Prevention Research Update No. 5, pp. 1–28). Portland, OR: Northwest Regional Educational Laboratory.

Ball, J. C., & Lau, M. P. (1966). The Chinese narcotic addict in the United States. *Social Forces, 45*(1), 68–72.

Chi, I., Lubben, J. E., & Kitano, H. L. (1989). Differences in drinking behavior among three Asian-American groups. *Journal of Studies on Alcohol, 50*(1), 15–23.

Chin, K.-L., Lai, T.-F. M., & Rouse, M. (1991). Social adjustment and alcoholism among Chinese immigrants in New York City. *International Journal of the Addictions, 25*(5A, 6A), 709–729.

Chu, G. (1972). Drinking patterns and attitudes of rooming-house Chinese in San Francisco. *Quarterly Journal of Studies on Alcohol* (Suppl. 6), 58–68.

Department of Health and Human Services, Substance Abuse and Mental Health Services Administration. (1998). *Uniform facility data set (UFDS): 1998 data on substance abuse treatment facilities.* Rockville, MD: Author.

Gaw, A. C. (1993). Psychiatric care of Chinese American. In A. C. Gaw (Ed.), *Culture, ethnicity and mental illness* (pp. 245–280). Washington, DC: American Psychiatric Press.

Hong Kong Committee Against Narcotics. (1993). *Hong Kong Narcotics Report 1993*. Hong Kong: Government Information Services.

Johnson, R., & Nagoshi, C. (1990, January/March). Asians, Asian Americans and alcohol. *Journal of Psychoactive Drugs, 22*(1), 45–52.

Johnson, R. C., Schwitters, S., Wilson, H. L., James, R., Craig, T., & McClearn, G. E. (1985). A cross-ethnic comparison of reasons given for using alcohol, not using alcohol or ceasing to use alcohol. *Journal of Studies on Alcohol, 46*(4), 283–288.

Lee, E. (1996). Chinese families. In M. McGoldrick, J. Giordano, & J. K. Pearce (Eds.), *Ethnicity and family therapy* (2nd ed., pp. 249–267). New York: Guilford Press.

Lee, J. A. (1987). Chinese, alcohol, and flushing: Sociohistorical and biobehavioral conditions. *Journal of Psychoactive Drugs, 19*(4), 319–327.

Lin, C. L. (1991). *How to prevent your children from drug abuse* [Chinese]. Taiwan: World Health Journal Press.

Lin, T. Y., & Lin, D. T. C. (1982). Alcoholism among the Chinese: Further observations of a low risk population. *Culture, Medicine and Psychiatry, 6,* 109–116.

Makimoto, K. (1998). Drinking patterns and drinking problems among Asian Americans and Pacific Islanders. *Alcohol Health and Research World, 22*(4), 270–275.

Mark, D. M. L., & Chih, G. (1993). *A place called Chinese America*. Dubuque, IA: Kendall/Hunt.

McLaughlin, G., Raymond, J., Murakami, S. R., & Goebert, D. (1987). Drug use among Asian Americans in Hawaii. *Journal of Psychoactive Drugs, 19*(1), 85–94.

Miller, S. C. (1969). *The unwelcome immigrant*. Berkeley: University of California Press.

Singer, K. (1972). Drinking patterns and alcoholism in the Chinese. *British Journal of Addiction, 67,* 3–14.

Singer, K. (1974). The choice of intoxicant among the Chinese. *British Journal of Addiction, 69,* 257–268.

Singer, K., & Wong, M. (1973). Alcoholic psychoses and alcoholism in the Chinese: A study of 100 consecutive cases admitted to a psychiatric hospital in Hong Kong. *Quarterly Journal of Studies on Alcohol, 34*(3), 878–886.

Sue, S., Kitano, H. H. L., Hatanaka, H., & Yeung, W. T. (1985). Alcohol consumption among Chinese in the United States. In L. A. Bennett & G. M. Ames (Eds.), *The American experience with alcohol: Contrasting cultural perspectives* (pp. 359–371). New York: Plenum Press.

Sue, S., & Nakamura, C. Y. (1984). An integrative model of physiological and social/psychological factors in alcohol consumption among Chinese and Japanese Americans. *Journal of Drug Issues, 14*(2), 349–364.

Tan, T. T. (1987). *Your Chinese roots*. Union City, CA: Heian.

Trimble, J. F., Padilla, A., & Bell, C. S. (Eds.). (1987). *Drug abuse among ethnic minorities* (DHHS Publication No. ADM 87–1474). Rockville, MD: National Institute on Drug Abuse.

Tseng, W. S., & Hsu J. (1969) Chinese culture, personality formation and mental illness. *International Journal of Psychiatry, 16*(1), 5–14.

U.S. Bureau of the Census. (1990) *Census of the Population: Supplemental Report.*

Race of the Population by States. Washington, DC: U.S. Government Printing Office.

U.S. Bureau of the Census. (1995). *The nation's Asian and Pacific Islander population—1994* (Statistical Brief SB-95–24). Washington, DC: U.S. Government Printing Office.

Wong, H. A. (1985). *Substance use and Chinese American youth*. Unpublished manuscript.

Yamamoto, J., Yeh, E. K., & Lee, C. K. (1986, September). *Alcohol abuse/dependence among Koreans and Chinese*. Paper presented at the annual meeting of the Society for the Study of Culture and Psychiatry, Baltimore.

18

Ethnocultural Background and Substance Abuse Treatment of Asian Indian Americans

Daya Singh Sandhu
Ruby Malik

India, called *Bharat* or *Hindustan*, is a land of contradictions. It is a place of immense beauty, wealth, and history, yet it is also a place afflicted with poverty, political strife, and corruption. As one drives through the streets, one sees Ford Escorts on one side of the street and rickshaws on the other. On the one hand, women are revered in the scriptures as goddess Durga or Kali, Mother Vaishnu Devi, and so forth; on the other, they are expected to be subservient to the men in their daily lives (Almeida, 1996). Sodowsky and Carey (1987) present a picturesque description of contradictions about India:

> A positive stereotype about Asian Indians is that they come from the land of Mahatma Gandhi, Indira Gandhi, Mother Teresa, and mathematical and philosophical geniuses; the land that is decked with shimmering silks, gold, and the Taj Mahal; and the land that excited E. M. Forster and Kipling. . . . [Yet] Americans see the Hindu as a turbaned person who comes from a land of child marriages, widow immolation, snake worshipers abounding filth and misery, and with an enslaving caste system. (p. 137)

In regard to the attitudes toward alcohol and/or drug use, the contradictions continue. The use of alcohol and/or drugs is promoted as a means of achieving internal peace, specifically with such drugs as cannabis or hashish, which are also viewed as *prasad,* the holy food disseminated after a religious ceremony. On other occasions, drug and alcohol abuse is condemned as an unnatural way to alter one's internal state, particularly in Sikhism and in the Muslim religion. This chapter examines the use of alcohol and drugs in India. It also delineates treatment issues likely to emerge when treating the Indian substance abuser in the United States. Lastly, it provides suggestions for treating the chemically dependent Indian patient.

CULTURAL BACKGROUND OF INDIA

India is the largest democracy in the world, with recent estimates of 960 million people. Although Hindi is spoken by the majority of the Indian population (55%), there are 16 major languages and hundreds of dialects spoken throughout the country. Each region in India has its own language, and the language embodies the unique feel, way of life, and cultural mores of that region. India's religions and values have an impact on the use of substances among its population and have implications for treatment of substance abusers of Indian descent in the United States.

Indian Religions

India is thought to be the motherland of several religions, including Hinduism, Jainism, Buddhism, and Sikhism, all of which are practiced throughout the country today. According to *The World Almanac and Book of Facts* (1991), the population of India consists of 83% Hindus, 11% Muslims, 3% Christians, 2% Sikhs, and 1% others.

    Diversity and tolerance for diversity are values that are critical to Indian culture (Almeida, 1990) and are certainly critical features of Hinduism, Sikhism, and the Muslim religions. The very essence of tolerance for diversity is expressed in the following *shaloka* (psalm) of *Sri Guru Granth Sahib,* the holy book of the Sikhs (translated and annotated by Gopal Singh, 1978),

> *Aval Allah noor upaya, kudrat ke sabh bande.*
> *Ek noor te sabh jag upjiya kaun bhale ko mande.*
> God is the Father of us all; His reflection is in everyone of us
> hence do not grade any person as inferior or superior.
> (*Sri Guru Granth Sahib,* p. 1349)

The Caste System

Much has been written about the caste system in India. The caste system was designed primarily for economic reasons and as a way to make sure that Indian society would always have scholars, educators, warriors, traders, businessmen, and people to provide unskilled labor.

> The Hindu belief about the division of society is that there are four caste categories, called *varna*. The *varna* are ranked according to their ritual purity, which in turn is based on their traditional occupations. The Brahmins, who are ranked highest, are priests and scholars; the Kshatriyas, or warrior caste, are second; the Vaishyas, or merchants, are ranked third; and the shudras, or menial workers and artisans, are ranked fourth. (Nanda, 1991, pp. 314–315)

There has been much talk by many Indian politicians about abolishing the caste system. Progress has certainly been made toward that end, but it has been slow. An example of the progress is that India currently has its first president from the untouchable caste a fifth group below the four *varna*. The caste system has been difficult to eliminate because, as is true in other nations, the people who possess the power and wealth do not give it up without a struggle.

Common Characteristics of Indians

It is worth stating the obvious, that there is no such thing as an Indian way of being. There are individual differences that are based on temperament, upbringing, psychopathology, and one's innate physiology. We are describing trends and attitudes that reflect a way of life in India. Within each region, cultural group, and family, vast differences exist.

Indian Belief Systems

India is a nation with a strong emphasis on spirituality and on destiny. There is a belief in *kismet,* or predeterminism, that has great bearing on people's lives. It is believed that things happen for a reason that has to do with one's fate and that certain challenges are preordained. This attitude is in sharp contrast to the Western notion of *nemesis*, wherein all positive and negative events are a result of one's behavior (Ibrahim, Ohnishi, & Sandhu, 1997).

Hindus and Sikhs also believe in reincarnation and, as such, believe that one's behavior in this life has great bearing on the next life. This belief certainly influences attitudes toward morality but also has an effect on reactions to one's caste. People born to one of the lower castes find comfort in the possibility that in their next life they may be born into a higher caste. Indians are often viewed as passive and complacent about their fate. What might be seen as passivity to the Western eye might be seen by an Indian person as accepting one's destiny and making the best of a situation. The belief in *kismet* leads to a relaxed style that permeates all aspects of life in India, positively and negatively. American society is based on a very different premise, a belief that one can alter one's life by simply working hard enough. This can result in a fast-paced life with a great deal of pressure that can be difficult for an Indian immigrant to adjust to.

Communication Styles

Indians tend to communicate in ways that would be considered indirect in the Western world. Much is communicated through disguise, innuendo, hinting, suggestions, and the use of metaphors or stories meant to convey meaning. To many in the United States, this can be frustrating, because so much of what is conveyed is unspoken and must be deciphered. A person raised from a very young age with this style of communicating learns to place a great deal of attention on interpersonal sensitivity and empathic attunement so as to minimize misinterpretations. A high premium is placed on being able to figure out what is important to others by watching them and looking for cues. Critics of this style claim that it results in Asian Indian children and adults who are externally rather than internally focused.

Role of Family

Family life is central to life in India. Nothing is as prized as one's commitment to one's family. The "family first" concept lays a sound foundation for the family cohesiveness and stability in Asian Indian families. Within the family, there is a great deal of sacrifice for one another. People make unusual requests of others and expect such requests to be reciprocated by family members. For example, instead of getting a loan from the bank, family members might borrow money from one another. A marriage in India is considered as the permanent alliance between two families, not just a union between individuals (Prathikanti, 1997). These two families are expected to build a mutual support system. The elderly play a prominent role in keeping the families together. They are treated as wise people who embody the family's history and as such are revered.

Johnson and Nagoshi (1990) suggest that the extended-family system in Asian Indians serves as a safeguard against mental health problems. A common criticism of the United States by Indians is that family is not as important as it should be. In other words, the American emphasis on individualism, or one's commitment to oneself, hurts the role of the family. By Western standards, the Indian family is enmeshed and lacks appropriate boundaries. By Eastern standards, the American family is too separate and disenfranchised.

Gender Roles

Gender roles in India are quite defined and specific. The adult male shows his love for the family by providing for them while also maintaining loyalty and strong ties to his family of origin, particularly his mother. A young boy's connection to his mother is typically quite intense. Men traditionally maintain a strong connection and attachment to their mothers even when they are married and have children of their own. Newly married couples are likely to live with the husband's family (Das & Kemp, 1997), and a wife's commitment to family is shown in the ways she adjusts to her husband's family. This patrilocal pattern of family residence is changing these days as more couples live on their own when they get married.

Competitiveness and jealousy between a man's wife and his mother are quite common. Married women sometimes report feeling that they are second in importance to their mothers-in-law, although this perception obviously depends on the actual family. Male children are thought to be a blessing bestowed on a family and are given a great deal of importance in the Indian family. Once the couple has children, all the women in the household are instrumental in child rearing.

Role of Women

As stated previously, Indian women are revered as mythical creatures and goddesses in ancient writings but are also considered to be inferior to men in daily life. In the past, much has been written about the practice of *Satti*, which involves a wife throwing herself, or being thrown against her will, into burning flames upon the death of her husband. This practice is now quite rare. Another controversial practice is the dowry system. Depending on the family's economic status, a bride's family is expected to lavish the groom's family with jewelry and gifts at the time of her engagement and marriage. For many Indian families, the parents begin planning for the dowry at the time of the girl's birth. For those families who do not have the money, the dowry is a source of tremendous anxiety because of the fear that the daughter will not be able to marry. In the most extreme of cases, infant girls are left to die because of these fears.

A large, decade-long survey (1985–1995) about culture and living habits of the people of India revealed that in most communities the women make crucial economic contributions to the family but have only a small role in making decisions, such as marriage and career choices for their sons and daughters (Jha, 1998). According to this survey, only one fourth of the communities allow women some role in decision making. The survey also noted that education for boys is favored by 75% of the Indian people, whereas only 55% favor educating girls. Among the low castes, less than 50% of the communities favor education for girls (Jha, 1998).

The recurring themes in Indian women's lives center on their powerlessness in a male-dominated society as reflected in arranged marriages, the inhibiting influences of patrifocal ideology, the dowry custom, and the expected obedience to their husbands (Mukhopadhyay & Seymour, 1994). Yet, despite their narrow role and power in the domestic sphere, a significant number of women have enjoyed an incredible degree of equality in some public areas of life (Prathikanti, 1997). Many women from the middle and upper classes tend to receive the same level of education as men. Jayakar (1994) noted that since 1947, after the independence of India, the number of women physicians in most medical specialities has been virtually equal to that of men. Moreover, India was one of the first nations in the modern world to be ruled by a woman when Indira Gandhi was named prime minister in 1966. There is tremendous irony in the fact that a country known to devalue women was one of the first to be ruled by one.

INDIAN IMMIGRANTS IN THE UNITED STATES

Partly due to internal political and religious conflicts and partly due to the exploitation of natural resources by the foreign invaders, especially during the 200 years of British colonialism, Asian Indians have often sought livelihood in foreign lands (Gupta, 1979; Minocha, 1987; Prathikanti, 1997; Sheth, 1995). As was true with other ethnic groups, Indian people saw the United States as a place for political asylum, freedom, and greater economic rewards. The first Indian to travel to the United States may have been a man from Madras who visited Massachusetts in 1790 (Sheth, 1995). As Salem, Massachusetts, developed its trade with India, young Indian men would occasionally come to the United States as ship workers. Others followed suit, and in 1900 the census reported 2,050 people from India in the

CLIENTS OF ASIAN BACKGROUND

United States, including Anglo-Indians. Most of those arriving during the 1800s were farmers or other laborers.

The idea of granting citizenship to people of Asian descent was not seriously discussed by Congress until the 1880s, at which time the legal scholar James Kent stated in his "Commentaries on the American Law" that "tawny races of Asia" could not be given citizenship under the term White. "The U.S. Supreme Court ruled in 1923 that Indians were not considered Caucasians and therefore not eligible for citizenship" (Sheth, 1995, p. 188). In spite of this ruling, there was much enthusiasm about Indian immigration, and Americans such as Ralph Waldo Emerson, Henry David Thoreau, and Walt Whitman, all of whom had studied India's history and spirituality, felt that the wisdom and art of India could be a model for Americans (Jensen, 1988).

Due to the United States immigration preference category, Indians who immigrated to the United States in the early to mid-20th century were people with higher education who typically came for the promise of upward mobility and economic rewards. Doshi (1975) found that more than 50% in a sample of 46,000 Asian Indian immigrants were working as scientists, engineers, or medical doctors. Compared with other Asian immigrants, the percentage of professionals, particularly physicians (Kamen, 1992), among Indian immigrants is quite impressive. For instance, Duleep (1988) noted that 90% of new immigrants from India held professional degrees, compared with 75% of Korean, 67% of Philippine, and 46% of Chinese immigrants.

The 1965 McCarran Immigration Act and the more recent Family Reunification Act opened the door to Asian immigrants and gave immigration priority to the relatives of earlier immigrants. As a result, there has been a stunning 200% increase in Asian Indians, from 361,544 in 1980 (U.S. Bureau of the Census, 1983) to 815,447 in 1990 (U.S. Bureau of the Census, 1993). An average of almost 20,000 Asian Indians entered the United States annually (U.S. Bureau of the Census, 1992). Many of the more recent immigrants come from rural areas, are less educated, and are less fluent in English than the previous immigrants. Many of these new immigrants are working as taxi drivers, small motel operators, and convenience store clerks.

The Model-Minority Myth

In the past, Asian Indians have been considered a model minority because of their high level of achievement in education, economic successes, and few overt social problems. With the third wave of Asian Indian immigrants under the Family Reunification Act and a more recent fourth wave of illegal immigrants entering the United States, the model-minority image of the Asian Indians warrants a new consideration (Sandhu, 1997). Mental health professionals need to reconsider that Asian Indians may be more psychologically maladjusted than the popular model-minority stereotype may suggest. Moreover, alcohol and drug abuse among Asian Indian Americans may be more prevalent now than ever in the past (Joe, 1996; Yen, 1992).

Indian Women in the United States

Nandan and Eames (1980) noted a striking difference between women in India and Indian women in the United States in the degree to which women take on employment outside the home. Contrary to the strong expectations for women to be housewives and mothers in traditional Asian societies, a higher percentage of Asian women in the United States than in India have to work to supplement their spouses' incomes (True, 1990). Such employment has served to enhance Indian women's increased independence. Compared with their ancestors, the second-generation Indian women in America have almost closed the gender gap in education and occupation (Sheth, 1995). Helweg and Helweg (1990) state that the proportion of female to male wage earners among South Asians is 45 to 55.

Despite higher education and professional careers, life for many Indian professional women in the United States tends to be quite stressful. Nayak (1997) voiced their anguish:

> These professional women married well. Many married colleagues and came to live in this country. Did their lives change? Outside the home there was much change, inside the home not much change at all.
>
> In the home they returned to their Indian routine. The grueling labor of cooking, cleaning and taking care of the kids was exhausting and often made them feel that they were less than and inferior to, their husbands. The trappings of success—large homes, and fancy cars—rarely helped overcome this inner struggle of living in contented conformity. (p. 3)

In a similar vein, Dhaliwal (1995) spoke about the fact that in addition to household duties, Indian-owned businesses generate additional work and related stress for Asian Indian women. This is particularly disturbing, as many Indian businesses are built on the backs of women. A common scenario for family-owned businesses is that the wife and children manage the store while the husband maintains other employment in order to supplement the family's income. The role of women in business is often unacknowledged, and the special needs of these overworked women, who have no rest or leisure, remain unaddressed.

ALCOHOL AND OTHER DRUG USE IN INDIA

Historical Context

Indians are confronted with numerous contradictions about the use of alcohol and other drugs. On the one hand, the scriptures condemn the use of alcohol and other drugs, whereas paradoxically their use in religious rituals is encouraged. Ritual use of hallucinogens for religious practices in India dates back to time immemorial. The hymns from Rig-Veda, written prior 1000 B.C., mention the use of *soma*, an intoxicating drink of the gods (Furst, 1990). Similarly, the resin of cannabis, popularly called *vijaya*, is known as god Indra's favorite drink. Drinking *bhang*, a mixer of cannabis resin, sugar, and water, on the conclusion of *Durga Pooja* (worship of Goddess Durga) is a customary religious practice among Hindus. It is also a Hindu religious tradition to distribute cannabis as a prayer food, *prasad*, to the congregation on *Shivratri,* celebration of Lord Shiva's birth night. Ancient Indian folklores also encourage the use of cannabis in the worship of Lord Shiva. Certain types of cannabis such as *bhang, charas,* and *ganza* have been used by priests and other religious figures to facilitate meditation. Cannabis juice, called *sukha shardai* (mixture of cannabis leaves, sugar, almonds, and milk) is used for spiritual meditation by some members of a sect of the Sikhs called *Nihangs.* Some devotees in India believe that cannabis intoxication can help to increase concentration, whereas others think that it allows one to better fix one's eyes on the Eternal and thus serve as the "heavenly guide" (Furst, 1990). Some Indian *Sadhus* (ascetics) use *datura,* a powerful intoxicant from the seeds of a flowery plant grown in northern India, to seek spiritual bliss.

In 1508, the Portuguese brought tobacco to Goa, and by the time it reached northern India, it was described as an "evil weed." Arab traders introduced opium to India in the ninth century. Initially, it was used for medicinal purposes. During the Moghul period, its use increased, and it was used for sedating purposes and as an analgesic. The use of cocaine to induce euphoria became popular in the late 1800s (Chopra, 1971). There are numerous references to *som ras* in the epics of Mahabharata and Ramayana, suggesting that this intoxicating juice was drunk by kings and their couriers in ancient India.

Sikhism and the Muslim religions contain a clear recommendation that the use of intoxicants, particularly alcohol, be prohibited. For instance, the holy book of the Sikhs, *Sri Guru Granth Sahib* (Singh, 1978), admonishes the followers again and again that

> One should "drink" the nectar of His Name, and not the useless alcohol. Drinking alcohol means losing the valuable life in gambling. (p. 360)

> If one wants to enjoy ecstasy, he should "drink" the Name of God, and that is the way to realize Him. One should strictly avoid alcohol by drinking of which one loses one's control of faculties. (p. 554)

The abuse of alcohol, tobacco, and other substances among *amirtdhari* (baptized) Sikhs is rare. Similarly, the Hindus wearing the sacred thread, *jeneeuu,* generally give up the use of tobacco, meat, alcohol, and drugs (Dorschner, 1983). Bhaktivedanta (1974) explains the importance of shunning the use of alcohol and drugs in achieving the spiritual ecstasy in Hinduism: "Propaganda that one can enjoy this life materially and at the same time spiritually advance is simply bogus. The principles of renunciation are four: 1) to avoid illicit sex life, 2) to avoid meat eating, 3) to avoid intoxication, and 4) to avoid gambling. These four principles are called *tapasya,* or austerity" (p. 137).

Using semistructured interviews, Dorschner (1983) found standard Hindu sanctions operative against intoxication. It is interesting to note that the least condemned practice is the use of hemp, particularly marijuana and hashish. It may explain why miles after miles of wild marijuana grows by sides of roads and railway tracks in India. At times, farmers have to burn marijuana to grow their crops.

Current Alcohol and Other Drug Use in India

Although drug usage is certainly prevalent in India, the most commonly abused substance is alcohol. Alcohol abuse exists in all groups, regardless of caste. Although Prashant (1993) did not find any correlation between alcohol abuse and marital status, caste, educational background, or religious affiliation, the problem appears to be more deleterious for the lower classes because of their struggle to take care of even the most basic needs.

The liquor that is consumed by the lower classes is usually distilled in the home and is called *sharab* (fired water) or *darru* (medicine). It is typically more potent and, as a result, more dangerous and deadly. The higher castes tend to drink imported liquors, and this practice is viewed as a status symbol. In fact, drinking is romanticized among business and upper classes as a sign of prosperity and status. A typical businessman, journalist, politician, or scholar gathers with friends in the evening for a few hours for cocktails and snacks, and excessive drinking is an integral part of such a ritual. In the affluent community, dinner is typically late (approximately 11:00 p.m.), and by then someone might have been drinking for 6 hours.

A study conducted by Prashant (1993) examined reasons for initial use of drugs and found that a large majority of people (72.7%) used drugs because of group pressure. The rest of the people in this study used drugs and alcohol for other reasons, such as to cope with loneliness, depression, and family discord. She also investigated various reasons for which people sought treatment and found that drug problems are the second most common reason for which people seek mental health treatment in India. Whereas in the past, alcohol, opium, and cannabis were the traditional substances of abuse, recently heroin and other injectable drugs, such as buprenorphine, are increasingly becoming common (Basu, Malhotra, & Varma, 1990; Chowdhury & Chowdhury, 1990). Moreover, the abuse of pemoline, an amphetamine used to aid with weight loss, is relatively high in India. India is also one of five countries that legally produce ephedrine, a precursor used in the production of amphetamine-type stimulants. Recently, Jha (1998) reported that, in 77% of communities across the country, chewing *paan* (betel leaf) and, in more than 80% of communities, smoking *beedies* (hand-rolled Indian cigarettes) are the most common addictions.

Substance Use and Abuse by Adolescents

India is experiencing an increasing use of drugs and alcohol among adolescents. Possible reasons for this include peer pressure, curiosity and experimentation, and a way to rebel and establish an identity separate from the family. Adolescent drug use can be traced to the 1960s and 1970s, when "hippies" and "flower children" from Western countries came to India and used drugs, particularly cannabis and hashish, that they associated with the traditional Indian values of internal peace, tranquility, and spirituality. Indian adolescents consequently associated drug use with the glamorized life of Westerners (Ali, 1988). Lather (1993) found that adolescent drug use in India includes barbiturates, amphetamines, LSD, tranquilizers, heroin, and pathedrine and heroin, rather than just alcohol or cannabis. Adolescents also abuse the synthetic drug carisoprodol, initially used to combat opiate withdrawal, which they romanticized and associated with heightened sensuality, enhanced interpersonal experiences, yoga, and meditation (Sikdar, Basu, Malhotra, Varma, & Mattoo, 1993).

Substance Abuse by Women

Substance abuse problems in India predominantly affect men. A study by Prashant (1993) found that 99.6% alcohol or drug abusers in India are male, and 75% of those are between the ages of 10 and 30. It is rare for women from the lower castes in India to drink or use drugs. Women from the upper classes are more likely to drink, but not nearly in the same way as men. Women who abuse a substance are kept hidden because it is viewed as a shameful disgrace to one's family.

DRUGS AND ALCOHOL ABUSE BY INDIANS IN THE UNITED STATES

National databases that survey alcohol and other drug abuse in the United States ignore or aggregate data for all Asian Americans and Pacific Islanders (Ja & Aoki, 1993). Thus there is no information about the percentages of substance-abusing Asian Indians in the United States. Moreover, cultural factors discourage or inhibit the admission of substance abuse problems among Asian Indians. Even in the United States, most Asian families tend to associate mental illness and substance abuse problems with shame, guilt, and stigma and keep them within the family (Sue, 1987). An open admission of such problems is considered a disgrace.

But having no readily available statistics does not mean that Asian Indians do not have problems related to alcohol and substance abuse. Although Lal and Singh (1979) found that the rate of alcohol abusers in a rural village in Punjab, India, was 4.7% ($N = 127$), a study conducted by United Communications (1989) on a similar population in Vancouver estimated that almost 25% of the males had alcohol problems. It seems that Indian immigrants are more prone to use alcohol and drugs after their migration to foreign countries than their counterparts in India. The following factors might contribute to this increased use of drugs and alcohol:

1. *Acculturative stress.* Several authors have identified acculturation and assimilation processes as painful experiences for immigrants (Bromley, 1988; Portes, 1996; Sandhu, 1997; Sandhu & Asrabadi, 1994). Sandhu, Portes, and McPhee (1996) assert that as a result of these processes, "threats to cultural identity, powerlessness, feelings of marginality, a sense of inferiority, loneliness, hostility, and perceived alienation and discrimination become major mental health concerns" (p. 16). Adapting to a novel social milieu, new culture, and assimilation of different lifestyles becomes a

source of personal stress and interpersonal conflicts for many Asian Indian immigrants (Ashcraft, 1986). Such stressors could lead to the abuse of alcohol or drugs as a coping mechanism (Harvey, 1985; Rebach, 1992; Yee & Thu, 1987; Zane & Sasao, 1992).

2. *Loneliness in the United States.* Due to a decline in primary group contacts, new immigrants generally experience a sense of loneliness in the United States (Saxton, 1986). Such primary groups include close friends, relatives, and family members with whom one may have interacted face-to-face on a regular basis (Medora, Woodward, & Larson, 1987). Raised in an extended family, Asian Indians are prone to loneliness after migrating to the United States. Turning to alcohol and drugs is one way of numbing the pain of loneliness and homesickness.

3. *Freedom from cultural restrictions and taboos.* Cultural mores and norms regulate an individual's behaviors in India. As indicated previously, alcohol and drug abuse is strictly prohibited for certain castes, religious sects, and women. For example, while living for 26 years in India, I (D. S. S.) only once saw an elderly lady smoking a tobacco pipe, and only at a wedding ceremony did I ever see a few young adult women sipping wine. Such cultural restrictions are not maintained abroad. Because life in the United States is a lot more individualized and free, Asian Indians in America, particularly young men and women, are more likely to smoke, drink, and use drugs than in India. This is particularly true of second-generation Asian Indians, who are more free from the cultural restrictions and taboos against alcohol and drugs that their parents observe. The gender gap between the second-generation men and women is also closing. It is not shocking to see second-generation women drinking, although the percentage of Indian American women who drink is still low compared with that of women from other ethnic groups.

4. *Easy access and financial feasibility.* Alcohol and other drugs, with the exception of marijuana, are more readily available in America than in India. Moreover, with a better financial situation, Asian Indians can easily afford to purchase them. This combination of both availability and affordability increase the rate of alcohol and drug abuse.

These various factors are responsible for the increase in alcohol and drug abuse found among Asian Indian Americans. However, it appears that a large number of Indian substance abusers are not getting into substance abuse treatment programs. One explanation for this situation may be a greater tolerance for pathological behavior within the family, so that the individual is often sheltered from the consequences of his or her drug use until the family can no longer deal with the problem. Moreover, as is true with most groups of immigrants, there is a trend initially to move to a relatively homogeneous neighborhood composed of other Indian people and Indian shops. People who live in such Indian communities typically rely on the elders of the community for help with all matters, including help with alcohol- and drug-related problems, and rarely turn to professional help.

TREATMENT APPROACHES FOR ASIAN INDIANS IN THE UNITED STATES

Substance abuse centers are now seeing Indian patients with greater frequency. All of the principles that apply to chemical dependency treatment in this country should apply to Indian patients as well. However, some of the typical treatment approaches may need to be slightly modified in order to provide effective treatment for this population.

Abstinence-based models certainly have the highest efficacy. Utilizing motivational enhancement techniques, clinicians need to talk to patients about the benefits of total abstinence and the consequences of continued use. If a client's family members are supportive of sobriety, they should be enlisted, as they likely exert a powerful influence over the patient. It is often the case that a client's success in treatment has a great deal to do with the family members' posture regarding the substance use. When a family member is opposed to treatment, extra effort should be made to include that person in the intake process so that he or she has an opportunity to air concerns. To the degree that it is possible, there should be agreement at the outset of treatment about the treatment goals. The client should also be helped to understand his or her patterns of drinking and drinking triggers. When patients are unwilling to commit to long-term abstinence, it is often helpful to have them attempt short-term abstinence, if only for 1 week or 1 month. Indian clients will likely be compliant with the initial treatment plan, and many are willing to continue with treatment once they begin to reap the benefits of it.

Harm-reduction strategies focus more on attempting to minimize the potential hazards associated with the substance rather than the use itself (Duncan, 1994). The harm-reduction strategies are considered an alternative to the moral, criminal, and disease models of drug use and addiction (Cronin, 1996; Des Jaralais, 1995; Marlatt, 1996; Samarasinghe, 1995). Such strategies can be used with clients of Indian descent. As is true with other patient groups, use of harm-reduction principles depends on the patient's level of functioning, duration of use, degree to which use had become out of control, and level of motivation. One of us (R. M.) has used harm-reduction techniques with clients who were unwilling to attempt total abstinence but willing to cut back on their consumption. With some, reduction of their intake resulted in a willingness to go to the next level and attempt total abstinence; for others, it did not. Of the patients who used harm-reduction principles, some were able to effectively control their use; those who were not ultimately dropped out of treatment.

Many Indian clients oppose attending 12-step groups such as Alcoholics Anonymous (AA) or Narcotics Anonymous (NA). The most common criticism has been that they are too public and that people talk about their personal problems in front of total strangers. This is something that would be considered shameful for many Indian clients. Language problems and cultural barriers also make it difficult for Asian Indian clients to engage in AA meetings and group therapy sessions. Clients should be encouraged to attend AA meetings, even if they do not talk. These clients can benefit a great deal even if they do not share their own stories. If, ultimately, they report feeling out of place at meetings and are unwilling to go, they should be educated about the 12-step principles. Clinicians working with Asian Indian substance abusers can enhance their therapeutic efficacy if they keep in mind the following cultural dynamics:

Dominant Family Figure

The father's authority is preeminent in Asian Indian families. As the head of the family and a decision maker, his authority remains unquestioned (Ramisetty-Mikler, 1993). Therefore, therapeutic efforts without the father's participation are likely to fail. Consequently, the father or the husband of a substance abuser needs to be involved in the therapeutic alliance (Lee, 1996). Because a husband is more likely to be the substance abuser, an Indian wife must have familial support from her adult children or in-laws before she will encourage her husband to enter treatment.

Generally speaking, family therapy is the therapy of choice because Asian Indian clients expect their family's active involvement in their problems. However, higher social class and greater acculturation to U.S. norms weaken the allegiance to traditional family roles (Dhruvarajan, 1993). In such cases, individual therapy might be a better choice for initial intervention. For Indian clients struggling to adapt to a Western lifestyle, it might be preferable to engage the family in treatment after an initial alliance has been formed with the client. It is therefore very important to assess the acculturation level of Asian Indian clients.

Shame and Guilt

Asian Indian patients with drug and alcohol problems face a double menace. In addition to their drug- and alcohol-related problems, these clients may experience deep feelings of shame, guilt, and humiliation. Such feelings result in enormous reluctance to seek professional treatment. Consequently, substance abuse problems may be kept secret until an emergency requires hospitalization or the person gets into legal difficulties. In addition, once in treatment, Asian Indian clients may not maintain eye contact with the therapist and may not demonstrate much enthusiasm and interest in the therapy session due to their feelings of shame and guilt. Clinicians must assess and address these feelings of shame before initiating any other therapeutic measures.

Focus on Somatic Problems

Because psychological or mental health problems are socially stigmatized among Asian Indians, clients are likely to discuss physical complaints more candidly than they are ready to discuss emotional or psychological issues relating to their drug and alcohol abuse. Consequently, during the first phase of substance abuse treatment, when building rapport, it may be helpful to offer clients some medical help or to focus on their physical problems before exploring the impact of addiction on other aspects of their lives.

Practical Solutions and Concrete Advice

Asian Indian clients equate therapy with medical services and expect practical solutions to their problems. They generally have not had any prior experiences with talk therapy, nor have they heard of such therapeutic practices in their home country. These clients are interested in solving their problems rather than discussing them for the sake of exploration. In Asian cultures, "wearing your heart on your sleeve" is considered shallow. Thus it is important that therapists spend some time explaining the nature of therapy. Brief solution-focused and cognitive-behavioral approaches should receive precedence over affective therapeutic approaches. Therapy with Asian Indian clients should be goal oriented, symptom relieving, and short term (Berg & Jaya, 1993). Long-term psychotherapy intended to explore inner conflicts and insights is not recommended unless a client expresses an interest in that kind of treatment.

Avoidance of Intimate Topics

During the initial stages of treatment, clinicians should avoid discussing topics that are viewed as too personal, such as sexual or religious matters. Asian Indian clients may not see the relevance of such discussions in the context of alcohol and drug problems. They may feel shy and ashamed and may perceive such discussion as unbecoming of a therapist who is considered a respected authority figure. Therapists should wait to discuss sexual issues until a good rapport is built or until clients initiate such inquiries themselves. If questions regarding sexual matters are part of the standard intake questionnaire, the clinician should prepare the client for the intimate nature of the questions and explain that it is part of the standard intake. The clinician also needs to educate the client about the connection that exists between drug or alcohol use and sexual behavior.

Use of Group Therapy

Therapists need to consider the pros and cons of group therapy with their Asian Indian clients before placing them in a group. Generally, Asian Indian clients are reluctant to participate in group therapy for various reasons. They may be reluctant to discuss their alcohol and drug problems with strangers or they may feel guilty about dishonoring their family in the presence of others. They may also be overly conscious of their skin color, national origin, and, especially, of their accent and language problems.

Lack of Verbal, Emotional, and Behavioral Expressiveness

Sue and Sue (1977) pointed out that Asian clients lack verbal, emotional, and behavioral expressiveness. It is not always the case that the client cannot express feelings; rather, they are not accustomed to doing so verbally. Moreover, Indian clients find it culturally unacceptable to express their anger directly. Adults may deal with psychological conflicts somatically, whereas children and adolescents may act them out behaviorally. Therefore, it is not uncommon for a substance-abusing patient or a family member to come to a clinician's office through a referral from a school or a physician.

Clinicians who place a high premium on self-disclosure would most likely be disappointed with Asian Indian clients. In the first few sessions, such clients are likely to be mostly silent, passive, and ingratiating. If allowed, an Asian Indian client may sit for a long time in silence, waiting for the clinician to find the solution for his or her problems. The best way of handling such clients is to be didactic in the early phase of treatment, to structure the treatment by asking questions, and to provide a model for talking about one's feeling states.

Because feelings are often expressed indirectly, clinicians working with an Indian client would need to approach issues regarding the client's family members gingerly. The client would most likely react with strong protectiveness if he or she thought the therapist was criticizing a family member.

Engaging Clients in Treatment

During an intake, it is critical that the clinician work to establish a good rapport or a working alliance with the client. Although this is important with all clients, with an Indian client such a relationship will provide the leverage needed to ask the patient to make changes in his or her life. The client will become more engaged in the recovery process if the relationship is the driving force. One way for the therapist to establish rapport with an Indian patient is to express some understanding or interest in the Indian culture. Indian patients are often fearful that a non-Indian clinician will view India as a backward or uncivilized nation. A clinician's curiosity will go a long way to help a patient feel secure in the therapeutic environment. Clinicians working with Asian Indian clients should avoid taking a stance of therapeutic distance and may need to become more open or self-revealing. It is not uncommon for Indian clients to ask about the clinician's age, family background, marital status, or religious faith. Although it is imperative to inquire about the reasons the patient is asking, at times it may be advisable to provide the client with limited information. The client may be asking such questions because he or she feels selfish for being the exclusive focus of attention. Moreover, the concept of reciprocity is also quite important for Indians; thus a client may ask questions about the clinician just to be polite, not necessarily to find out the information. The way to determine the client's true motivation is obviously through a detailed inquiry.

With all substance abuse treatment, there is a need for greater structure in the beginning. As the length of treatment increases, the treatment approach can become more psychodynamic and exploratory. However, in the early phases, a strong emphasis on psychoeducation is most helpful. The critical issue when treating Indian clients is to make the education appear as a natural outgrowth of the relationship rather than as an academic effort.

Treatment Compliance and Noncompliance

Indian clients are likely to show initial compliance with treatment suggestions, but such compliance can be deceptive. As is true in most Asian countries, there is a strong emphasis on teaching children to treat authority figures (e.g., parents, teachers, and doctors) with respect and to comply with their requests. Although this can enhance patient cooperation initially, it can also lead the clinician to underestimate patient resistance and ambivalence. The patient will not mention this ambivalence unless he or she is invited to do so. It is not unusual to encounter patients of Indian background who were superficially compliant with all requests but who had no intention of maintaining sobriety. Because of respect for the clinician, they may not reveal this to the clinician unless asked directly.

When exploring a patient's ambivalence, clinicians must avoid direct confrontation of denial. That would likely cause an Indian client to feel attacked and shut down the process of therapy. The clinician should exercise this cautious style until a therapeutic alliance has been established. As is true with other substance abusers, the degree to which a clinician can encourage or help a client talk about his or her own concerns about the substance use will likely determine how much the client will benefit from the treatment. Moreover, as pointed out earlier, it might be quite difficult for the Indian client to express direct anger toward the clinicians. The clinician needs to be vigilant to detect signs of anger and help the client talk about these feelings. The therapist must convey that he or she can tolerate angry feelings. Given the traditional Indian communication style discussed earlier, these clients will be quite sensitive to the therapist's cues and are quite skilled at hearing the spoken and unspoken messages. They will be looking for signs that indicate that the therapist accepts them.

Some Asian Indian cultural behaviors may encourage patients to continue their abuse of drugs and alcohol and defeat treatment efforts. Understanding the following dynamics can be useful in understanding noncompliant clients and helping them in their recovery process.

Drinking as a Status Symbol

Among upper classes, drinking is viewed as a symbol of one's standing in the community, and evening cocktails are often an integral part of personal and professional dealings. The clinician needs to convey to the client that he or she understands the difficulty patients will have when they attempt to be totally abstinent. For example:

> Mr. S, a 54-year-old business man, struggled a great deal with the fact that people would suspect that something was wrong with him if he was not drinking. He feared their disdain and was concerned that it would render him less effective in business if people lost respect for him because he was not drinking. He spent much of his individual sessions talking about how others might view him and about how to answer questions about why he was not drinking. He was quite concerned about saving face within his community and viewed his need

for treatment as an admission that he had failed. His community and lifestyle were an integral part of his existence, and he needed the clinician to empathize with the numerous losses he would be enduring. The clinician explored what it would mean for him to lose people's respect and examined ways in which Mr. S could present his change of lifestyle while still saving face, such as stating that he had a medical condition that required that he stop drinking. This approach helped him to feel less humiliated. Ultimately, Mr. S became less focused on what others were thinking and more comfortable with his abstinence.

Filial Piety

In some instances, filial piety, high respect for the family at the sacrifice of personal desires (Ho, 1992), may encourage an Asian Indian client to engage or continue in addictive behaviors just to comply with the wishes of the elders. For example, an interesting conversation between a father and son was witnessed by one of us (D. S. S.) when, under the euphoria of opium, the father offered some opium to his 17-year-old son:

FATHER: Son, have this miracle thing with hot tea. It will save you from the cold.

SON: No, Daddy, I better not take it. I will get addicted.

FATHER: Come on son, I have been taking it for the past ten years. I am not addicted yet, how would you get addicted so soon?

Fatalism

Many Asian Indians believe that their lives are predestined (Ibrahim, Ohnishi, & Sandhu, 1997). Thus they may perceive that alcoholism and drug-related problems are preordained and have to be sustained and that addiction is the result of their bad luck. It might be necessary to educate such clients about addiction, its deleterious nature, and treatment options.

Family Involvement

Given the Indian focus on family, it is clear that a critical component to a person's recovery is family involvement. Family members typically will not attend Al-Anon meetings. Airing family problems in public is seen as distasteful and thus not done. Yet a client may find it almost impossible to establish abstinence without family support. For example, Mr. S's wife and adult daughter objected to his efforts to become totally abstinent from alcohol. They feared the impact his sobriety would have on their family standing, and because they did not understand his alcoholism, they expected that he should be able to drink moderately. Mr. S, who had not been able to moderate his drinking in the past, felt torn between doing what he felt was in his own best interest and what his family wanted. Because the good of the family is always primary to the personal desires and needs of the individual in Asian families, Mr. S drank whenever he was in a social situation with his family. The task facing the clinician was to engage the family members to support the patient's treatment. Because shame plays a prominent role in the interpersonal relationships of Asians, the clinician had to be very sensitive not to embarrass the family members in the presence of one another (Berg & Jaya, 1993). The clinician encouraged Mr. S's entire family—his wife, an adult daughter, and his parents—to attend a few sessions with the patient to define treatment goals and to air their concerns. It took some prodding to help the family members admit to their fears about Mr. S becoming totally abstinent. In their minds, he would be acknowledging weakness or failure if he accepted the belief that he needed to stop drinking completely. The family's support was facilitated by focusing on the disease concept and delineating the ways the family would benefit from the client's sobriety.

CONCLUSION

The model-minority myth established by the first wave of Asian Indian immigrants who tended to be medical doctors, scientists, and educators and whose personal problems did not attract the attention of mental health professionals discouraged clinical and research focus on this population. During the recent wave of immigration, the number of Asian Indian immigrants has been increasing, and the demographics are changing. Anecdotal and clinical evidence suggests that serious alcohol and substance abuse problems exist in this population. Yet there is a real paucity of alcohol and drug abuse literature focusing on Asian Indians. Culture-specific practices prevalent in traditional Asian Indian families also discourage help-seeking behaviors outside the family due to shame and guilt. For this reason, there are more questions than answers for researchers and practitioners interested in helping Asian Indian patients. There is a growing need for more empirical investigations of Asian Indian that can facilitate effective prevention and treatment of substance abuse problems. Such lack of cultural considerations can lead to serious problems in assessment, and faulty conclusions can lead to detrimental outcomes (Sue & Sue, 1987).

REFERENCES

Ali, S. (1988). South Asian paradise: Business is booming for illegal trade in drugs and goods (Indian subcontinent). *Far Eastern Economic Review, 142*(52), 18–19.

Almeida, R. (1990). Asian Indian mothers. *Journal of Feminist Family Therapy, 2,* 33–40.

Almeida, R. (1996). Hindu, Christian, and Muslim families. In M. McGoldrick, J. Giordano, & J. K. Pearce (Eds.), *Ethnicity and family therapy* (2nd ed., pp 395–423). New York: Guilford Press.

Ashcraft, N. (1986). The clash of traditions: Asian Indian immigrants in crisis. In R. H. Brown & G. V. Coelho (Eds.), *Traditions and transformation: Asian Indians in America* (pp. 53–70). Williamsburg, VA: Studies in Third World Societies.

Basu, D., Malhotra, A. K., & Varma, V. K. (1990). Buprenorphine dependence: A new addiction in India. *Disabilities and Impairments, 3,* 142–146.

Berg, I. K., & Jaya, A. (1993). Different and same: Family therapy with Asian American families. *Journal of Marital and Family Therapy, 19*(1), 31–38.

Bhaktivedanta, A. C. (1974). *Srimad Bhagavatam.* New York: Bhaktivedanta Book Trust.

Bromley, M. A. (1988). Identity as a central adjustment issue for the Southeast Asian unaccompanied refugee minor. *Child and Youth Care Quarterly, 17*(2), 104–113.

Chopra, I. C. (1971). Drug addiction in India. *Journal of Pharmacy, 3,* 43.

Chowdhury, A. N., & Chowdhury, S. (1990). Buprenorphine abuse in India. *British Journal of Addiction, 85,* 1349–1350.

Cronin, C. (1996). Harm reduction for alcohol-use-related problems among college students. *Substance Use and Misuse, 31*(14), 2029–2037.

Das, A. K., & Kemp, S. F. (1997). Between two worlds: Counseling South Asian Americans. *Journal of Multicultural Counseling and Development, 25*(1), 23–33.

Des Jaralais, D. C. (1995). Harm reduction: A framework for incorporating science into drug policy. *American Journal of Public Health, 85*(1), 10–12.

Dhaliwal, A. K. (1995). Gender at work: The renegotiation of middle-class womanhood in a South-Asian owned business. In W. L. Ng, S.-Y. Chin, J. S. Moy, & G. Y. Okihiro (Eds.), *Reviewing Asian America: Locating diversity* (pp. 75–85). Pullman: Washington State University Press.

Dhruvarajan, V. (1993). Ethnic cultural retention and transmission among first generation Hindu Asian Indians in a Canadian prairie city. *Journal of Comparative Family Studies, 24*(1), 63–79.

Dorschner, J. P. (1983). *Alcohol consumption in a village in North India.* Ann Arbor, MI: UMI Research Press.

Doshi, M. (1975). *Who is who among Indian immigrants in North America.* New York: B. K. Verma.

Duleep, H. O. (1988). *Economic status of Americans of Asian descent.* Washington, DC: U.S. Commission on Civil Rights.

Duncan, D. (1994). Harm reduction: An emerging new paradigm for drug education. *Journal of Drug Education, 24*(4), 281–290.

Furst, P. T. (Ed.). (1990). *Flesh of the gods: The ritual use of hallucinogens*. Prospect Heights, IL: Waveland Press.

Gupta, S. N. (1979). *British, the magnificent exploiters of India*. New Delhi: Chand.

Harvey, W. B. (1985). Alcohol abuse and the black community: A contemporary analysis. *Journal of Drug Issues, 15*, 81–91.

Helweg, A. W., & Helweg, U. M. (1990). *An immigrant success story: East Indians in America*. Philadelphia, PA: University of Pennsylvania Press.

Ho, M. K. (1992). *Minority children and adolescents in therapy*. Newbury Park, CA: Sage.

Hoffman, M. S. (Ed.). (1991). *World almanac and book of facts*. New York: Scripps-Howard.

Ibrahim, F., Ohnishi, H., & Sandhu, D. S. (1997). Asian American identity development: A culture specific model for South Asian Americans. *Journal of Multicultural Counseling and Development, 25*(1), 34–50.

Ja, D. Y., & Aoki, B. (1993). Substance abuse treatment: Cultural barriers in the Asian-American community. *Journal of Psychoactive Drugs, 25*(1), 61–71.

Jayakar, K. (1994). Women of the Indian subcontinent. In L. Comas-Díaz & B. Greene (Eds.), *Women of color: Integrating ethnic and gender identities in psychotherapy* (pp. 161–181). New York: Guilford Press.

Jensen, J. M. (1988). *Passage from India: Asian Indian immigrants in North America*. New Haven, CT: Yale University Press.

Jha, L. K. (1998, January 2). The rediscovery of India. *India Abroad, 28*, 14–18.

Joe, K. A. (1996). The lives and times of Asian-Pacific American women drug users: An ethnographic study of their methamphetamine use. *Journal of Drug Issues, 26*(1), 199–218.

Johnson, R. C., & Nagoshi, C. T. (1990, January/March). Asians, Asian Americans and alcohol. *Journal of Psychoactive Drugs, 22*(1), 45–52.

Kamen, A. (1992, November 16). After immigration, an unexpected fear: New Jersey's Indian community is terrorized by racial violence. *The Washington Post*, p. A1.

Lal, B., & Singh, G. (1979). Drug abuse in Indo-Pakistani. *British Journal of Addiction, 74*, 411–427.

Lather, A. S. (1993). *Drug abuse among students*. Chandigarh, India: Arun.

Lee, E. (1996). Asian American families: An overview. In M. McGoldrick, J. Giordano, & J. K. Pearce (Eds.), *Ethnicity and family therapy* (2nd ed., pp. 227–248). New York: Guilford Press.

Marlatt, G. A. (1996). Harm reduction: Come as you are. *Addictive Behaviors, 21*(6), 779–788.

Medora, N., Woodward, J., & Larson, J. (1987). Adolescent loneliness: A cross-cultural comparison of Americans and Asian Indians. *International Journal of Comparative Sociology, 28*(3/4), 204–211.

Minocha, U. (1987). South Asian immigrants: Trends and impacts on the sending and receiving societies. In J. T. Fawcett & B. V. Carino (Eds.), *Pacific bridges: The new immigration from Asia and the Pacific Islands* (pp. 347–374). Staten Island, NY: Center for Migration Studies.

Mukhopadhyay, C. C., & Seymour, S. (Ed.). (1994). *Women, education, and family structure in India*. San Francisco, CA: Westview Press.

Nanda, S. (1991). *Cultural anthropology* (4th ed.). Belmont, CA: Wadsworth.

Nandan, Y., & Eames, E. (1980). Typology and analysis of the Asian Indian family. In P. Saran & E. Eames (Eds.), *The new ethics: Asian Indians in the United States*. New York: Praeger.

Nayak, J. (1997, November 14). Need to change home environment [Letter to the editor]. *India Abroad*, p. 3.

Portes, P. R. (1996). Ethnicity in education and psychology. In D. Berlinger & R. Calfee (Eds.), *The handbook of educational psychology* (pp. 331–358). New York: Macmillan.

Prashant, S. (1993). *Drug abuse and society: The Indian scenario*. Springfield, VA: Nataraj Books.

Prathikanti, S. (1997). East Indian American families. In E. Lee (Ed.), *Working with Asian Americans: A guide for clinicians* (pp. 79–100). New York: Guilford Press.

Ramisetty-Mikler, S. (1993). Asian Indian immigrants in America and sociocultural issues in counseling. *Journal of Multicultural Counseling and Development, 21*, 36–49.

Rebach, H. (1992). Alcohol and drug use among American minorities. In J. E. Trimble, C. S. Bolek, & S. J. Niemcryck (Eds.), *Ethnic and multicultural drug abuse: Perspectives in current research* (pp. 23–57). New York: Haworth Press.

Samarasinghe, D. (1995). Harm reduction in the developing world. *Drug and Alcohol Review, 14*(3), 305–309.

Sandhu, D. S. (1997). Psychocultural profiles of Asian and Pacific Islander Americans: Implications for counseling and psychotherapy. *Journal of Multicultural Counseling and Development, 25*, 7–22.

Sandhu, D. S., & Asrabadi, B. R. (1994). Development of an acculturative stress scale for international students: Preliminary findings. *Psychological Reports, 75*, 435–448.

Sandhu, D. S., Portes, P. R., & McPhee, S. A. (1996). Assessing acculturation adaptation: Psychometric properties of the Cultural Adaptation Pain Scale. *Journal of Multicultural Counseling and Development, 24*(1), 15–25.

Saxton, L. (1986). *The individual, marriage, and the family*. Belmont, CA: Wadsworth.

Sheth, M. (1995). Asian Indian Americans. In P. G. Min (Ed.), *Asian Americans: Contemporary trends and issues* (pp. 169–198). Thousand Oaks, CA: Sage.

Sikdar, S., Basu, D., Malhotra, A. K., Varma, V. K, & Mattoo, S. K. (1993). Carisoprodol abuse: Report from India. *Acta Psychiatrica Scandinavica, 88*, 302–303.

Singh, G. (1978). (Trans.). *Sri Guru Granth Sahib* [English]. Chandigarh, India: World Sikh University Press.

Sodowsky, G. R., & Carey, J. C. (1987). Asian Indian immigrants in America: Factors related to adjustment. *Journal of Multicultural Counseling and Development, 15*(3), 129–141.

Sue, D. (1987). Use and abuse of alcohol by Asian Americans. *Journal of Psychoactive Drugs, 1957–1966.*

Sue, D., & Sue, S. (1987). Cultural factors in the clinical assessment of Asian Americans. *Journal of Consulting and Clinical Psychology, 55*(4), 479–487.

Sue, D. W., & Sue, D. (1977). Barriers to effective cross-cultural counseling. *Journal of Counseling Psychology, 24,* 420–429.

True, R. H. (1990). Psychotherapeutic issues with Asian American women. *Sex Roles, 22*(7, 8), 477–486.

United Communications Research. (1989). *Alcohol and drug abuse study: Focus group report.* Vancouver, British Columbia, Canada: Author.

U.S. Bureau of the Census. (1983). *1980 census of population, general population characteristics, United States summary (Publication No. PC80–1-B1).* Washington, DC: U.S. Government Printing Office.

U.S. Bureau of the Census. (1992). *Statistical abstract of the United States, 1990.* Washington, DC: U.S. Government Printing Office.

U.S. Bureau of the Census. (1993). *1990 census of population, general population characteristics, the United States* (Publication No. CP-1-1). Washington, DC: U.S. Government Printing Office.

Yee, B. W. K., & Thu, N. D. (1987). Correlates of drug use and abuse among Indo-Chinese refugees: Mental health implications. *Journal of Psychoactive Drugs, 19,* 77–83.

Yen, S. (1992). Cultural competence for evaluators working with Asian/Pacific Island American communities: Some common themes and important implications. In M. A. Orlandi, R. Weston, & L. G. Epstein (Eds.), *Cultural competence for evaluators: A guide for alcohol and other drug abuse prevention practitioners working with ethnic/racial communities* (pp. 261–291). Rockville, MD: U.S. Department of Health and Human Services, Public Health Service, Alcohol, Drug Abuse, and Mental Health Administration, Office for Substance Abuse Prevention, Division of Community Prevention and Training.

Zane, N., & Sasao, T. (1992). Research on drug abuse among Asian Pacific Americans. In J. E. Trimble, C. S. Bolek, & S. J. Niemcryk (Eds.), *Ethnic and multicultural drug abuse: Perspectives on current research* (pp. 181–209). New York: Haworth Press.

19

Substance Abuse Interventions for Japanese and Japanese American Clients

Jun Matsuyoshi

The Japanese population in the United States is made up of several different groups with differing rates of acculturation into the mainstream American culture. Like all ethnocultural groups, Japanese Americans have specific characteristics that could put them at risk for substance abuse. These characteristics are related to biological, cultural, historical, and personal factors. There are few culturally specific treatment facilities for Japanese clients, and working with Japanese clients may present challenges to clinicians unfamiliar with the Japanese culture. This chapter discusses the cultural variables unique to Japanese clients and suggests ways in which interventions might be tailored to serve these clients.

JAPANESE IMMIGRANTS IN THE UNITED STATES

The 1990 census reported that Japanese Americans represent 12% of Asians and Pacific Islanders, making them the third largest subgroup of Asians after the Chinese and Filipinos (Ong & Hee, 1993). The Japanese population in the United States usually falls into three categories: descendants of the early immigrants, immigrants who arrived after World War II, and visiting businessmen and their families. Each group is at risk for substance abuse for different reasons.

The largest category, comprising 75% of the persons of Japanese ancestry, are the descendants of those who emigrated between 1900 and 1924. The Japanese first migrated to the United States during the Meiji Era, 1868–1912, when Japan, reacting to the threat of colonization by the West, transformed itself from an isolated feudal country to an industrialized nation. To finance this modernization, Japan levied increased taxes on farms. Many farmers, who found these taxes burdensome, left for Hawaii and the mainland United States in hopes of making enough money to offset the tax burdens before returning to Japan (Matsui, 1996). The descendants of this first group have been in America for more than five generations, considerably longer than many other Asian populations. In many cases, these Japanese Americans have become so acculturated that they may lack awareness of Japanese cultural influences that affect their behavior, and their use of substances reflects their acculturation to the mainstream American values and norms.

The second group of Japanese in the United States includes Japanese wives of American servicemen who were in Japan during the Allied occupation after World War II. These women, known as "war brides," numbered about 25,000 in 1960. Many of their marriages ended in divorce, which stigmatized the women and led to increased vulnerability to mental health and substance abuse problems (Marden, 1992).

The third group consists of Japanese businessmen and their families who are here on temporary assignments of 3 to 5 years and who want to retain their traditional ways in order that their families may reenter their culture upon their return. These people continue their traditional way of socializing, which includes regular drinking after work, and thus may be at risk for alcohol abuse or dependence. Other Japanese in this group include those who came seeking opportunities available in the American culture that were not available in the closed Japanese society. These immigrants included those who experienced difficulties in professional advancement, as well as those seeking a lifestyle that is possible in a country that emphasizes individual freedom to a greater degree than does Japan. Some individuals in this group may have had difficulties with substance abuse in Japan or may have turned to substance abuse as a way of coping with problems related to the immigration process.

The Early Settlers and Their Descendants

The experiences of the first groups of migrant workers, called *Issei*, or first-generation, settled in Hawaii and on the West Coast of the United States.

The experiences of these two groups differed greatly. The Japanese in Hawaii made up more than one third of Hawaii's population and established themselves as the largest group in the local ethnic landscape. During World War II, the Japanese in Hawaii closed down all Japanese institutions and had their "Americanized" children represent their families in public. In 1942, when the War Relocation Authority interned persons of Japanese ancestry in camps, only 1% of the Japanese in Hawaii were interned (Marden, 1992). Many sought to prove their loyalty to the United States by volunteering for combat in European theaters and were among the most highly decorated soldiers (Kimura, 1988).

Although many families suffered the impact of having their young men killed or injured in the course of wartime duties, Japanese in Hawaii enjoyed a more cohesive family life than Japanese on the West Coast. Following World War II, the Japanese in Hawaii became politically active and continue to exert influence in national and local politics to this day (Marden, 1992).

In contrast to the Japanese in Hawaii, the Japanese on the West Coast, who numbered less than 1% of the local population, were frequent targets of anti-Japanese sentiment. These Japanese laborers, who were willing to take low-paying jobs, were resented by labor unions as unfair competition. Decades of agitation and animosity against mainland Japanese, who were deemed unassimilable and anti-American, resulted in the Johnson–Reed Act of 1924, which effectively barred immigration from Asia until it was rescinded in 1952.

Because many *Issei* men migrated to the United States with the intention of staying for only a few years and then returning home to marry, there were many more Japanese men than women among the immigrants. The 1924 Johnson–Reed Act curtailed Japanese immigration, and many *Issei* men never married. By 1940 there were 131 Japanese males for every 100 females (Marden, 1992).

With the passage of the War Relocation Authority in February 1942, more than 90% of mainland Japanese, over 100,000 people, including 77,000 who were born in the United States, were interned in camps. The internment took a psychological as well as economic toll on the mainland Japanese, as they were forced to abruptly abandon their homes and businesses. Families experienced disruption in many aspects of family life. *Issei* men lost status in the eyes of their families, because leadership roles in the camps were assigned only to the American-born *Nisei* (second generation). *Issei* men who were not married suffered additional difficulties as a result of lack of family structure and support and were especially susceptible to depression and problem drinking (Marden, 1992). The deprivation and traumatic impact of internment during World War II was eventually ac-knowledged by the United States government when the Civil Liberties Act, usually referred to as the Reparations Act, was signed in 1988.

The *Sansei,* or third-generation Japanese Americans, born into a mid-dle-class society and spared the blatant racial discrimination experienced by their forebears, felt freer to choose between retention of traditional cul-tural values or further assimilation. Succeeding generations are undergoing further assimilation, as shown by such indicators as a high level of inter-marriage with other ethnic groups (Sue & Sue, 1990) and reduced ability to speak Japanese (Kitano, Lubben, & Chi, 1988).

TRADITIONAL CULTURAL TRAITS

The early Japanese immigrants displayed traditional cultural traits that combined those of feudal Japan and the industrialized Meiji Era. The tradi-tional feudal characteristics included the precedence of group loyalty over individual desires, maintenance of harmony, emotional reservedness, post-ponement of gratification, endurance of hardship, and respect for superi-ors. These characteristics, expressed in prescribed behavior in social situa-tions, continue to shape the behavior of Japanese Americans even today.

Following Japan's defeat in World War II and the resulting Allied oc-cupation, Japan underwent profound changes. With the adoption of de-mocratization and universal suffrage, many cultural changes have been tak-ing place, including in the notion of the traditional family led by the dominant male (Roland, 1988). Nonetheless, many traditional values are still evident in Japan and among many Japanese Americans.

Traditional Gender and Family Roles

In Japanese society, gender and family roles are hierarchical and well de-fined. Affection is displayed not by emotional demonstrativeness but by ad-herence to the strictures of one's role. The father, as leader of the family, is expected to provide for the economic welfare of the family and to enforce family rules. "He is frequently seen as somewhat stern, distant, and less ap-proachable than the mother" (Shon & Ja, 1982, p. 212). The role of the mother is that of homemaker and emotional center of the family. She man-ages all aspects of the home, including family finances and the children's education.

The Japanese are group oriented, and each individual feels loyal to his or her school, family, or company group. Prior to World War II the primary group was the *ie*, a kind of corporate household to which people belonged who were related by kinship or who had certain occupational ties to the family. Following the Allied occupation, business corporations replaced the *ie* system, and men transferred their loyalty to the company or the bureaucracy in which they were employed (Roland, 1988). Consequently, the role of the father in the home has diminished.

Whereas in the United States the marital relationship is considered primary, in Japan the parent–child relationship takes precedence, so married couples relate to each other as parents rather than as partners. Older members of the family, even siblings who are only slightly older, are addressed with terms signifying respect, such as "older brother" or "older sister." The most important child in the family is traditionally the oldest son, who is the most privileged and is expected to set an example for younger siblings (Uba, 1994).

In general, young children are shown much affection and may even be viewed as spoiled by Western standards. As children get older, they are more likely to be praised for obedience than to be shown affection. For adults, affection is manifested in expressions and expectations of good will. This good will, roughly corresponding to the warm feelings a child might have for someone who takes care of him or her, is called *amae* (Doi, 1985).

Traditionally, Japanese social behavior is determined by a code of obligation and shame. Obligation is known as *giri* and seen not just as a burden but as an opportunity to display affection and gratitude. Love and affection may be expressed through *giri*. The child is obligated to the parents, who provide for him or her. The businessman is obligated to the company, which protects him or her with continued employment and benefits. The citizen is obligated to his or her country, which provides security and identity. When shame is incurred, it means support is withdrawn and obligatory relationships are suspended. Inability to fulfill one's obligation results in loss of face and may lead to self-imposed isolation or social ostracism. An individual accused of wrongdoing or labeled a misfit, such as a substance abuser, brings shame not only to him- or herself, but also to his or her family.

Current Family Dynamics

In modern Japan, men have become even more disconnected from their families because they spend many hours commuting, working, and socializing with peers. In urban areas, many men spend only Sundays with their families, leaving women to raise families on their own. It is not uncommon for Japanese women to think of their husbands as eldest sons for whom they provide care (T. Shibusawa, personal communication, February 15, 1998).

Japanese mothers transmit to their children the importance of skillful negotiation of human relationships and high academic achievement. Women often make sacrifices to help their children excel and derive self-esteem from their children's success. Consequently, children experience feelings of guilt and shame if they cannot live up to their mother's expectations (Roland, 1988; Straussner & Matsuyoshi, 1995)

Communication Styles

The Japanese values of interpersonal harmony, the precedence of group over individual interests and of duties over rights, and the importance of reciprocating acts of kindness are manifested in communication styles. Communication is indirect, with a reliance on nonverbal signals. Japan is largely an ethnically homogeneous country in which 99.4% of the population is composed of Japanese (Dolan & Worden, 1994). Roland (1988) describes Japan as a society in which nonverbal communication and empathic sensing are highly developed, with "shared cultural meanings that have remained remarkably homogeneous over many centuries" (p. 88). Japanese children are taught from an early age that they must be sensitive to what others are thinking and feeling. Emphasis is on cooperation and conciliation rather than confrontation. Conflicts are suppressed and discussions are carried out in a nonthreatening, seemingly superficial way. In ambiguous situations, the proper behavior is withdrawal, silence, and watchfulness (Uba, 1994).

There is a dualistic relationship between what is outside and inside (who is in the group versus who is not), what is revealed and concealed (what is articulated and what remains unspoken), and what is social convention and what is individual behavior. Roland (1988) observes that individuality is maintained by keeping a private self. Rather than revealing themselves, individuals engage in indirect communication. Such communication ensures that individual desires do not interfere with group functioning. Indirectness also preserves self-esteem by preventing conflicts or confrontations.

Thus, in contrast to the Western way of expressing emotions, the Japanese experience their emotions without necessarily expressing them (Doi, 1985). To the Japanese, emotions are not located within individuals but are experienced in the context of interactions with others. For example, a grandmother experiences joy when she is with her grandchild, but she does not have to demonstrate her joy. The restrained behavior of the Japanese, which may be deemed as repression by Westerners, is viewed by Japanese as simply good manners and modesty.

SUBSTANCE ABUSE IN JAPAN

The primary substances used in Japan are alcohol, tobacco, solvents, amphetamines, tranquilizers, and analgesics. Historically, alcohol and tobacco have enjoyed benign regard, whereas other substances are considered harmful. The most widely used illicit substances are amphetamines, which are popular among the young and the criminal population. Use of opiates, cocaine, or marijuana is much lower than in Western countries (Suwaki, 1989; Tamura, 1992; Wada & Fukui, 1993).

Use of Alcohol

Among the substances used in Japan, none is more imbued with cultural meaning or more positively accepted than alcohol. The use of alcohol must be examined in its biological and cultural context in order to understand the Japanese attitudes toward alcohol.

Physiological Aspects of Drinking

There is a physiological aspect of drinking that is unique to certain ethnocultural groups, including the Japanese. An "atypical" form of the enzyme aldehyde dehydrogenase is considered to play an important role in what is known as the "flushing response." Some individuals with this enzyme deficiency display marked physiological and psychological changes when drinking. Such changes may include facial reddening (known as flushing), accelerated heartbeat, heightened blood pressure and other circulatory system changes, dizziness, drowsiness, anxiety, headaches, sweating, nausea, and feelings of weakness and malaise (Higuchi et al., 1991; Johnson & Nagoshi, 1990; Nagoshi, Dixon, Johnson, & Yuen, 1988). These physiological changes appear to affect drinking patterns. A 1982 study in Hawaii (Johnson & Nagoshi, 1990) found that in Japanese men, flushing seems to lessen drinking, partly because it relieves them of the social pressure to drink. Substantial family resemblances between generations in flushing and in alcohol use patterns were found to exist among Japanese men (Johnson & Nagoshi, 1990).

Cultural Aspects of Drinking

Japanese cultural attitudes toward drinking evolved in feudal times, when society was based on an agrarian economy. A clear distinction between routine workdays and festival days was essential for survival. There was no drinking during workdays, whereas on festival days the citizenry drank *sake*, or rice wine, which was considered a gift from the gods. Today, the Japanese continue to keep a clear distinction between work and leisure hours. They have difficulty understanding practices that include alcohol consumption during a workday, such as having wine with lunch (Smith, 1988).

Use of Alcohol by Men

Drinking is viewed as positive and almost socially compulsory for men. They regard alcohol as a good way to relieve stress, and some even consider it to be part of a good diet.

Drinking at company parties and after work serves to bind people together. As in the larger culture, Japanese businesses emphasize consensus building, through formal communication based upon rules of proper conduct. In order to access each other's views and to get information that may not be obtained through formal channels at work, groups of men often go drinking after work. A man who does not drink is looked upon as an outsider and thus may lose access to information. Some men spend so little time with their families that their reduced roles may contribute to their tendency to drink with other men (T. Shibusawa, personal communication, February 15, 1998).

With such importance placed on the role of alcohol in business and social relationships, it is not surprising that drinking norms are considered to be permissive. Because many executives believe that the advantages of alcohol use far outweigh the disadvantages, alcohol-related problems of businessmen rarely are identified in the workplace. As noted by Izuno and colleagues (1992), "It is often said, but not documented, that Japanese society is tolerant of public inebriety" (p. 1397). These culturally sanctioned attitudes toward drinking make it difficult for many Japanese people to associate drinking with negative consequences or to seek treatment for alcohol abuse (Nakamura, Tanaka, & Takano,1993).

Use of Alcohol by Women

Whereas in the past alcohol problems were found primarily among men, they are now increasing among women. A 1991 survey found that 61%

of Japanese women drink, compared with 13% in 1954 (Hada, 1991; Higuchi & Kono, 1994). The increase in women drinkers seems to coincide with the increased participation of women in the workforce and in social activities outside the home. Some Japanese consider it a sign of masculinity if men drink large quantities of alcohol and even go so far as to excuse the behavior of inebriated men. Most people, however, consider it unfeminine for women to show a loss of control while drinking. Consequently, women who have drinking problems tend to conceal their drinking in what has been termed "kitchen drinking" (Higuchi & Kono, 1994). Many women, who are caretakers of their elderly parents as well as their children, find it difficult to seek help for themselves if they have problems.

Japanese society has been slow to acknowledge that alcohol use is problematic for some women. Families of women who have drinking problems are ashamed of them and try to conceal the problems as long as possible. It is only when the family has exhausted its coping resources that the woman alcoholic is turned over to professionals. At that point it is not uncommon for their husbands to divorce them and for their children to be taken into custody by others. The stigma of women's alcoholism is so great that even medical providers are apt to give a vague diagnosis, such as "loss of consciousness for unknown reason," to women who are referred for medical attention because of drinking problems (Gotoh, 1994).

Use of Stimulants

The controlled substances most widely abused in Japan are amphetamines and other stimulants. The use of stimulants is synchronous with the Japanese view that it is important to be a "doer," one who works hard, rather than a "dreamer" (a common view of one who uses opiates, such as heroin; Tamura, 1992). Stimulants also may relieve boredom in a society in which most behavior is circumscribed.

Use of Other Substances

Although as many as 100 young Japanese die annually from sniffing paint thinner, glue, and other solvents (Tamura, 1989), law enforcement has not been successful in curbing usage because solvents are commercially available materials. The number of arrests for solvent use has averaged 45,000 annually (Wada & Fukui, 1993), with 90% of those arrested under age 20.

In recent years there have been reports of cough syrup abuse among urban adolescents and abuse of tranquilizers and analgesics by older people, usually in conjunction with medical treatment. Many elderly individuals receive prescriptions for these drugs from physicians and pharmacists who are not aware of the risks of multiple prescriptions and drug abuse.

SUBSTANCE ABUSE AMONG PERSONS OF JAPANESE ETHNICITY IN THE UNITED STATES

Several studies have shown significant use of alcohol and other drugs among individuals of Japanese descent. Kitano and Chi (1985), in their study of alcohol consumption by Chinese, Japanese, Koreans, and Filipinos in Los Angeles, found that the Japanese had the highest percentage of heavy drinkers. Sasao (1991), in a study of drug use by Asian and Pacific Islander groups in California, also found that Japanese Americans reported the highest level of lifetime alcohol use (69%), compared with Koreans (49%), Vietnamese (43%), Chinese (42%), Filipinos (39%), and Chinese Vietnamese (36%). This study also found that the Japanese had the highest percentage of reported use of tobacco products (45%) compared with the other Asian Pacific groups.

Some research indicates that the Japanese also have high prevalence of use of other drugs besides alcohol (Zane & Sasao, 1992). McLaughlin and colleagues (as cited in Zane & Kim, 1994), in a 1987 study, found that compared with other Asian Pacific groups, Japanese and Chinese had a higher prevalence of tranquilizer use. Findings in California showing the Japanese community to have the highest prevalence of marijuana and cocaine use among the six Asian groups (Sasao, 1991) correlates with anecdotal reports in New York.

Demand for Treatment Services

Despite the preceding findings, clients of Japanese background are underrepresented in treatment settings. There are several reasons for the low demand for substance abuse services among Japanese populations. These include lack of knowledge about the hazards of substance use, cultural inhibitions about seeking help, lack of knowledge about treatment services, and lack of culturally sensitive services.

In community forums among various Asian populations in California, it was found that shame and the stigma of seeking help were key factors that prevented persons of Japanese ethnicity from obtaining treatment

(Kuramoto, 1995). Although the forums reported that the most prevalently used substances were alcohol, marijuana, tobacco, crack cocaine, and amphetamines, the relative absence of problem behavior contributed to denial of the impact of substance abuse (Kuramoto, 1995). Moreover, studies of newly arrived Japanese nationals in the United States showed that they had less knowledge about substance abuse and less concern than more acculturated individuals, indicating that newer immigrants may not realize the dangers of alcohol and tobacco use until such use becomes severely problematic (Sasao, 1991).

TREATMENT INTERVENTIONS FOR JAPANESE AND JAPANESE AMERICAN CLIENTS

There are numerous explanations for substance abuse with various implications for clinical intervention. In 1984 Sue and Nakamura (as cited in Kuramoto, 1995) proposed the reciprocity model that suggests that alcohol consumption is a phenomenon in which the physiological, social, and psychological factors interact with one another. This hypothesis assumes that consumption of alcohol and other drugs is influenced by such factors as one's native culture, the mainstream culture, and the generational status of individuals (Kuramoto, 1995). Similarly, Straussner (1993) states that substance abuse stems from a combination of factors, including "biochemical, genetic, familial, environmental, and cultural ones, as well as personality dynamics" (p. 11). Thus clinicians must take into account the historical and cultural context of their clients and adapt their treatment approaches to meet the needs of clients of Japanese background. The following discussion focuses on the use of modified clinical approaches during the engagement, assessment, and treatment phases when working with Japanese and Japanese American clients.

The Engagement Phase

During the engagement phase with individuals of Japanese background, it is important to establish credibility with clients and to give them a "gift" in the form of a direct benefit from treatment. The gift is a gesture of caring on the part of the clinician. Particularly when working with traditionally oriented Japanese, it is important for clients to perceive direct benefits from treatment in order to allay skepticism about Western forms of treatment (Zane & Kim, 1994). Gift giving may take the form of alleviation of stress or anxiety. By helping clients develop clarity and by normalizing their experience as one that is shared by others, the clinician can convey a sense of relief that will be perceived as a gift. Additionally, helping clients to talk may lessen feelings of isolation, shame, and "loss of face," and may also be perceived as a gift. In turn, clients may wish to reciprocate with their own gift at a later point in the treatment.

When working with traditionally oriented clients, especially with more recent Japanese immigrants, the clinician would do well to show respect for those who are older or of elevated status by addressing them by their last name, by allowing them to walk ahead, and by deferring to their schedules when making appointments. To establish credibility as an expert, the clinician may impart certain information, such as his or her experiences in working with Japanese clients, his or her educational background, or information about the clinician's family origins if his or her background is Japanese. During the encounter the clinician should observe the client's nonverbal cues, such as eye contact, body posture, smiles, and so forth (Suzuki, 1976, cited in Lebra & Lebra, 1986).

Clinicians should be aware of culturally influenced attitudes and behavior. For example, doctor–patient relationships in Japan are influenced by the tradition of respect for those of elevated status. Japanese clients expect doctors to make a quick diagnosis and to give them concrete instructions to cure the problem (Munakata, 1986). Often, they expect the doctor to prescribe medication. Therefore, the non-Japanese clinician has to educate clients about his or her role and the services that will be provided, and why certain questions are asked. The clinician might point out that in a fairly homogeneous society such as Japan's, people can make certain assumptions about each other, but in a heterogeneous society such as the United States, which comprises many ethnocutural groups with different levels of acculturation, it is difficult to operate under assumptions. Clients need help in understanding that thorough assessments are necessary to determine the course of treatment.

If interpreters are used who are not mental health or substance abuse professionals, certain guidelines should be observed. The clinician should meet with interpreters prior to client interviews and provide information about substance abuse issues, review the issues that are to be addressed, and emphasize the need for confidentiality. Relatives of clients should not be used as interpreters (Lee, 1996).

The Assessment Phase

An accurate assessment will shape interventions in the treatment phase. Assessments should include family history and immigration history. Japanese Americans, like other immigrants, may be affected by immigration and acculturation stressors, which may be risk factors for substance abuse (Uba, 1994). Acculturation to American values includes acceptance of social drinking by both men and women and the acceptance of alcohol and drug experimentation by adolescents. Thus greater acculturation may put Japanese women (Tsunoda et al., 1992) and adolescents in the United States at higher risk for substance abuse than in Japan. Kitano and colleagues (1985) found that more recent Japanese immigrants have a much higher proportion of heavy drinkers than Caucasians. In addition to coping with stressors due to adjustment to new work and home environments, immigrants may experience pronounced intergenerational conflicts. Children may acculturate more rapidly than their parents (Montalvo & Gutierrez, 1990), which may upset the authoritarian structure of Japanese families. Furthermore, parent–child conflicts may be due to parental concerns that too much "Americanization" of their children will bring problems when the family returns to Japan. Individuals might choose to cope with these stressors through the accepted way of dealing with stress in Japan—the use of alcohol.

Complete assessments include the client's perceptions of the problem. Although it is important to maintain cultural sensitivity by avoiding the use of direct and confrontational approaches or premature discussions of taboo topics such as sex, clinicians may find that clients are usually willing to explain their view of the problem (Lee, 1996). Much information may be gained by asking clients about their perception of the problem, how such a problem would be handled in the country of origin, how they have attempted to deal with the problem, and what they expect of treatment. In addition, questions about holidays and cultural events as occasions for use of alcohol and questions about familial flushing responses may yield information about substance use.

In Japan, the way to maintain mental health is to keep busy, refraining from dwelling upon one's problems (Munakata, 1986). A certain amount of unhappiness is viewed as normal and something that should be stoically endured (Lebra, 1976). Physical illness is the only acceptable reason to exempt someone from responsibilities, and, as in other countries, there is public prejudice about mental illness. Strong emotions, especially anger, are unacceptable. Rather, they are often manifested as somatic symptoms. Not surprisingly, the Japanese have more somatic complaints than psychological ones (Munakata, 1986).

Japanese society prefers to view mental and behavioral anomalies as departures from the norm that the individual may correct with help from his or her family; thus the inclination is not to seek professional treatment but to shore up the person with encouragement. The role of the wife is to offer emotional support to her husband, so women often help men cover up the effects of drinking by helping them get work. Culturally permissive attitudes toward drinking also make it difficult for alcohol-related problems to be identified.

In contrast to the American medical model of substance abuse as a disease, the Japanese view of substance abuse is that of loss of will power. No matter how severe the effects of alcohol may seem, a man is usually not considered an alcoholic if he can maintain his job (Smith, 1988). The behavior of individuals affects the social position of the entire family, so stigma tends to dampen efforts to seek treatment until the situation is so unmanageable that family members give up. As mentioned earlier, treatment is sought often as a last resort. Family members feel that seeking treatment is equivalent to abdicating their responsibility, and they experience a great deal of guilt and shame. They expect social criticism (Munakata, 1986). In addition, substance abuse treatment is limited by lack of training of professionals. Doctors, even psychiatrists, receive little instruction in substance abuse-related disorders (Higuchi & Kono, 1994; Kono, 1988). Even when substance-related problems are evident, treating professionals are reluctant to make a substance abuse diagnosis because they wish to protect patients from the resulting stigma.

In accordance with cultural expectations, the clinician may wish to take an authoritarian stance as the expert and define concrete goals, such as education on the health consequences of heavy drinking. Goals must be mutually agreed upon so that the client does not prematurely drop out of treatment (Lee, 1996; Uba, 1994). Clinicians may demonstrate respect for the family's authoritarian structure by allowing adults, particularly fathers, the opportunity to discuss their problems in private rather than in front of their children.

As previously mentioned, individuality in Japan is preserved by keeping a very private self (Lebra, 1992). Feelings of vulnerability arise in situations in which the inner world may be revealed, so clients may feel more comfortable with an object such as a small table between themselves and the clinician to serve as a symbolic barrier against intrusion (Roland, 1988).

The Treatment Phase

During the treatment phase, it is important to continue using techniques that are culturally acceptable. Such interventions include reinforcing the importance of roles and values such as obligation and loyalty to one's family, employing psychoeducational approaches, and using an intermediary to allow clients to accept help without direct confrontation (Lee, 1996; Uba,

1994; Zane & Kim, 1994). The clinician can support clients by using reframing techniques to emphasize the positive aspects of their efforts to cope with problems, such as praising them for enduring as much as they have and for working together to preserve the family's good name. Approaches used by Japanese therapists include assuming an "inferior" position or questioning attitude, using humor, or verbally reflecting what the clinician senses the client is feeling in order that the client may confirm or correct the clinician (Roland, 1988). When working with clients of Japanese background, it is as necessary for clinicians to listen carefully for what is not said as it is to listen to what is expressed. Clients may resist "spelling out" their issues and concerns and may communicate in an indirect manner. If the clinician insists on directness and verbalization, clients may feel they are not understood or may feel that they are losing face in front of others.

Group treatment may be an option for clients of Japanese background, especially if they have had previous group treatment experience. Morita therapy is a form of group therapy practiced in Japan. Patients are treated in groups to encourage them to interact with others to help them "accept things as they are" and "let nature take its course" (Lebra, 1992, p. 116). It is believed that a person's problems stem from rumination on the gap between present reality and an idealized state; therefore, the Morita patient is instructed to "submit to his symptom" and to "unite with his illness" (Lebra, 1992, p. 124). Japanese clients may have had group experiences in Japan through involvement in Alcoholics Anonymous (AA) or Danshukai, a self-help support group without the emphasis on anonymity. Even clients without group experience may favor the AA approach, in which they can listen and observe without revealing themselves. Japanese clients may also value participation in a group with a specific agenda, such as a psychoeducational group focused on the impact of substance abuse on physical health.

During the process of termination, clients who have difficulty verbalizing feelings sometimes acknowledge their gratitude by reciprocating with a gift or by inviting the clinician to dinner. Clients also may want to continue some association with the clinician even after the treatment ends. The clinician may want to accept such gestures as being culturally appropriate (Lee, 1996).

Working with Families

As indicated previously, families are expected to control the behavior of their members, so seeking professional help is a last resort after other efforts have failed. Japanese pride themselves on their ability to endure hardship or suffering without complaining, as expressed in the phrase *gaman suru*. Families who seek help may feel it is an admission of failure, may experience shame in their inability to handle family problems, and may fear criticism. Clinicians can offer support to families in the form of reframing techniques, such as reminding family members of all they have done to take care of the problem and how much they have endured (Shibusawa, 1996).

Case Illustrations

The following case examples illustrate clinical work with a substance-abusing man, a woman, and an adolescent.

Working with Substance-Abusing Men

Mr. K is a Japanese businessman who lived in a New York suburb with his wife and two young children while temporarily assigned to his company's New York branch. In addition to experiencing stress in unfamiliar business situations, he had to function without the daily support of his colleagues back in Japan. He complained of fatigue and insomnia. Believing that drinking was a way to combat fatigue and deal with stress, he began drinking more in the late evenings after the family was asleep. He gruffly rebuffed his wife's attempts to engage him in conversation about these matters. She wanted to improve the situation but felt that a good wife must defer to her husband and should endure a certain amount of suffering. She experienced conflict between wanting to talk to someone about the situation and wanting to remain loyal to her husband. Further, she felt that seeking help was an admission of her failure as a wife and a sign of disloyalty to her husband. Failure as a wife would not only reflect upon her but also on her family in Japan. Eventually she confided in a friend in her cooking class, who suggested that she speak to a Japanese physician. The physician, who was familiar with the drinking patterns of Japanese men, suggested that Mr. K come to see him for a physical examination to ensure his continuing health. Although the physical exam was normal, the physician, by engaging Mr. K in talking about his efforts to cope with work pressures, elicited information about Mr. K's increased drinking. In asking about Mr. K's family, the doctor discovered that Mr. K was concerned about whether the children would be able to do well in the United States and still readapt upon the family's return to Japan. The doctor told Mr. K that these were normal concerns that he had observed in other Japanese clients. He praised Mr. K for his concern about his children in the midst of his business pressures. He pointed out that because Mr. K's family looked to him for leadership, he had to maintain his health. The doctor educated Mr. K about the effects of drinking on health and recommended exercise as a way to relieve stress and help with his insomnia. Mr. K agreed with the doctor that he had to maintain his health to ensure that he would be able to help his children succeed in the United States and upon their return to Japan.

It was evident that Mr. K used alcohol as a way of coping with stress. Although the family system was involved, the doctor in this situation worked only with the father, allowing him to remain in his role as the head of the family. The doctor used culturally syntonic techniques, such as emphasizing health concerns and the importance of the client as a parent, rather than focusing on the drinking itself. He reframed Mr. K's anger at home as a sign of caring in spite of the business pressures the client was experiencing.

Working with Substance-Abusing Women

Clinicians working with Japanese and Japanese American women must be aware of the special problems of substance-abusing women in general.

Biological factors that contribute to women's vulnerability to alcohol drinking include not only the flushing factor but also women's physiology. It is documented that women, with smaller body sizes and more fatty tissue than men, are more vulnerable to the effects of alcohol (Pape, 1993). Caring for others is the guiding principle in the lives of Japanese women and compromises their ability to seek help for themselves. Child-care concerns may also prevent women from accessing help. Additionally, it has been noted that women tend to feel more guilt and shame about substance abuse than do men (Pape, 1993). The shame-based Japanese culture may put an added burden on women who have substance abuse problems. They may feel shame about their behavior while under the influence of alcohol or drugs and shame about their inability to maintain role functioning as wives and mothers. Japanese women may be influenced by cultural attitudes, such as enduring hardship without complaint, and may use alcohol as a coping mechanism. In the following case example, cultural attitudes influenced the woman's ability to seek and receive help.

Mrs. S, who was raised in Tokyo, married an American who conducted business in Japan. She and her husband moved to the United States and settled in California in 1970. At first Mrs. S was homesick because she had few occasions to associate with Japanese-speaking people, but she listened to Japanese-language radio programs and soon became proficient enough in English to get a job as a bank teller. She was proud of her job performance and of her children's success, but was deeply ashamed when her marriage ended after 22 years. She felt the divorce was her fault because her native culture decreed that good wives kept their marriages together. Also, she had been warned by her relatives in Japan about the difficulties of a bicultural marriage. Her children were on their way to becoming professionals; one was in medical school and the other was finishing college. Although pleased by their success, Mrs. S felt that she was no longer needed as a mother.

Feeling isolated and lonely, she began to drink at night and began to show up late to her job at a local bank. Although Mrs. S was friendly with Japanese American coworkers, they did not speak with her about her difficulties but tried to offer face-saving help by sharing special foods or inviting her to their homes. Her supervisor, a Caucasian man, tried to talk to her, but she denied that she had problems. Finally, when it was obvious that her work was suffering, he told her that she would have to go to the company's Employee Assistance Program (EAP). The EAP counselor referred her to a local AA group, but after attending one meeting, she did not continue going, as she felt stigmatized as the only Japanese woman there. After a follow-up call, the EAP counselor referred Mrs. S to a Japanese American social worker in private practice who was familiar with substance abuse issues. The therapist persuaded her to get involved in activities sponsored by the local Japanese-language radio station. Mrs. S made new female friends and felt less isolated. With these gains, Mrs. S began to trust her therapist, who started to inquire about Mrs. S's family history. The therapist helped Mrs. S deal with her unresolved feelings about leaving Japan and marrying outside her ethnic group. The therapist found that Mrs. S's family had a history of flushing in reaction to the use of alcohol and educated her about the dangers of alcoholism. She asked Mrs. S how she would feel if her family in Japan knew of her problems. Mrs. S, who up to this point had minimized her drinking, began to reflect on feelings of obligation to her family and became more open to looking at her drinking behavior.

This case illustrates the impact of cultural factors on a client's receptivity to treatment. Using an intermediary, appealing to cultural ideals, and getting women with common interests to support each other are interventions tailored to the cultural context of persons of Japanese ancestry. Rather than directly confronting Mrs. S in the beginning, which might have led to increased feelings of shame and low self-esteem, the therapist waited until Mrs. S had received a "gift" in terms of her new friends before asking about her family. Not only was Mrs. S experiencing the "empty nest syndrome," but also her children's acculturation created a wider gap between the two generations. These difficulties were compounded by culturally influenced factors. Mrs. S's feelings of failure as a wife and shame about her drinking behavior made it difficult for her to talk to people about her problems. Her Japanese peers, acting in accordance with cultural constraints that precluded confrontation, could not speak directly to her about her problems.

Working with Substance-Abusing Adolescents

Parents of substance-abusing adolescents face special challenges. They may want their children to succeed in this country but may feel conflicts beyond the usual generational ones. Success may mean increased acculturation and assimilation, as demonstrated not only by the younger generation's adaptability to the mainstream culture but also by their limited ability to speak Japanese and their scorn for "old-fashioned" ideas and customs, such as removing one's shoes before entering the home.

The following case example illustrates a family's generational conflicts, which are complicated by cultural expectations.

Mr. M, a *Sansei* (third-generation) father, was concerned about his 16-year-old son, Michael, because he suspected that the son smoked marijuana. As a youth, Mr. M had worked after school in his father's dry-cleaning business. He had never talked to Michael about the material deprivation his family had suffered during post-World War II, trying instead to put the memories behind him and hoping that his son would be spared such experiences. He expected that Michael would enter the family business and was delighted when the son helped out there after school. Recently, however, Michael had refused to work at the business, refused to attend family gatherings, and had arguments with his father about his interest in going to art school upon graduation from high school. Worse, Michael had talked back to his father. Asked about smoking marijuana, he had replied that his father relaxed by drinking beer with his friends, so he, Michael, should be allowed to relax in the way those of his generation preferred. Mr. M was shocked that his son spoke to him in this way, something he would never have dared to do with *his* father. He ordered Michael to spend more time at home, which the son refused to do. The father felt ashamed that he could not control his son's behavior. Michael's academic performance, previously very high, began to plummet, and the parents were asked to meet with the school's counselor. Mr. M met with the counselor, who, sensitive to cultural issues, supported his efforts to be a good father. He framed the father's ability to provide for his family as evidence of his caring. By doing this, the counselor helped decrease the father's sense of shame and build trust. With the father's permission, the counselor included Michael in the next meeting and suggested that he join an after-school youth group. Among the group's activities were peer education about alcohol and other drugs and sports activities. These teenagers felt it was "not cool" to use drugs and lose control, and they tried to influence their peers. When they needed posters to advertise a fund-raising car wash, Michael proudly filled the need with his art talent. As his peer group changed, Michael stopped smoking marijuana. His grades improved, and he argued less with his father. Although Michael no longer helped out at the family business, Mr. M was glad to see the improvements and began to reconcile himself to "the younger generation."

In this case, the father's uneasiness about seeking help was mollified by the counselor's understanding of cultural values, such as filial piety. According to Zane and Kim (1994) in their report on the Asian Youth Substance Abuse Project (AYSAP), a San Francisco consortium of agencies that collaborated in youth drug abuse prevention efforts, it is important to link peer- and family-oriented approaches. The statewide alcohol needs assessment in California conducted by Hatanaka (as cited in Sasao, 1991) found that outreach and education to community groups, such as schools and churches, was necessary in order to reach Japanese and other Asian populations.

Community-Based Treatment and Preventive Services

In the community forums conducted by the statewide drug services needs assessment in California in 1991, the Japanese American community emphasized the need for education and outreach conducted by bilingual and bicultural professionals. Preventive educational efforts based on health needs were considered important (Sasao, 1991).

In communities with large Japanese populations, independent services based on existing substance abuse treatment models may be established. Such programs must include bilingual and bicultural service providers. For example, in Scarsdale, a New York City suburb that includes many Japanese business executives and their families, two medical practices have been opened by major New York hospitals, Beth Israel Medical Center and Mount Sinai Medical Center. These medical practices employ American doctors and dentists, with periodic visits by a Japanese doctor and a dentist. The medical practitioners are trained to be alert to certain disorders that are common among Japanese patients, such as stomach cancer. The assistants and administrators, who are Japanese, provide a bridge between patients and doctors and their respective cultures. Not only do they provide translation skills that are important in obtaining medical histories, but they also explain Japanese expectations of medical treatment to doctors and educate patients on Western medical practices. Incorporating substance abuse screening and referral services into such medical practices, with administrators and medical practitioners trained in the provision of substance abuse services, would be beneficial. Medical doctors would need to be alert for signs of substance abuse, such as changes in liver function tests or patients' reporting of somatic symptoms.

Another way of providing services is establishing new agencies and programs specifically designed to serve a Japanese clientele. Such centers might be modeled after Japanese corporations, which take on a somewhat paternal role with their employees. Integrated, multicare service centers might provide such amenities as legal assistance with documentation issues, educational assistance with language skills, and health care services offering annual physical examinations and substance abuse services. Service providers trained in assessments of substance abuse would be alert to such complaints as occupational stresses, academic problems, or somatic symptoms; all of these may be manifestations of substance abuse problems for Japanese clients.

In traditional substance abuse treatment facilities, training sessions to increase clinicians' cultural sensitivity or hiring bilingual staff knowledgeable about Japanese culture are ways of improving services to such clients. For clients who are reluctant to seek treatment, accessing services in privacy may be easier on the Internet. For example, the Pacific Asian Alcohol Program (1998) on the Internet gives comprehensive information and offers publications in Japanese and other Asian languages. This same website offers information on the Asian American Residential Recovery Services, a 24-month drug and alcohol rehabilitation program; the Asian Youth Substance Abuse Project; and the Asian American Drug Abuse Program Special Deliveries Perinatal Program for women and their children.

Community-based approaches to education and prevention of substance abuse can be used to empower Japanese communities to seek solutions to problems. Community participation is important in understanding residents' perception of problems, in increasing their awareness of substance abuse as a problem, and in eliciting culturally congruent pride in solving their problems (Sasao, 1991). Some approaches that may be useful are peer education in youth groups, training in after-school Japanese programs, and speeches by community leaders.

CONCLUSION

Although myths and stereotypes of a model minority exist about Japanese people, it is clear that they are at risk for substance abuse. Statistics of service utilization belie the need for services, partly because of the impact of cultural factors that inhibit Japanese clients from seeking services and partly because of the ignorance of the hazards of substance abuse. There are dangers in accepting the low statistics of service utilization at face value. The majority of statistics are garnered from too few studies to provide an accurate account of the reasons for the low demand for services. Japanese people and others may unwittingly take comfort in stereotypes and perpetuate the myth that substance abuse rarely exists among the Japanese. Unfortunately, low statistics of service utilization also may translate into low funding for services.

Substance abuse services must include comprehensive assessment and treatment that is delivered by clinicians trained in delivering culturally acceptable services. For recent immigrants, such services may include bilingual and bicultural providers within mainstream treatment facilities or near business establishments at which Japanese clients seek legal, medical, and other services. Services must address education and prevention issues, as well as treatment needs. These services may be provided by clinicians who adapt strategies sensitive to cultural attitudes and values. Community support through institutions and individuals is necessary to reach the largest number of people.

REFERENCES

Doi, T. (1985). *The anatomy of the self*. Tokyo: Kodansha.

Dolan, R. E., & Worden, R. L. (Eds.). (1994, January). Society. In *Japan: A Country Study* [Online]. Available: lcweb2.locgov/cgi-bin/query/r?frd/cstdy:@field (DOCID+jp0006)

Gotoh, M. (1994). Alcohol dependence of women in Japan: Comments on Ikuesan's "Drinking problems and the position of women in Nigeria" and Mphi's "Female alcoholism problems in Lesotho." *Addiction, 89*(8), 953–954.

Hada, A. (1991). Alcohol dependency. In T. Inoue & Y. Ehara (Eds.), *Women's data book* (pp. 60–61). Tokyo: Yukihaku.

Higuchi, S., & Kono, H. (1994). Early diagnosis and treatment of alcoholism: The Japanese experience. *Alcohol and Alcoholism, 29*(4), 363–373.

Higuchi, S., Muramatsu, T., Yamada, K., Muraoka, H., Kono, H., & Eboshida, A. (1991). Special treatment facilities for alcoholics in Japan. *Journal of Alcohol Studies, 52*(6), 547–554.

Izuno, T., Miyakawa, M., Tsunoda, T., Parrish, K., Kono, H., Ogata, M., Harford, T. D., & Towle, L. H. (1992). Alcohol-related problems encountered by Japanese, Caucasians, and Japanese-Americans. *The International Journal of the Addictions, 27*(12), 1389–1400.

Johnson, R. C., & Nagoshi, C. T. (1990, January/March). Asians, Asian-Americans and alcohol. *Journal of Psychoactive Drugs, 22*(1), 45–52.

Kimura, Y. (1988). *Issei: Japanese immigrants in Hawaii* (pp. 215–240). Honolulu: University of Hawaii Press.

Kitano, H. H. L., & Chi, I. (1985). Asian Americans and alcohol: The Chinese, Japanese, Koreans, and Filipinos in Los Angeles. In D. Spiegler, D. Tate, S. Aitken, & C. Christian (Eds.), *Alcohol use among U.S. ethnic minorities* (pp. 373–382). Washington, DC: National Institute on Alcohol Abuse and Alcoholism.

Kitano, H. H. L., Lubben, J. E., & Chi, I. (1988). Predicting Japanese American drinking behavior. *International Journal of the Addictions, 23*(4), 417–428.

Kono, H. (1988). Drinking patterns, problems, and treatment in Japan. In L. H. Towle & T. C. Harford (Eds.), *Cultural influences and drinking patterns: A focus on Hispanic and Japanese populations* (pp. 53–62). Washington, DC: U.S. Government Printing Office.

Kuramoto, F. H. (1995). Asian Americans. In J. Philleo & F. Brisbane (Eds.), *Cultural competence for social workers: A guide for alcohol and other drug abuse prevention professionals working with ethnic/racial communities* (pp. 105–155). Washington, DC: U.S. Department of Health & Human Services, Public Health Service, Substance Abuse and Mental Health Services Administration, Center for Substance Abuse Prevention.

Lebra, T. S. (1976). *Japanese patterns of behavior.* Honolulu: University of Hawaii Press.

Lebra, T. S. (1992). Self in Japanese culture. In N. R. Rosenberger (Ed.), *Japanese sense of self* (pp. 105–120). Cambridge, England: Cambridge University Press.

Lebra, T. S., & Lebra, W. P. (1986). (Eds.). *Japanese culture and behavior.* Honolulu: University of Hawaii Press.

Lee, E. (1996). Asian American families: An overview. In M. McGoldrick, J. Giordano, & J. K. Pearce (Eds.), *Ethnicity and family therapy* (2nd ed., pp. 227–248). New York: Guilford Press.

Marden, P. W. (1992) Japanese Americans. In C. F. Marden, G. Meyer, & M. Engel (Eds.), *Minorities in American society* (pp. 393–433). New York: HarperCollins.

Matsui, W. T. (1996). Japanese families. In M. McGoldrick, J. Giordano, & J. K. Pearce (Eds.), *Ethnicity and family therapy* (2nd ed., pp. 268–280). New York: Guilford Press.

Montalvo, B., & Gutierrez, M. J. (1990). Nine assumptions for work with ethnic minority families. In G. W. Saba, B. M. Karrer, & K. V. Hardy (Ed.), *Minorities and family therapy* (pp. 35–52). Binghamton, NY: Haworth Press.

Munakata, T. (1986). Japanese attitudes toward mental health and mental health care. In T. S. Lebra & W. P. Lebra (Eds.), *Japanese culture and behavior* (pp. 369–378). Honolulu: University of Hawaii Press.

Nagoshi, C. T., Dixon, L. K., Johnson, R. C., & Yuen, S. H. L. (1988). Familial transmission of alcohol consumption and the flushing response to alcohol in three oriental groups. *Journal of Studies on Alcohol, 49*(3), 261–267.

Nakamura, K., Tanaka, A., & Takano, T. (1993). The social cost of alcohol abuse in Japan. *Journal of Alcohol Studies, 54,* 618–625.

Ong, P., & Hee, S. J. (1993). The growth of the Asian Pacific American population: Twenty million in 2020. In *The State of Asian Pacific America* (pp. 11–24). Los

Angeles: Leadership Education for Asian Pacifics, Asian Pacific American Public Policy Institute and UCLA Asian American Studies Center.

Pacific Asian Alcohol Program. (1998). *Office of Minority Health Resource Center Database Record* [Online]. Available: http://www/omhrc.gov/mhr2/progs/88CO851.htm

Pape, P. A. (1993). Issues in assessment and intervention with alcohol- and drug-abusing women. In S. L. A. Straussner (Ed.), *Clinical work with substance-abusing clients* (pp. 251–269). New York: Guilford Press.

Roland, A. (1988). *In search of self in India and Japan.* Princeton, NJ: Princeton University Press.

Sasao, T. (1991). *Statewide Asian drug service needs assessment: A multimethod approach.* Sacramento: California Department of Alcohol and Drug Programs.

Shibusawa, T. (1996, October 11). *Psychotherapy with families in the context of Asian cultures.* Paper presented at the second annual Asian American Mental Health Training Conference, Resoled, CA.

Shon, S. P., & Ja, D. Y. (1982). Asian families. In M. McGoldrick, J. Giordano, & J. K. Pearce (Eds.), *Ethnicity and family therapy* (pp. 208–228). New York: Guilford Press.

Smith, S. R. (1988). *Drinking and sobriety in Japan.* Unpublished doctoral dissertation, Columbia University, New York.

Straussner, S. L. A. (1993). Assessment and treatment of clients with alcohol and other drug abuse problems: An overview. In S. L. A. Straussner (Ed.), *Clinical work with substance-abusing clients* (pp. 3–49). New York: Guilford Press.

Straussner, S. L. A., & Matsuyoshi, J. (1995). The impact of familial alcoholism on Japanese American college students. In R. Morimoto (Ed.), *Asians in America 1995 Conference Proceedings* (pp.74–78). New York: New York University.

Sue, D. W., & Sue, D. (1990). Counseling Asian Americans. In S. W. Sue & D. Sue (Eds.), *Counseling the culturally different: Theory and practice* (2nd ed., pp. 189–208). New York: Wiley.

Suzuki, T. (1976). Language and behavior in Japan: The conceptualization of personal relations. In T. S. Lebra & W. P. Lebra (Eds.), *Japanese culture and behavior* (pp. 142–157). Honolulu: University of Hawaii Press.

Suwaki, H. (1989). Addictions: What's happening in Japan [Editorial]. *International Review of Psychiatry, 1,* 9–11.

Tamura, M. (1989). Japan: Stimulant epidemics past and present. *Bulletin on Narcotics, 41*(1, 2), 83–93.

Tamura, M. (1992). The Yakuza and amphetamine abuse in Japan. In H. H. Traver & M. S. Gaylord (Eds.), *Drugs, law and the state* (pp. 98–117). Hong Kong: Hong Kong University Press.

Tsunoda, T., Parrish, K. M., Higuchi, S., Stinson, F. S., Kono, H., Ogata, M., & Harford, T. C. (1992). The effect of acculturation on drinking attitudes among Japanese in Japan and Japanese Americans in Hawaii and California. *Journal of Studies on Alcohol, 53*(4).

Uba, L. (1994). *Asian Americans: Personality patterns, identity, and mental health.* New York: Guilford Press.

Wada, K., & Fukui, S. (1993). Prevalence of volatile solvent inhalation among junior high school students in Japan and background life style of users. *Addiction, 88,* 89–100.

Zane, N., & Kim, J. H. (1994) Substance use and abuse. In N. W. S. Zane, D. T. Takeuchi, & K. N. J. Young (Eds.), *Confronting critical health issues of Asians and Pacific Islander Americans* (pp. 316–343). Thousand Oaks, CA: Sage.

Zane, N., & Sasao, T. (1992). Research on drug abuse among Asian Pacific Americans. *Drugs and Society, 6,* 181–209.

20

Substance Abuse among Korean Americans: A Sociocultural Perspective and Framework for Intervention

Young Hee Kwon-Ahn

Many Korean immigrants arriving in the United States experience hardships in learning a new language and adjusting to a culture so different from their own. Although Korean immigrants and their American-born children utilize a variety of coping mechanisms, some, particularly males, begin to use and abuse substances to deal with life's stress. Although the number of Korean Americans needing help for their substance abuse problems appears to be increasing, statistics show that few of them seek assistance from formal treatment facilities or clinicians. This chapter describes available data on substance use and abuse among Korean Americans and familiarizes clinicians with treatment issues particular to this group. In order to better understand the root of their substance use and abuse, it is essential first to examine the Korean historical background, national character, and cultural values, as well as the unique dilemmas facing Korean Americans.

GEOPOLITICAL CONTEXT OF KOREA

Korea is a peninsula located on the East Asian continent that is surrounded by three powerful nations: China, Russia, and Japan. Although its location allowed Korea easy access to continental culture, it brought with it hazards as well. Throughout its long history of over 4,000 years, Korea was overshadowed and often attacked by its neighboring nations. The incessant aggression from its adjacent countries forced Korea to take the position of a "hermit nation" for almost a century and to isolate itself from other nations in the world. In fact, it was only in 1882 that, for the first time in Korean history, the government officially opened its doors to Western nations (Kyo Yang Kook Sa Yeun Koo Whe, 1994).

Between the years 1910 and 1946, Japan took over the peninsula and held it as a colony for 36 years. Although it was liberated from Japan after World War II, the Korean peninsula was divided by two diametrically opposing worlds: the communist in the North and the democratic republic in the South. In 1950 North Korea suddenly invaded the South, beginning the 3-year-long Korean War.

Over the years, the social and political upheavals have been aggravated by economic instability and a lack of adequate natural resources. Only recently has South Korea experienced rapid industrialization, modernization and economic growth for the first time in its long history.

KOREANS IN THE UNITED STATES

Of the many ethnocultural groups, Koreans are one of the latest to join the American social fabric. The majority of Koreans arrived after passage of the Immigration and Naturalization Act of 1965. Although the number of Koreans in the United States is small, the population has grown rapidly in the past decade, more than doubling in size from 357,393 in 1980 (U.S. Bureau of the Census, 1980) to 797,300 in 1990 (U.S. Bureau of the Census, 1990).

According to the 1990 census, Korean Americans made up 11% of the Asian and Pacific Islander population. They are found all over the United States but are largely concentrated in Los Angeles (72,097), New York (69,718) and Chicago (13,863).

Reasons for Immigration

Historically, many Koreans left their country for the United States primarily because of political instability and a fear of outbreak of war. More recently, however, Koreans have found that an equally compelling reason to leave is that the American educational system offers wider access to higher education.

The Korean educational structure has its roots in Korean tradition and culture, in which there is an enormous emphasis on education. In fact, educational achievement is considered the sole means to success, status, and power. Parents and children alike must endure many years of difficulty in order to attain the "right" education for the children. Parents start preparing their children for college entrance as early as kindergarten, and teachers and parents place overwhelming pressure upon young children to succeed in school. Consequently, children forego many of the childhood activities enjoyed by their American counterparts. For parents, the cost of sending their children to the reputable universities is so high that many exhaust most of their assets. Moreover, the recent changes in the occupational structure of the South Korean economy and its rapid urbanization have prompted a population explosion in the major cities and with it fierce competition for jobs. As a result, college admission has become even more competitive and represents one of the most difficult challenges for children and their parents. Aware that the Korean educational system is structured so that only the very top students will gain admission to college, some Korean parents migrate to America with the expectation that their children will have a much wider opportunity to pursue college and a successful career.

Immigration History

The initial immigration from Korea to the United States occurred between 1902 and 1905, mostly from the rural areas. The roots of Korean immigration can be traced to particular needs existing within Korea and the United States at the turn of the century. The sugar market was rapidly expanding throughout the world, and this necessitated the importation of cheap labor, especially to the Hawaiian Islands, which had become a United States territory in the 1900s. At that time, European labor was too costly to consider, and inexpensive labor supplied by Chinese immigrants was no longer available as a result of the 1882 Chinese Exclusion Act. The United States thus had to look elsewhere. Numerous meetings were held between the representatives of the Hawaiian Sugar Planters' Association and Horace N. Allen, the chief of the U.S. Legation in Seoul, Korea. As a result, the Korean government was persuaded to allow Koreans to emigrate as laborers to Hawaii, and about 7,000 Korean male laborers arrived in Hawaii to work on sugar plantations (Kim & Patterson, 1974).

Following the early wave of Korean immigrant laborers, a small number of students and political exiles arrived. The restraints of the Japanese government, which ruled over Korea between 1910 and 1945, on the one hand and the restrictions of American immigration on the other are the likeliest factors in explaining the sudden cessation of the immigration flow after 1910. Significant numbers of immigrants, however, began to arrive after the 1960s, following the 1965 amendments to the Immigration and Naturalization Act.

It is estimated that fully 90% of Korean immigrants entered the United States after the 1965 act. In accordance with the act's categories of preference, which mainly consisted of relatives of U.S. citizens and skilled workers, a large proportion of Koreans entering the United States in the 1970s were professionals such as doctors, pharmacists, and nurses. However, as of the mid-1980s, the United States began experiencing an increasingly tight job market, and domestic competition for jobs became fierce. As a result, the immigration of Korean professionals and skilled workers became more restricted. At the same time, Korea was undergoing rapid economic and industrial growth, providing its professionals with ample work opportunities at home. Because of these dynamics, recent Korean emigres consist mainly of relatives of earlier emigres. Many of the newer immigrants are not as well educated as their relatives who migrated previously.

By and large, recent Korean immigrants, unlike the early settlers, arrived together with their immediate family members. For the Koreans, entering the United States in family groups has had both positive and negative aspects. The advantages include the fact that the family is spared experiencing the trauma of separation among its members. In addition, the family forms a powerful economic unit, as members may work together to establish a family business. However, for some, intrafamilial problems begin to emerge soon after the move. As each individual must learn to adapt to a new culture and language, all family members are simultaneously affected by adjustment issues, and each member experiences his or her own unique strains. For example, the parents may feel overwhelmed as they attempt to secure housing, enroll their children in school, and seek to obtain a job or establish a business immediately in order to support the family. The parents often find themselves feeling inept and unintelligent due to lack of knowledge of the culture and the language skills of the adopted land. At the same time, the children tend to feel lost, as they cannot turn to their parents for help with their schoolwork or emotional support (Castex, 1996).

The language barrier affects all members of the family. As the head of the household, the Korean father perhaps feels the most frustration in trying to cope with the new language. Regardless of his preemigration occupational status, he is often forced to accept any available job in the ethnic community, where there is always a demand for labor-intensive work, such as grocery store clerk, warehouse worker, and transporter of goods. These jobs typically require little or no use of English, but they call for long hours, pay little, and provide neither challenge nor personal satisfaction (Drachman, Kwon-Ahn, & Paulino, 1996). It should be noted that the language difficulty generally persists among many Korean immigrants regardless of their length of residency in the United States. This fact is attributed to the unusual dissimilarities between Korean- and English-language structures, because the way in which words are put together to form sentences in Korean is antithetical to that in English (Nah, 1993). As a result, many have little choice but to remain in the small-scale, low-status service sector, particularly in occupations such as dry cleaning, operation of fruit and vegetable stands, beauty salons, and other small businesses.

KOREAN CULTURE AND CHARACTER TRAITS

A discussion of Korean culture and pertinent character traits is particularly relevant, as they play a decisive role in the way Koreans view alcohol consumption. As noted, incessant acts of aggression by its neighboring countries affected Korea's political stability throughout its history. Nevertheless, Korea has survived and retained its physical boundaries, its language, and its unique national character and culture.

Cultural Traits

Many Korean cultural traits can be said to have evolved out of four religions: two indigenous religions—Shamanism and Taejonggyo—and two imported ones—Buddhism and Taoism. These four religions taught Koreans the values of patience and self-discipline. They also helped to establish the basic national character, described as having the strength to overcome difficulties, to endure pain, and to maintain calm regardless of circumstances.

Although Confucianism is not, strictly speaking, a religion, it too had a great impact upon Korean society and became a strong component of the sociopolitical system. The central themes of Confucianism were filial piety, benevolence, a respect for learning, and a strict moral and ethical code regarding human relationships in order to maintain an orderly society. A primary appeal of Confucianism was its stress on family unity. Confucian philosophy assumes the family as a basic unit and center of all other social institutions. Likewise, the family is the core of Korean culture, to an extent even greater than for other Asian nations (Lee, 1977). Within the family, there exists a strong sense of loyalty, obligation, and collectivity. These notions are reflected in the Korean language, in which one uses the plural possessive form, such as "our father," "our home," and so forth, instead of the singular possessive form when referring to his or her family members.

Central to family unity is the Confucian influence of maintaining a hierarchical family structure. Each person's status and role is clearly distinct from that of every other, based on age, sex, and birth order. The husband's status is superior to his wife's. The oldest sibling's status is superior to that of the younger ones; he or she is entitled to respect from the younger siblings and in turn is responsible for their welfare. The family also socializes the child to submit his or her will to the will of the group. The child is taught to be tactful in dealing with others. He or she also learns how to disguise his or her emotions so as not to injure others' feelings.

Character Traits

Through the centuries, the Korean character has developed out of diverse influences and events—among them, as mentioned previously, several religions, geographical circumstances, political history, cultural exchanges, and the innate characteristics of the people. The following traits and values reflect the general characteristics of many Korean Americans.

Inner Strength and the Intense Will to Achieve "Success"

Koreans generally yearn for success in order to live better earthly lives. This desire for achievement and power might be attributed to the Korean history of economic and psychological deprivations caused by foreign invasions, as noted earlier. Both forms of deprivation most likely fueled the Koreans' desire to attain prestige and economic bliss throughout the generations.

To become successful and economically prosperous, a child must be able to postpone immediate gratification and develop inner strength. This concept of inner strength is often reflected in the choice of boys' names, such as Chadori ("Hardest Rock") and Saedori ("Rock of Iron"). Similarly, many girls' names begin with Bok ("Bliss"), such as Bok Soon and Bok Hee, as with boy's names, symbolizing the dream of luck and happiness. One may notice that the Chinese character for bliss is frequently embroidered on Korean pillowcases and cushions and carved on furniture.

Through Buddhism's teachings of patience, self-discipline, and the achievement of enlightenment, together with the experience of hardship, Koreans in general may not have renounced their desires, but they have learned to accept and overcome externally derived hardships. They have developed the inner strength to cope with and to adapt to whatever circumstances come their way. Pearl S. Buck illustrated this point in her book, *The*

Living Reed (1963). Here she pointed out that although Korean women appear to be frail on the outside, they are rock-like on the inside. Koreans call it "Korean spirit" or *Ul*—the ability to face adversity yet maintain tranquillity. The concept of the *Ul* is a powerful aspect of Korean American character—manifested mainly in the way Koreans seldom disclose personal problems or their weaknesses to others (Lee, 1977).

Korean immigrants in America, particularly those in large urban areas, are frequently stereotyped by non-Koreans as people who engage in "routine killing" of themselves through overwork and their willingness to start small businesses in the most dangerous areas of the inner city. Such risk taking and determination in the face of hardship are a reflection of *Ul*.

Face

To Koreans, face involves a multitude of meanings other than the merely physical. There are many expressions associated with the word *face*—usually conveying shame: "I cannot lift my face," "I've lost face," or " . . . face is smudged with ink." Although the definition of face is vague and intangible, it is very real to Koreans. Traditionally, face was more valued than anything else, particularly among men. Men were forbidden to express their feelings openly. Mustering all his might, a Korean man would resist showing any feelings of sadness, excitement, and especially tears. Aggressive emotions also had to be concealed because they might create a negative impression. Hence, showing a tranquil facade represented a person's inner strength and had to be cultivated at all costs.

When making requests, Koreans seldom directly say, "I need your help with. . . . " Rather, they tend to speak at a metacommunicative level designed to make the other person respond immediately with: "Let me help you." On the surface, or to a Westerner's view, it might seem like manipulation or forcing the other to offer help. It is, however, a very natural, spontaneous, and culturally rooted polite way to behave related to the notion of face.

Koreans tend to have dual faces—one private, the other public. The public face projects a formal, polite, and ceremonious façade, whereas the private face represents one's genuine feelings. The private face emerges only when a relationship is established. By switching between these two faces, Koreans are able to maintain a harmonious social life (Lee, 1977). The maintenance of these dual faces is associated with Confucian teaching, which stresses harmonious interpersonal relationships, rituals, formality, and decorum.

Nonverbal Communication

Koreans in general tend to be very sensitive to nonverbal cues (*noon chi*). During the socialization process, Korean children are discouraged from directly expressing their differences of opinion with others in the family. Rather, they are taught to respect and follow the ways of their parents and older siblings. They are also taught to be sensitive to the nonverbal expressions of others and to be careful with their own. For Koreans, it is more natural to use facial expressions and gestures to express their feelings than to express them verbally. In personal conversation, the ability to listen is more highly valued than speaking. Particularly among men, verbosity is considered frivolous.

SOCIAL ATTITUDES REGARDING
SUBSTANCE ABUSE IN KOREA

Drinking alcoholic beverages during times of celebration and social gatherings is as much a part of Korean history and tradition as it is in many other countries. Among Korean adult males, drinking rice wine is very common, and wine is not viewed as a serious alcoholic beverage. According to Korean history, during fall harvest season, the entire populace thronged together for the October harvest festival ceremony. Drinking rice wine, along with eating and dancing, was a vital part of the ceremony. Even today in rural parts of Korea, farmers celebrate the harvest festival by drinking the flavorful wine. It is natural to become inebriated as part of the festival; there is no stigma attached to this behavior during these special occasions.

Males and females, particularly elderly women, also drink home-brewed coarse rice wine after worshipping their ancestors, an important ceremony still practiced by many Koreans today in which rice wine and traditional dishes are offered to the dead (Lee, 1974).

Moreover, during social occasions, offering rice wine to guests represents a showing of hospitality. Such drinking helps Korean males to become more open and verbally expressive, especially at dinner gatherings with other men after a hard day's work. During such gatherings, it is considered polite to "force" wine on a person and to exchange glasses with one another; generally speaking, it is impolite to refuse a drink.

In addition to strong cultural sanctions toward drinking, there is a great tolerance toward outward drunken behavior. Alcoholism is not viewed as a medical or social problem. Thus there are no national, state, or local laws regulating the sale of alcoholic beverages to minors. It was only in 1989 that the government passed laws making it a crime to drive while intoxicated (Health and Welfare Department of Korea, 1990). An intoxicated man who engages in disorderly conduct is detained by the police overnight and released the next morning.

Korean alcoholics are rarely referred for treatment because, on the one hand, alcoholism is not viewed as a disease, and on the other, there are no alcohol treatment programs widely available in public or private city hospitals. Currently, there are only a handful of outpatient clinics in Korea staffed by professionals who are knowledgeable about alcoholism. These clinics are usually run by religious institutions, and they often provide counseling services for families and individuals.

Whereas the government does not seem very concerned about alcohol-related problems, it is very strict about the use of other drugs. Since 1946, the South Korean government has established law after law prohibiting the possession or use of drugs, including marijuana. The law imposes a 10-year prison term for those convicted of drug-related involvement. According to a report by the Health and Welfare Department of Korea (1990), the number of people selling, using, and/or possessing drugs such as marijuana, cocaine, heroin, and crack has been increasing rapidly. As Korea has entered the world economy, the Health and Welfare Department has attributed the prevalence of drugs to the increase in foreign travelers; many of them involved in drug trafficking. For example, 1,101 Koreans were convicted of drug-related offenses during 1983, whereas more than 3,897, three times as many, were imprisoned in 1989. The report further indicated that among the drug users, 34% were unemployed, 13.5% were involved in the agricultural business, 10.4% were cocktail lounge and bar employees, and 4.2% were medical professionals. Male drug abusers outnumbered females by four to one, reflecting the stronger stigma attached to female drug users. Although more recent drug-related statistics were unavailable, substance abuse problems in Korea appear to be escalating every year, whereas the lack of adequate treatment facilities persists (Kim, 1992).

SUBSTANCE ABUSE AMONG KOREAN AMERICANS

Few studies have been done on substance use and abuse among Korean Americans. According to available literature, the use of substances of any kind is less frequent among Asian Americans than non- Asian Americans (Johnson, Nagoshe, Ahern, Wilson, & Yuen, 1987; Trimble, Padilla, & Bell, 1987; Tucker, 1985). The lower level of alcohol consumption among Asian Americans is said to be associated with their higher alcohol-related sensitivity, which results in flushing of the face and body, a rapid heart rate, and a drop in blood pressure (Ewing, Rouse, & Aderhold, 1979; Goodwin, 1979).

One of the earliest surveys of alcohol problems among Asian Americans was conducted by Cahalan and Cisin (1976), who explored the drinking patterns of Chinese, Japanese, Korean, and Filipino males. They found that the alcohol drinking patterns of these men were similar to those found in a national sample of adult male respondents. The study also indicated that the Japanese (25.4%) and Filipino (19.6%) populations had a higher percentage of heavy drinkers than the Koreans (14.6%) or the Chinese (10.4%).

The overall lack of empirical research studies, combined with an underutilization of service programs by the Korean community, obscures the scope of substance abuse problems among Korean Americans. Clinical and anecdotal evidence from Korean community services in Los Angeles and New York reveal that Korean American males are more inclined to use alcohol than other drugs, probably reflecting the strong stigma attached to the use of drugs and the social acceptability of drinking.

Alcoholism and driving while intoxicated presents a growing problem for Korean Americans. The *Korea Times of New York*, one of five major Korean newspapers in the United States, reported that during the early 1990s the number of Korean male drunk drivers has increased, and that 30 intoxicated drivers had been prosecuted between June and August of 1994 in Queens, New York, alone ("Alcoholism Among Koreans" 1994). The problem has been attributed both to the plethora of Korean bars in Queens and to the stressful lives of Korean immigrants who drink to cope with daily pressure. The annual report of the Asian American Drug Abuse Program, Inc., in Los Angeles (1992–1993) indicated that 19% of all drug-abusing clients who participated in their residential program were Korean men aged between 25 and 34 (Asian American Drug Abuse Program, 1992–1993). According to Pastor Shi Hwan Kim of the Hahn-Barck Presbyterian Independent Church of New Jersey, his 1995 survey of several junior and senior high schools with a high concentration of Korean Americans (six schools in Queens, New York, one in Brooklyn, New York, and four in New Jersey) found that approximately 13–16% of Korean teenagers ages between 13 and 19 experimented with various substances and that 5% were heavily involved with drugs such as marijuana, heroin, cocaine, and crack (S. H. Kim, personal communication, August 15, 1995). Many of them also abused alcohol, and most have required some kind of residential treatment. According to Pastor Kim, 60% of these youngsters obtained drugs through their connections with gangs. He also noted that the parents of these teenagers worked 7 days a week and spent little or no time with their children. Feeling rejected by their parents and isolated in school, these youngsters become easy targets of Korean gangs, who, displaying warmth, acceptance, and "brotherly" support, often provide them with a sense of belonging. This alarming trend is depicted in the following case:

> J is a 14-year-old ninth grader at a local junior high school. J came to the United States with his family at age 12. His 42-year-old father had worked as a pharmacist in Korea, and his 40-year-old mother had been a homemaker. One year after their arrival in New York, the parents opened a delicatessen and, from the start, worked from 6:30 A.M. until 10:00 P.M. every day, including weekends.
>
> The oldest of three boys, J was expected to succeed in school and to be the role model to his younger brothers. Initially, he worked very hard toward becoming academically superior and gaining respect among his peers. J believed that in so doing, he would bring honor to his family name. At home, J was responsible for caring for his younger brothers, ages 10 and 8, until his parents finished work.
>
> Although J had been a top student in Korea, his limited knowledge of English affected his learning. After several months, J found himself overwhelmed by his responsibilities at home and by trying to maintain his schoolwork at the same time. Furthermore, J had few friends and became increasingly frustrated and lonely. J's grades and school attendance began to descend over the course of the school year.
>
> In the meantime, J's parents were pouring all of their energies into establishing their new business, all the while unaware of their son's difficulties. J's teacher finally contacted his mother and informed her that J had been associating with a gang whose members tended to use drugs. When confronted by his mother, J admitted that he had been using marijuana regularly. J's mother immediately stopped working and brought him to the pastor at their church. The pastor saw the boy for pastoral counseling and got him involved with the church youth group.

HELP SEEKING AMONG KOREAN AMERICANS

Although there has been a rise in both gang-related drug use and drunk driving among Korean Americans, particularly in cities such as Los Angeles and New York in which large clusters of Korean Americans reside, substance abuse and community service agencies report that Korean Americans generally do not seek outside help for themselves. For example, the Korean Youth and Community Center, the largest community service agency for Koreans in Los Angeles, disclosed in its client summary reports that between October 1991 and March 1994 substance abuse problems made up only 5–6% of its total caseload (Korean Youth and Community Center, 1991–1994). According to a personal communication from the executive director of the Korean Family Counseling and Research Program in New York, Koreans tend to delay counseling and generally will avoid and/ or deny the problem altogether until it becomes so severe that it is virtually impossible to handle at home (R. Kim, personal communication, September 2, 1995).

With regard to substance abuse problems among adolescents, Korean parents will often resort to "geographical escape," hoping that moving away will eliminate the problem. In cases of substance- abusing adults, it is usually the wives who will seek help for their heavily drinking spouses. The husbands, however, invariably resist professional help. Moreover, because there are virtually no bilingual/bicultural treatment programs or support groups available to Korean Americans, help options are limited.

The one common source of help that is found in the Korean community is the local pastor. A majority of Korean Americans are members of a local Korean church and view the church not only as a place for spiritual enhancement but also as a personal social service provider (Kwon-Ahn, 1987). As seen in the case of J, when facing individual or family problems, Korean Americans tend to first reach out to their church leaders. A 1987 study on the Korean Church's role as a provider of social service to new immigrants found that Koreans utilize the Korean Protestant Church for housing and legal matters, as well as for individual and family counseling. However, although their congregants relied upon them for counseling, many of the pastors interviewed did not feel that they possessed the knowledge or skills to counsel their parishioners about family and personal problems (Kwon-Ahn, 1987). This lack of skill is especially apparent when providing counseling for substance abuse problems and points out the need for the provision of appropriate training for local pastors.

ASSESSMENT ISSUES

In order to provide effective substance abuse treatment for people of Korean background, it is imperative that the therapist has both a general and specific knowledge of Korean American clients. A general knowledge of the culture and national character offers a framework for broad-based understanding. On the other hand, a specific knowledge of the individual's pre- and postimmigration experience provides data on important issues such as changes in socioeconomic status, impact and status of immigration, educational aspirations, physical and mental health, family relations (current family and family of origin), life goals, support systems, and relationship to substance abuse.

The entire experience of resettlement—facing language and cultural barriers, experiencing social isolation, downward occupational mobility, unemployment, and racial discrimination—is extremely stressful. In addition, resettlement often results in changes within the traditional Korean family structure, as heretofore-successful husbands and fathers may experience a shift in their role as their wives become more independent and their children less obedient. Such changes increase the levels of anxiety, stress, and "loss of face" among men (Sue & Sue 1990). Excessive alcohol consumption may be the result, as can be seen in the following vignette.

Mr. C, aged 35, came to the United States with his wife and 4-year-old son, S, in the mid-1990s. In Korea, he had worked at a large business firm after graduating from a reputable college. The purpose of emigrating was to obtain a professional degree in the field of political science and eventually to work for the Korean government. Mrs. C also intended to study in the United States toward a master's degree in special education and then to resume her teaching career in Korea.

However, because of unanticipated financial difficulties due to economic problems at home, the couple found that they were unable to continue their graduate education. Mrs. C could no longer afford to pay a babysitter or to put her child in day care, so she stayed home, while Mr. C, who did not have a work visa, took the first available job he could find, as an off-the-books laborer in a Korean vegetable and fruit stand.

Having achieved a high level of education and success in Korea, Mr. C's loss in status left him frustrated, angry, and bitter. After enduring 1 year of what he considered monotonous, labor-intensive, and demeaning work, he began to drink, at first two or three cans of beer after work. Gradually he began coming home later, each day intoxicated. As Mr. C's drinking increased, his temper grew worse. Mrs. C began to live in fear of Mr. C's outbursts and uncontrollable drinking episodes. Mr. C eventually started having various physical problems, such as insomnia, stomachaches, and difficulties in walking. He refused Mrs. C's suggestions that he seek help and insisted that he could take care of himself. Mrs. C then called a Korean friend who worked as a physician at a nearby hospital, hoping that he would advise Mr. C to stop drinking. Instead, the friend called Mr. C to suggest that he schedule a physical examination. Only after a couple of visits to evaluate his physical problems did the physician address Mr. C's drinking by educating him about the connection between his drinking and his physical problems.

COUNSELING IMPLICATIONS

One should anticipate a number of difficulties in counseling Korean clients. In general, Koreans are reluctant to enter counseling, not only because they find it unfamiliar but also because it is strongly stigmatized. Instead, they try to solve problems on their own or within the family or with close friends. As indicated earlier, if the severity of the problem requires outside help, Koreans will often turn first to their clergy for practical advice. Another reason for their inhibitions toward therapy is their fear of "losing face" and bringing shame upon the family. Consequently, even when they do seek help, they tend not to fully disclose their most vulnerable or shameful experiences or feelings.

As pointed out, Korean Americans rarely seek therapy on their own initiative. Rather, it is only after the problem becomes sufficiently severe that it is recognized by others, such as teachers or other school officials, the police (as in the case of battered women), or the legal or medical system, that they obtain outside help. Typically, it is through these settings that Koreans are referred for substance abuse treatment. Even then, they tend to delay and may need to have the clinician reach out and initiate phone contact. For example, in numerous instances school guidance counselors have referred Korean parents of problem children to me for help with their children's problems. However, it is usually only after I have made repeated attempts to contact the family that an initial interview is finally established.

In the case of alcohol-related problems in adults, it is not unusual for the wives of alcoholic husbands to call a counselor and request that he or she contacts their husbands in order to schedule an appointment. Given this dynamic, clinicians and agencies wanting to reach Korean substance abusers may need to reevaluate their traditional treatment approach of waiting for the substance abuser to initiate treatment.

In treating Korean clients, it is advisable to start with concrete, tangible issues in order to help clients acclimate themselves to the counseling process and setting and also to set the basis for a positive, trusting relationship. As was seen in Mr. C's case, one might initially ask the client to describe his physical condition or any physical complaints. During this initial phase, direct confrontation or even discussion with the client of his substance abuse problem is not advised. The therapist could engage the client by focusing on the physical consequences of substance abuse, such as changes in sleeping and eating habits, memory problems, headaches, stomach or leg pains, and so forth. Indeed, the clinician should make a proper recommendation for physical assessment before focusing on the substance abuse.

Only after the clinician–client relationship has been established can the counselor focus on how these physical problems relate to substance abuse and how drinking or drug use may relate to family conflicts, loss of status, loss of hope, difficulties in learning a new language and adjusting to a new culture, and so forth. Discussions should also address the client's feelings of shame, anger and hopelessness resulting from being in treatment.

In general, most Koreans give deference to authority figures and anticipate receiving clear "how to" advice. Thus the traditional substance abuse treatment approach, in which the clinician assumes an active role in the treatment process and takes initiative in the interaction by, for example, explaining the nature of alcoholism or drug addiction and providing clear and direct advice, is well suited for Korean clients.

Generally speaking, Korean Americans are encouraged to be sensitive to nonverbal communication and discouraged from being verbally expressive. They will thus expect the clinician to pick up the nonverbal communication through their facial expression, tone of voice, and body gestures (Uba, 1994). If clients sense that the clinician does not promptly recognize the nonverbal cues, they may falsely judge the clinician as incompetent or incapable of solving their substance-related problems and thus abandon treatment after the initial interview.

Another common assumption that Korean Americans have regarding substance abuse is that the problem is due to a lack of will power and that will power can be fostered by listening to advice, admonition, or reproach from others, particularly authority figures such as pastors, teachers, doctors, or clinicians. As this view may only exacerbate the problem, it is crucial that Korean American clients and their family members be educated regarding symptoms of addiction and the best treatment approaches in dealing with substance-abusing family members. Such psychoeducation should be provided through Korean mass media, churches, or various community organizations, as well as by clinicians.

Although family therapy can be employed as an effective treatment modality, the clinician must be constantly careful not to degrade the authoritative roles of Korean parents in front of their children or of the husband in front of his wife. In the case of J, for instance, whose parents left most of the domestic responsibilities to him while they worked, the clinician could help the parents devise a plan to divide the house chores among J's brothers. In this way, the parents could allow J more time to concentrate on his schoolwork while helping the brothers to become more independent.

When working with Korean substance-abusing clients or their family members, the clinician may need to utilize translators. In such cases, the translators should be not only proficient in the respective languages but also biculturally competent. It is important that they also have some understanding of addiction so that they may be able to translate the client's messages as accurately as possible and not add their own subjective thoughts, feelings, and perceptions. Some translators may have a need to distort important information in order to protect their and their client's "face" in the presence of the clinician (Amodeo, Robb, Peou, & Tran, 1996).

Use of Groups and 12-Step Programs

Group counseling and utilization of 12-step groups, as well as other self-help groups, are not generally recommended for Korean American substance abusers. Koreans tend to believe that those who succumb to substance abuse lack the inner strength and will power to succeed. Disclosing and acknowledging their problems in a group setting, let alone admitting their substance abuse, can thus be a torturous experience. Furthermore, their feelings of failure may be reinforced through associating and identifying with other substance abusers, which may lead to even greater feelings of loss of face and self-hatred and possibly to the resumption of alcohol or drug use.

Working with Adolescents

Many Korean Americans assume that the substance abuse problems of their youngsters are due to their association with "bad kids" and that simply moving and separating their sons from the undesirable crowd will solve the problem. This "geographical escape" may lead to further negative consequences because such relocation leads to additional disruptive changes in their and their children's lives. Thus it is important to educate parents regarding such dynamics.

Although Koreans may attach a strong stigma to psychological or substance abuse counseling when considering possible treatment for their adolescents, they value most advice or consultation concerning their children's academic or educational interests. Therefore, it is more appropriate to focus initially on school-related issues, such as the adolescent's school attendance, grades, extracurricular school activities, and so forth. Such an approach facilitates the initial rapport and trust with both parents and the youth. Only once such trust is established can the issue of substance abuse be broached.

CONCLUSION

Treating Koreans with alcohol- and drug-related problems presents a number of great difficulties. Most significant is a lack of systematized research regarding the full extent of alcohol and drug problems among people of Korean background. There is also a community-wide lack of understanding with respect to the nature and severity of the problem. Added to these obstacles is the current dearth of Korean bilingual/bicultural professionals who are knowledgeable about substance abuse issues. Moreover, there are no available facilities or self-help groups in the United States aimed at providing substance abuse treatment for Korean speaking individuals and their families.

To begin awareness of and intervention for the problem, help must be offered to Korean American families and individuals.

REFERENCES

Alcoholism among Koreans. (1994, August 30). *The Korea Times of New York*, p. 1A.

Amodeo, M., Robb, N., Peou, S., & Tran, H. (1996). Adapting mainstream substance-abuse interventions for Southeast Asian clients. *Families in Society, 77*(7), 403–412.

Asian-American Drug Abuse Program, Inc. (1992–1993). *Annual report.* Los Angeles, CA: Author.

Buck, P. S. (1963). *The living reed.* New York: John Day.

Cahalan, D., & Cisn, I. H. (1976). Drinking behavior and drinking problems in the United States. In G. Kissin & H. Begleiter (Eds.), *Social aspects of alcoholism* (pp. 77–115). New York: Plenum Press.

Castex, G. M. (1996). Immigrant children in the United States. In N. K. Phillips & S. L. A. Straussner (Eds.), *Children in the urban environment* (pp. 43–60). Springfield, IL: Thomas.

Drachman, D., Kwon-Ahn, Y. H., & Paulino, A. (1996). Migration and resettlement experiences of Dominican and Korean families. *Families in Society, 77*(10), 626–638.

Ewing, J. A., Rouse, B. A., & Aderhold, R. M. (1979). Studies of the mechanism of Oriental hypersensitivity to alcohol. *Currents in Alcoholism, 5*, 45–52.

Goodwin, D. W. (1979). Protective factors in alcoholism. *Journal of Drug and Alcohol Dependency, 4*, 99–100.

Health and Welfare Department of Korea. (1990). *Report on substance abuse.* Seoul, Korea: Korean Government Printing Office.

Johnson, R. C., Nagoshe, G. T., Ahern, F. M., Wilson, J. R., & Yuen, S. H. L. (1987). Cultural factors as explanations for ethnic group differences in alcohol use in Hawaii. *Journal of Psychoactive Drugs, 19*, 67–75.

Kim, H., & Patterson, W. (1974). *The Koreans in America, 1882–1974.* New York: Oceana.

Kim, K. B. (1992). *Substance abuse of the adolescent.* Seoul, Korea: Korean Health Association.

Korean Youth and Community Center. (1991–1994). *Quarterly client profile summary report.* Los Angeles, CA: Author.

Kwon-Ahn, Y. H. (1987). *The Korean Protestant Church: The role in service delivery for Korean immigrants.* Unpublished doctoral dissertation, Columbia University School of Social Work.

Kyo Yang National History Research Association. (1994). *Korean history.* Seoul, Korea: Chung Ah.

Lee, K. T. (1977). *The Korean way of thought.* Seoul, Korea: Moolisa.

Nah, K. H. (1993). Perceived problems and service delivery for Korean immigrants. *Social Work, 38*(2), 289–296.

Sue, D. W., & Sue, D. (1990). *Theory and counseling: The culturally different practice.* New York. Wiley.

Trimble, J. E., Padilla, A., & Bell, C. S. (Eds.). (1987). *Drug abuse among ethnic minorities* (FDHHS Publication No. ADM 87–1474). Rockville, MD: National Institute on Drug Abuse.

Tucker, M. B. (1985). U.S. ethnic minorities and drug use: An assessment of science and practices. *International Journal of the Addictions, 20*(6/7), 1021–1047.

Uba, L. (1994). *Asian Americans: Personality patterns, identity, and mental health.* New York: Guilford Press.

U.S. Bureau of the Census. (1980). *General characteristics of the population.* Washington, DC: Author.

U.S. Bureau of Census. (1990). *Asian and Pacific Islanders in the United States: Social characteristics.* Washington, DC: Author.

Index

Abstinence movements
  in Czarist Russia, 255–256
  Pioneer Total Abstinence
    Association (Ireland), 204
Acculturation, 146
  as painful process, 15–16
Adolescents and substance abuse,
    African Americans, 41–42
African Americans
  cultural norms and values, 33
    extended view of family/focus
      on children, 34–35
    mutual aid concept. See Seven
      principles
    present orientation/spiral
      concept of time, 35
    value of oneness with nature/
      spirituality, 33–34
    worldview, 33
  explanations for contemporary
    substance abuse patterns, 35
    advertising, 38, 48
    "double consciousness," 37
    economic frustration, 36
    emotional consequences of
      racism, 36
    racism and internalized
      oppression, 36–37
    historical patterns, 36
    ideology of conspiracy, 39
    lack of positive role models, 38
    overabundance of availability,
      36
    poverty and violence, 37–38

historic use of alcohol
  migration to urban inner–cities
    after World War I, 32
  in period of slavery, 32
  in West Africa, 32
history of slavery influence, 31
Muslims, and life–sustaining
  community services, 35
patterns of substance use and
  abuse, 39. See also AIDS/
  HIV
  adolescents, 41–42
  lesbians and gay men, 42
  women, 40–41
sources of cultural/ethnic identity,
  58
substance abuse–racism
  connection, 31–32
See also Treatment issues/
  approaches; West Indian
  immigrants
AIDS/HIV, 11
  and African Americans, 43
    as consequence of maladaptive
      coping strategies for African
      American women, 40
  among Cuban Americans, 105
  among Mexican Americans,
    120
  in Ireland, 206–207
  in Italy, 223
  use of alcohol and drugs as
    cofactor in transmission, 42,
    158

437

DEMCO

SEP 2 9 2003